Contexts of nursing
An introduction

Contexts of nursing
An introduction
3e

Edited by

John Daly

Sandra Speedy

Debra Jackson

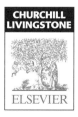

CHURCHILL
LIVINGSTONE

ELSEVIER

Sydney Edinburgh London New York Philadelphia St Louis Toronto

Churchill Livingstone
is an imprint of Elsevier

Elsevier Australia. ACN 001 002 357

(a division of Reed International Books Australia Pty Ltd)

Tower 1, 475 Victoria Avenue, Chatswood, NSW 2067

This edition © 2010 Elsevier Australia
2nd edn 2006; 1st edn 2000

National Library of Australia Cataloguing-in-Publication Data

_____

Daly, John.

Contexts of nursing : an introduction/John Daly,
Sandra Speedy, Debra Jackson.

3rd ed.

978 0 7295 3925 8 (pbk.)

Includes index.
Bibliography.

Nursing--Australia.
Nursing--Social aspects--Australia.
Nursing --Study and teaching--Australia.
Nursing ethics.
Medical care--Australia.

Speedy, Sandra.
Jackson, Debra.

610.730994

_____

Publisher: Luisa Cecotti
Developmental Editor: Larissa Norrie
Publishing Services Manager: Helena Klijn
Editorial Coordinators: Andreea Heriseanu and Sarah Botros
Edited by Ruth Matheson
Proofread by Jon Forsyth
Cover and internal design by Trina McDonald
Index by Jon Forsyth
Typeset by TNQ
Printed in China by China Translation & Printing Services Ltd

CONTENTS

CONTRIBUTORS

Alan Barnard PhD MA BA RN
Member, Institute of Health and Biomedical Innovation; Senior Lecturer, School of Nursing and Midwifery, Queensland University of Technology

Sally Borbasi RN BEd(Nurs) MA(Educ) PhD MRCNA
Professor of Nursing, School of Nursing and Midwifery, Griffith University

Vicki Bradford M(IndigHlthStud) GradDip(IndigHlthStud) GradCertEducStud (HigherEd) RN
Faculty Advisor, Indigenous Health, Undergraduate Coordinator, Nursing and Midwifery, University of Sydney

Angela Brown RN PhD candidate MA(HealthCareEthics) PGDip(HlthServRes&Tech Assess) BSc(Hons)(Nurs)
Senior Lecturer and Associate Head, School of Nursing, Midwifery and Indigenous Health, Faculty of Health and Behavioural Science, University of Wollongong

Esther Chang RN CM DNE BAppSc(AdvNur) MEd(Admin) PhD FCN(NSW)
Professor of Nursing, Research Director Staff Development, School of Nursing and Midwifery, College of Health and Science, University of Western Sydney

Moya Conrick (deceased) RN RM DipApSc BN MClEd PhD
Lecturer, School of Nursing and Midwifery, Griffith University

Jane Conway RN BNurs(Hons) GradCertHRM DEd
Consultant in Health Professional Education and Training, Conjoint Senior Lecturer, School of Nursing and Midwifery, University of Newcastle

Debra K Creedy PhD MEd BA(Hons) RN FACMHN
Professor and Head, Alice Lee Centre for Nursing Studies, National University of Singapore

Patrick Crookes RN BSc(Nurs) CertEd RNT PhD
Professor and Head of School of Nursing, Midwifery and Indigenous Health; Dean, Faculty of Health and Behavioural Sciences, University of Wollongong

John Daly RN PhD FRCNA FCN
Professor and Dean, Faculty of Nursing, Midwifery and Health; Head, WHO Collaborating Centre for Nursing, Midwifery and Health Development, University of Technology, Sydney

Philip Darbyshire PhD MN RNMH RSCN DipN(Lond) RNT
Principal, Philip Darbyshire Consulting Ltd; Adjunct Professor, School of Nursing, College of Health and Science, University of Western Sydney

Christine Davey RN CM ECN MRHP(Nurs)
Nursing Coordinator, Central Australia Remote Health

Patricia M Davidson RN BA MEd PhD FRCNA
Professor of Cardiovascular and Chronic Care, Professorial Chair in Cardiovascular Nursing Research, St Vincent's and Mater Health; Curtin Health Innovation Research Institute, Curtin University of Technology, Sydney

Gay Edgecombe RN RM CHN BAppSc MS PhD FRCNA
Professor of Nursing, Community Child Health Nursing, RMIT University, Division of Nursing and Midwifery

Doug Elliott RN PhD MAppSc BAppSc
Professor of Nursing and Director of Research, Faculty of Nursing, Midwifery and Health, University of Technology, Sydney

Isabelle Ellis PhD MPH&TM MBA GradDipProfComm(Multimedia) CTCM&H RN RM
Professor, Rural and Remote Health Services, Combined Universities Centre for Rural Health, University of Western Australia

Jean Gilmour PhD DipSocSci BA RN
Senior Lecturer, School of Health and Social Services, Massey University, New Zealand

Madonna Grehan RN RM CertSexHlth&Reprod GrDipHlthEth PhD
Director, Australian Nursing and Midwifery History Project, School of Nursing and Social Work, University of Melbourne

Rhonda Griffiths AM DrPH MSc(Hons) BEd(Nurs) RN RM FRCNA FCN
Professor of Nursing, Head, School of Nursing and Midwifery, University of Western Sydney; Director, New South Wales Centre for Evidence Based Health Care

Desley Hegney PhD BA(Hons) DipNurseEd CertOccupHealthNursing CertNeurol&Neurosurg Nurs RN
Professor and Director of Research, Alice Lee Centre for Nursing Studies, Yong Loo Lin School of Medicine, National University of Singapore; Honorary Professor, School of Nursing and Midwifery, University of Queensland, Brisbane

Amanda Henderson PhD MScSoc GradDipNurs(Educ) BSc RN RM
Associate Fellow, Australian Learning and Teaching Council; Nursing Director (Education), Metro South, Queensland Health; Professor, Griffith Health, Griffith University

Colin Holmes PhD MPhil BA(Hons) TCert
Professor of Nursing, School of Nursing, Midwifery and Nutrition, James Cook University

Annette Huntington BN PhD FCNA(NZ)
Associate Professor, Director of Nursing Programmes, School of Health and Social Services, Massey University, New Zealand

Debra Jackson PhD RN
Director, Higher Degree Research, School of Nursing and Midwifery, University of Western Sydney

Megan-Jane Johnstone PhD BA RN FRCNA FCN
Professor of Nursing and Associate Head of School (Research), School of Nursing, Faculty of Health, Medicine, Nursing and Behavioural Sciences, Deakin University, Melbourne

Judith Mair PhD LLB DNE RN RM
Legal educator; casual lecturer, Faculty of Health Sciences, University of Sydney

Margaret McMillan PhD MCurrSt(Hons) BA RN DipNEd GradCertMg
Conjoint Professor, School of Nursing and Midwifery, University of Newcastle

Akram Omeri PhD RN RM BSN MN CTN FRCNA
Associate Professor, School of Nursing, University of Notre Dame, Australia

Judith M Parker AM RN BA(Hons) PhD MD(Hons)
Professor, School of Nursing and Midwifery, Victoria University

Steve Parker RN MHN DipT(NurseEd) BEd PhD
Associate Dean (Teaching and Learning), School of Nursing and Midwifery, Flinders University

Lynette Raymond RN RM BA MA DipAppCouns CertIV TAA40104 PhD(Nurs) MRCNA
Clinical Coordinator and Senior Lecturer, School of Nursing, University of Notre Dame, Sydney

Anthony C Smith PhD MEd BN RN
Senior Research Fellow, School of Medicine, Faculty of Health Sciences; Deputy Director, Centre for Online Health, University of Queensland, Australia

Sandra Speedy EdD MURP GradDip(Educ) BA(Hons) RN FACMHN MAPS
Emeritus Professor, Course Coordinator, Master of Public Health, School of Health and Human Sciences, Faculty of Health and Science, Southern Cross University

Ray Stephens MNurs(Research) BN RN
Lecturer, RMIT, Nursing and Midwifery

Kim Usher PhD DipHSc BA MNSt RN RPN FRCNA FACMHN
Professor, Director of Research and Higher Degree Students, Associate Dean Graduate Research Training, School of Nursing, Midwifery and Nutrition, Faculty of Medicine, Health and Molecular Sciences, James Cook University

Kim Walker PhD BAppSc(AdvNsg) RN
Professor of Nursing (Applied Research), St Vincent's Private Hospital, Sydney, Australian Catholic University; Adjunct Professor, University of Technology, Sydney; Clinical Associate Professor, University of Tasmania

Sarah Winch RN BA(Hons) PhD(Q)
Senior Lecturer Health Ethics, Mayne School of Medicine, University of Queensland

REVIEWERS

Anita Bamford-Wade DNurs MA DipBus RN MRCNA
Joint Head of Nursing, Faculty of Health and Environmental Sciences, AUT University, Auckland, New Zealand

Murray Bardwell RN PsychNurse DipApSc BN MN MACMHN
Course Coordinator, School of Nursing and Midwifery, Australian Catholic University, Ballarat

Sue Floyd RN BN MN MCNA(NZ)
Nursing Practicum Manager, Cervical Screening Coordinator, Faculty of Health and Sport Science, Eastern Institute of Technology

Karen L Jackson RN RSCN MSc PGDipAdEd
Lecturer, School of Nursing, Faculty of Health, Medicine, Nursing and Behavioural Sciences, Geelong Waterfront Campus, Deakin University

Helen Kelly RN BN(Hons) GradCertCardiacNursing MCN
Lecturer, School of Nursing, University of Notre Dame, Sydney

Annabel Matheson PhD candidate BNurs(Hons—1st class) DipHlthSci(Nurs) RN MRCNA
Lecturer and Course Coordinator of Bachelor of Nursing, School of Nursing and Midwifery, Charles Sturt University

Penny Paliadelis PhD MNurs(Hons) BNurs RN MRCNA MACCCN
Senior Lecturer, Deputy Head of School, Nursing Course Coordinator, School of Health, Faculty of the Professions, University of New England, Armidale, NSW

Marilyn Richardson-Tench PhD MEdStud BAppSc(AdvNsg) MACORN
Senior Lecturer, Coordinator—Teaching and Learning, School of Nursing and Midwifery, Faculty of Health, Engineering and Science, Victoria University

PREFACE

Welcome to the third edition of *Contexts of Nursing*! The discipline and profession of nursing continues to evolve, mature and develop within Australia and New Zealand and globally. As we write, we are aware that very big questions are currently being asked about the kind of health system Australia will require to meet population needs in the future, the kind of education that will be needed to prepare health professionals for the system, and the range of health professional roles which will ensure optimal healthcare (Bennett 2008). Debate and discussion of the issues is being facilitated by a number of leading organisations, including the National Health and Hospitals Reform Commission (www.nhhrc.org.au) and the National Health Workforce Taskforce (www.nhwt.gov.au). Human resources for health have become a serious challenge to provision of timely and adequate healthcare (World Health Organization 2006). Governments have recognised that the current health system is in crisis and this has implications for the provision of healthcare and the education of health professionals, including registered nurses.

A number of issues have come to the fore in healthcare, including quality and safety, access to care, management of diminishing resources in a context of increasing demand for and costs of care, adequacy of staffing levels and skill mix, quality of work-life and Indigenous health. All demand resolution. New trends are also emerging in response to some of these constraints, such as the use of clinical simulation environments to complement traditional approaches to clinical education in a number of health professions, and a renewed emphasis on the need for quality interprofessional approaches to health professional education to enhance team work and ultimately quality of care.

Clearly, it is impossible to predict outcomes of the review of the healthcare system currently underway. However, it seems likely that solutions to health service problems will require new models of care and changes in the roles and responsibilities of health professionals. This has potential for transformation in the role and expectations of registered nurses and for greater recognition of their sophisticated knowledge and skill base and capacity to manage increasing levels of responsibility in the provision of care. This will require of registered nurses a continuing commitment to the pursuit of excellence in knowledge acquisition and in application of this in practice. We will observe the progress of these critical debates and discussions with interest and their influence on changes in policy, practice and health professional roles.

As with the previous editions, this volume introduces students to the theory, language and scholarship of nursing. Our major objective has been (and remains) to provide a comprehensive coverage of key ideas underpinning the practice of contemporary nursing. This book is a collection of views and voices; consequently, the chapters are not all identical in nature. This reflects our position that it is important that students/readers engage with various (and sometimes conflicting) views to challenge and extend them.

We have specifically sought out a range of contributors who not only reflect the dynamic nature of nursing scholarship in Australia and New Zealand, but who are helping to shape contemporary nursing in this part of the world. These scholars have been chosen not only because of their expert knowledge, but also because of their professional standing, leadership, and the sometimes controversial stances they take on various contemporary issues. We have not sought to silence the controversies or quieten the debates; rather, we present them to you, the reader, as a stimulus for reflection, discussion and debate, and as a catalyst to further develop your own positions on various issues.

We have explained previously why the notion of 'contexts' has appeal for us in conceptualising nursing knowledge as a fabric comprised of theoretical threads. This 'knowledge-as-fabric' metaphor provides access to a number of other related ideas, such as weaving and tapestry. In this edition we have added chapters on new topics. Some new threads have been woven into the fabric of nursing knowledge presented in this work. Selection of these topics was based on extensive consultation with nurses who found the second edition useful in undergraduate and graduate courses and in their teaching and learning. Of course student evaluations of the work were also considered. In addition, a number of experienced nurse authors and editors provided useful critique and feedback, which has helped us in shaping this new volume. We hope that the new contexts and topics we have included in this edition will make the book truly comprehensive and contemporary.

Though we have updated and added new content to this edition of *Contexts of Nursing*, it is based on the same aims and objectives that underpinned the design and development of the first edition of the work. Nursing knowledge and its foundational elements are explored and considered in relation to professional nursing practice. Our emphasis on pedagogic strength and accessibility, and the use of reflective questions and exercises to stimulate critical thinking and learning, has been maintained.

The editors acknowledge Luisa Cecotti and Larissa Norrie, and the entire team at Elsevier, for their ongoing enthusiasm, encouragement, support and assistance in the preparation and production of this edition.

Most of all, we thank our contributors, who have risen again to the challenge of developing engaging, scholarly and teaching/learning-oriented work to stimulate reflection, discussion and debate.

John Daly

Sandra Speedy

Debra Jackson
Sydney, February 2009

REFERENCES

Bennett C 2008 A healthier future for all Australians: interim report. National Health and Hospitals Reform Commission, Canberra

World Health Organization (WHO) 2006 Working together for health: the world health report. WHO, Geneva

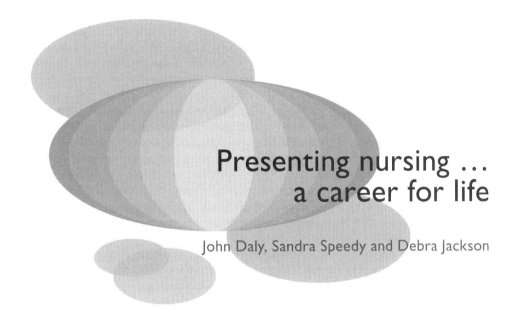

CHAPTER 1

Presenting nursing ...
a career for life

John Daly, Sandra Speedy and Debra Jackson

LEARNING OBJECTIVES

By reading and reflecting on this chapter, readers will be able to:

- list some of the myths, legends and stereotypes that surround nursing
- arrive at a personal beginning definition of nursing
- establish their passion for nursing
- describe the different types of nurse in Australia and New Zealand
- verbalise some of the choices that a nursing degree offers for graduates, and
- describe the meaning of the term 'professional conduct'.

KEY WORDS

Nursing, stereotypes, critical perspective, career codes of conduct, lifelong learning

WHY NURSING?

Nursing is a unique and wonderful career choice. It is a curious mix of technology and myth … of science and art … reality and romance. It blends the concrete and the abstract. It combines thinking and doing … 'being with' and 'doing for'. Nurses have privileged access to people's homes and share some of the most precious and highly intimate moments in people's lives—moments that remain hidden from most other people and professions. Nurses witness birth and death, and just about everything in between. Nurses share in people's most difficult moments of suffering and pain, and also bear witness to times of great joy and happiness. Because of the special place in society that nurses hold, nurses enjoy a high level of community trust. Indeed, in Australia and New Zealand, nurses continually rank very highly in surveys of public confidence.

Nursing can be a career for life. A degree in nursing provides a foundation for lifelong learning. It is the entry requirement to a fulfilling career, to a range of postgraduate courses in areas as diverse as paediatrics, midwifery, cancer care, community nursing, women's health, nurse education and nursing research. Age and experience are valued in nursing. Unlike many other professions and career choices in which people experience increasing difficulty in obtaining work as they get older, nurses can remain productively employed until retirement, and even post-retirement. Nursing is a career to which one can always return. Career interruption because of family responsibilities (or other reasons) can be extremely disadvantaging in some professions, but many nurses have effectively blended very successful careers with raising families. Nursing opens many doors. Internationally, Australian and New Zealand nurses are well respected and are eligible for registration in many other countries.

In this opening chapter, we aim to share what captured us and created our passion and enthusiasm for the career that is nursing—the passion and enthusiasm that has sustained and carried us successfully through our nursing careers. We also describe the different types and levels of nurse in Australia and New Zealand, and aim to introduce you to some of the ideas of interest to nurses and nursing, many of which are discussed in more detail in subsequent chapters of this book.

NURSING: MYTHS, LEGENDS AND STEREOTYPES

Perhaps more than any other professional group, nursing and nurses are the subject of myth and popular belief; there are also many romantic connotations. Certain of these myths and beliefs are almost folkloric, yet they strongly influence the ways in which nurses are perceived by the general public, and also in the ways that nurses see themselves. Through the media, nursing is often portrayed as a dramatic, exciting, glamorous and romantic activity, with nurses frequently represented in the role of handmaiden/helper to doctors.

Several of the almost legendary attributes that surround nursing are derived from myths about Florence Nightingale and her work in the Crimean War. For example, the romantic notion of the 'angel of mercy', the quiet, modest and self-effacing woman who, with a religious-like fervour, would tirelessly and uncomplainingly nurse the ill and injured back to full strength, and the image of the 'lady with the lamp' fearlessly working at the frontline of a war zone, and instilling calm, peace and tranquillity where only chaos and suffering had reigned, have become enduring and mythologised popular images of the nurse.

Because of her continued allure, much of Nightingale's life has been reconstructed and, in the process, subject to various forms of poetic licence. An excellent example of this poetic licence is explored by Jones (1988) in her critical examination of *The White Angel*, a motion picture released in 1936, which purported to be a biographical representation of the life of Florence Nightingale. On its release, this film was widely acclaimed, both within and outside the nursing profession, with influential professional nursing journals promoting the movie as 'a good educational picture', and commending it to the nursing profession, 'especially those concerned with information and education' (Jones 1988:222). However, although the movie was widely accepted as factual, even by the nursing community, Jones (1988) proposes that the screenplay contained a series of key errors, which served to trivialise major events in the life of Nightingale, and reinforced the myth that her decision to become a nurse was made in the manner of a religious calling.

> [S]he is dressed in white, thus fulfilling the image of the title [*The White Angel*], but the image does more than just show Nightingale in white. Her dress and veil are like a bridal gown and veil in style as well as color. The association of white with virginity and purity is important, as is the bridal association. At the same time she announces her decision to be a nurse, Nightingale announces to her parents that she will never marry. Because she is visually presented as a bride at the same time that she rejects marriage, the subliminal message is that her marriage is to her profession, just as a nun's marriage is to Christ (Jones 1988:225–226).

However, notwithstanding the influence of myth and legend, nursing does have a noble history, and there are many stories of the fortitude, bravery and courage shown by Australian nurses in wartime and other times of community hardship (e.g. Biedermann 2004, Hallett 2007, Scannell-Desch 2005). In Chapter 2 of this book, you will find an in-depth discussion of the history of modern nursing and, after reading it, you will have greater insights and understandings of the origins of some of the myths that surround nursing.

Nursing is endlessly fascinating to many people and this is reflected in the number of television shows, novels and movies that feature nursing and nurses as a major component. There is not the same level of interest in bank workers, or bus drivers or beauty therapists for example. Nursing is ripe with imagery. Many of the images associated with nursing are seemingly at odds with one another, yet all may be conjured up by the word 'nurse'. Images of selflessness (Fealy 2004), kindness, compassion and dedication, hard work, long hours, submission and low pay are among the things that come to mind for some people when they think of nursing. But though nursing has current or historical elements of all these things, there is so much more to nursing than these portray.

Nursing and nurses are subject to various entrenched stereotypes (Fletcher 2007), and some of these are at least partly derived from the myth that surrounds nursing. In the early 1980s, Kalisch et al (1983) identified some major ways that nursing and nurses were stereotyped, and though this work was undertaken in the United States more than two decades ago, it remains relevant to nurses in Australia today, as well as nurses in other parts of the world (see also Muff 1988). The media and popular literature also tend to present nurses as having stereotyped personal characteristics such as youth, femaleness, purity and naivety, altruism and idealism, compliance, and diminutive stature and 'good character' (Fealy 2004, Fletcher 2007).

Nurses are also credited with having certain qualities and virtues that are grounded in romanticism. De Vries et al (1995), in their study of images of nurses as portrayed in popular medical romances, found that nurses are almost always represented as youthful, pure, virginal, kind, petite, beautiful, subservient, sensitive, considerate, competent and able females. In addition to these personal characteristics, the heroines of these stories are typically presented as Caucasian, with blonde hair and green or blue eyes. They are also portrayed and represented as being emotional and hence not to be taken seriously (Ceci 2004).

Darbyshire (1995), in his exploration of the depiction of Nurse Ratched in the popular film *One Flew Over the Cuckoo's Nest*, discusses a counter image of nursing—the battleaxe/torturer. Unlike the nurses found in the medical romance genre, Nurse Ratched is not petite or subservient, and nor is she acquiescent or particularly beautiful. Hunter (1988), in her discussion of the book upon which the film is based, proposes that the Nurse Ratched character is but one example of misogynistic literary tendencies which, she argues, frequently satirically portray the battleaxe/torturer/oppressor nurse as female, and the tender, gentle carer nurse figure as male. Hunter (1988) supports this notion by exploring the images evoked in Tolstoy's description of the gentle hero, Gerasim (*The Death of Ivan Ilyich*, 1886), and Whitman's poem 'The wound dresser' (*Leaves of Grass*, 1891), and comparing them with those evoked by Kesey's Nurse Ratched (*One Flew Over the Cuckoo's Nest*, 1962). In Chapter 4 of this book, Philip Darbyshire scrutinises some current and past nursing stereotypes in more detail.

Though we still see nurses portrayed in various stereotypical and sometimes highly sexualised ways, which is exemplified in the myth of 'nurse as whore', these stereotypes coexist with some of the noble and romantic images of nursing. Failure to challenge these stereotypes is dangerous for nurses and nursing (Fletcher 2007): various stereotypes give the nurse the status of a worker–handmaiden rather than a health professional (Fealy 2004). Stereotypes of this nature perpetuate an anti-intellectual bias against nursing, which is manifest in the view that good nurses are practical people, rather than highly educated professionals.

Coexisting with the romantic myths and stereotypes surrounding nursing is the reality of nursing. This reality is that nurses become acquainted with the visceral and raw aspects of humanity that are usually hidden from the world, because of the illness, the incapacity, the frailty, the disability or other needs of those who are the recipients of nursing care. Nursing provides opportunities for human connectedness and growth that few other careers can offer.

But why is this significant? It is clear, as Fealy states, that it is:

> ... naive to assume that ideology will not continue to influence the development of nursing, and that factors such as class and gender relationships, power brokerage and economics, will not continue to reside at the heart of commentary on the nurse (Fealy 2004:655).

It is for this reason that nurses need to be aware of the danger lurking in latent meaning and rhetoric, and recognise that a reality is being created on behalf of nursing—a reality that is not necessarily theirs. It is important to recognise that the concept of 'nurse' is socially constructed, and that nurses may want to believe in their power and control, but the broader societal context situates nurses in a much more fragile position. Nursing exists within a male-dominated healthcare system, bound by authority and power of that class. The sense of 'self as nurse' is thus subject to what David (2000) refers to as 'received behaviours', which can result in 'horizontal violence' or bullying—behaviours of aggression towards other nurses—in order to maintain fragile perceptions of self. These behaviours are self-defeating, as they destroy collegial relationships, and 'limit freedom of thought and action, and preserves nurses' borderline status' (David 2000:84).

HOW TO DEFINE NURSING?

The urge to define nursing has attracted the attention of nurse scholars for a number of years. While defining a nurse is relatively simple, as you will see as you read further in this chapter, nursing itself has proved somewhat more challenging to define. Though you can probably describe what you think nursing is, the nature and breadth of activities that comprise nursing have contributed to the difficulties associated with defining nursing. Some definitions centre on the functions of a nurse, rather than offering an intrinsic definition of nursing. Henderson produced such a definition of nursing:

> The unique function of the nurse is to assist the individual, sick or well, in the performance of those activities contributing to health or its recovery (or to a peaceful death) that he [sic] would perform unaided if he [sic] had the necessary strength, will or knowledge. And to do this in such a way as to help him [sic] gain independence as rapidly as possible (Henderson, cited in Tomey & Alligood 1998:102).

What needs to be noted in passing is the sexist language that continues to be used when referring to nursing. Language is 'not a neutral information-carrying vehicle', but creates meaning; this meaning changes over time, which makes language very powerful (Fealy 2004:650); its importance cannot be underestimated. David (2000) provides a useful analysis of how nurses collude with their oppressors by uncritically accepting outsiders' social construction of nurses and nursing, suggesting that nurses need to socially construct themselves and their context in order to regain their identity and power.

The complexities and difficulties associated with defining nursing means that some definitions may seem cumbersome and quite ambiguous. But remember that this is more a reflection of the complex nature of nursing than any lack of clarity on behalf of those who have proffered a definition. The International Council of Nurses (ICN), a coalition of nurses' associations that represents nurses in more than 120 countries, has captured some of the complexities in its definition:

> Nursing encompasses autonomous and collaborative care of individuals of all ages, families, groups and communities, sick or well and in all settings. Nursing includes the promotion of health, prevention of illness, and the care of ill, disabled and dying people. Advocacy, promotion of a safe environment, research, participation in shaping health policy and in patient and health systems management, and education are also key nursing roles (www.icn.ch/definition.htm).

In 2003, the Royal College of Nursing (RCN) published a definition of nursing that was the culmination of 18 months' research, and included extensive consultation. The RCN proffered a definition and six key characteristics that capture the essence and varied activities of nursing. The six characteristics are quite detailed and cover issues such as values, relationships and interventions. The full statements can be seen at the

RCN website at www.rcn.org.uk/downloads/definingnursing/definingnursing-a5.pdf. The RCN definition reads as follows:

> Nursing is the use of clinical judgement in the provision of care to enable people to improve, maintain or recover health to cope with health problems and to achieve the best possible quality of life whatever their disease or disability, until death (www.rcn.org.uk/downloads/definingnursing/definingnursing-a5.pdf).

So what is it that excited us about becoming nurses? And, more importantly, what has sustained us on our journeys?

CHOOSING NURSING

Nursing was a gender choice given the societal and historical context of the time (early 1960s and 1970s). It was certainly viewed as an appropriate career choice for females, but also offered potential for achievement, growth and development. It was also a profession that attracted people motivated by altruism and the desire to make a difference to people suffering because of illness and disadvantage. Indeed, this is still a significant motivator of people who choose nursing today. Since the 1970s nursing has made stronger claims to a focus on health promotion, and this now has greater emphasis in construction of nursing knowledge and in conceptualisation of practice. But further to that, there was an overriding quest for understanding and caring for people. This was demonstrated in an egalitarian approach that proved to be unacceptable in nursing at the time (1963–77), when spending time with and caring about patients was viewed as naive and misguided. Such a view denied empathy and concern, and existed through the 1980s and 1990s (McVicar 2003). Currently, the concept of nurses distancing themselves from their patients has been superseded by recognition of the importance of the nurse–patient relationship or the 'therapeutic alliance' (Speedy 1999), which is now characterised as 'emotional labour' (McQueen 2004).

NURSING: WHAT SUSTAINS US

One of the most sustaining things about nursing and being a nurse is the opportunity to contribute a perspective that is informed by feminism. A feminist perspective is 'concerned with gender, power relations, patriarchy and hegemony in society, emphasising gender as a key factor in determining the experiences of women in … nursing' (Fealy 2004:650). Feminist theory can be used to examine power relationships in nursing and healthcare, resulting in the exposure of the 'doctor–nurse game', and more recently in the 'health administrator–nurse game' (Dendaas 2004), which elaborates on how nurses can be losers in the power stakes.

The issue of gender is important for nurses, and is an issue that continues to generate critical discussion in nursing (see, for example, Anthony 2004, Tracey & Nicholl 2007). Gender is critical to the maintenance of power relations, and the formation of an identity in nursing. This issue is discussed further in detail in Chapter 12. Nurses are socialised early in their development to adopt 'appropriate' behaviours and beliefs about how to behave as professionals, and how to, as women (predominantly), 'look, talk and feel' (Peter 2004). Their age, gender, family and life experiences all contribute to and influence the way they perceive the power structures and dynamics of the world that is nursing work (Roberts 2000). To be unaware of the impact of power relations and the oppression arising from these is to be locked in a cycle of relationships that serve to severely disadvantage nurses and nursing, perpetuating disunity and disempowerment.

It should be noted in passing that many young women of today appear to have an uneasy relationship with feminism; however, the real problem has been identified as: 'can I be who I am and be feminist?' (Baumgardner & Richards 2003:448). This confusion is understandable, since young women are unclear about what feminism requires of them (and does not require of them). For example, can they still like fashion, have boyfriends, and be who they want to be? They 'often think of feminism as telling them what they can't do, rather than as a philosophy that *shows them the potential for what they can do*' (Baumgardner & Richards 2003:448, emphasis added), and hence what they can contribute. This suggests that it is time to assist young women to develop clarity about this situation (see Ch 12).

A natural consequence of a feminist perspective was an interest in the theory and practice of feminist research, which demanded refocusing on the experiences of women. This required some fortitude and commitment, because at that time there was scepticism and ridicule directed towards those who advocated its usage, particularly from researchers who promoted a 'hard science' perspective as the only valid and reliable form of research. However, research that is informed by feminist (and other postmodern) perspectives is now more readily accepted as an appropriate methodology in many (but not all) research camps.

A sustaining factor within a nursing career is the opportunity to provide leadership in as many ways as possible, be it research, management or practice. Effective leadership requires particular attributes, such as high-level communication skills, awareness of one's beliefs, values, attitudes and emotions, respect for others, commitment, passion, flexibility and adaptability (Jackson 2008).

Transformational leaders are able to create shared visions, act as role models, inspire, motivate, intellectually stimulate and mentor others (Reinhardt 2004). In many ways, 'leadership is a process of drawing out rather than putting in' (Kitson 2004:211). This implicitly suggests that everyone has a responsibility to exercise leadership qualities. Acknowledging that nursing has many talented participants, Kitson implores us to desist from 'eating our young', or cutting our leaders down ('tall poppy syndrome'), and suggests that, as we work with patients, families, colleagues and managers, we:

> ... draw out our vision, our values and beliefs about nursing; our notion of service; our understanding of our own humanity and our ability to face pain, suffering, anxiety, anger and all the other human emotions that nurses face on a daily basis (Kitson 2004:211).

By developing these understandings, we can understand and accept ourselves, and see beyond to the dysfunctionality of organisations and workplaces in order to reform them. This requires nurse leaders to be political and astute (Antrobus 2004, Dendaas 2004, Donnelly 2003).

Women have specific leadership skills that can be harnessed, although these are typically disparaged. Research literature suggests that, in general, successful women leaders value interconnectedness, inclusivity and relationships, whereas male leaders value competition, dominance, ambition, aggression and decisiveness (Robinson-Walker 1999). Rudan (2003), in focusing on leadership in nursing, identified a warm demeanour, personal and professional interest in followers, nurturing behaviour, promotion of growth in others, and the use of humour and interpersonal talk as some of the characteristics that make for successful nurse leadership. These are all the skills that nurses at every level of the profession have, to a greater or lesser degree, which provides them with opportunities to assume leadership roles whatever the level and location of their work.

Over the years of our own nursing careers we have witnessed many changes—from changes in how students are prepared for registration as nurses, through to changes to the environment in which nurses work. Nurses work in climates of continual change, and are challenged by the demands of ageing and increasingly complex clients, as well as themselves. Elsewhere, Jackson notes:

> As nurses we are facing some of the greatest tests in the history of the discipline. In a climate of persistent international volatility and instability, and with ever diminishing resources, we are challenged to provide increasingly complex care to incredibly diverse and/or fractured communities. We are further challenged to provide inclusive, sensitive, accessible and user friendly services that defy entrenched, cumbersome sometimes inflexible health care cultures (Jackson 2003:347).

In addition to these challenges, nursing is currently making attempts to address an international widespread shortage of experienced nurses, particularly specialist nurses. Recruitment and retention issues have contributed to an ageing nursing workforce, increasing casualisation of that workforce, and increasing international recruitment (Jackson et al 2001). Furthermore, issues including bullying, abuse and violence, professional autonomy, imposed organisational change, occupational health and safety issues, and constant restructuring (Jackson et al 2001) have been associated with difficulties in retaining a viable nursing workforce in that they contribute to a working environment that can be experienced as hostile and difficult (Hutchinson et al 2008). However, despite these difficulties, nursing still offers the qualifications and skills upon which satisfying and rewarding careers can be built.

TYPES OF NURSE IN AUSTRALIA AND NEW ZEALAND

There are a number of entry points into nursing. In Australia and New Zealand, the title 'nurse' refers to someone who is either registered or enrolled by national or state-registering authorities. Nurses belong to a regulated professional group that is responsible to the community it serves for supplying healthcare to a constantly high standard, through the maintenance of professional standards and personal integrity. Currently, there are three types of nurse who practice in a wide range of health and community settings (see the box below for some examples). These are the assistant in nursing or nurse's aide, the enrolled nurse and the registered nurse. In Australia, enrolled and registered nurses are required to meet national competency standards, as explicated by the Australian Nursing and Midwifery Council (ANMC). Further details about these types of nurses are given below.

Assistant in nursing or nurse's aide

The *assistant in nursing* (AIN) or *nurse's aide* is a person who carries out some nursing duties under the direct supervision of a registered nurse. Most often, the duties are associated with activities of daily living, such as hygiene, feeding and personal care. Many undergraduate students undertake employment as an AIN while they are studying their undergraduate degree at university. In New South Wales, for example, it is estimated that in excess of 60% of graduates in nursing have gained clinical experience through AIN employment while engaged in undergraduate education (Bulter & Garvey 2003).

CLINICAL PRACTICE SETTINGS FOR NURSES

Nurses practise in a wide range of health and community settings, including:

- acute hospital settings
- day surgery nursing
- daycare clinics
- residential care facilities (such as nursing homes)
- school nursing
- drug and alcohol nursing
- general community nursing
- specialist community nursing (such as mental health nursing)
- occupational health nursing
- general practice (or practice) nursing
- justice health (including remand centres, prisons and juvenile justice settings), and
- rural and remote area nursing.

In recognition of the status of these undergraduate student AINs, provision has been made (in some areas) for them to perform more wide-ranging and advanced duties than those performed by those AINs who are not engaged in undergraduate nurse education (Bulter & Garvey 2003). According to 'New South Wales Health Circular 2001/80', student AINs are able to practise an 'extended role', with permissible duties varying according to the level of undergraduate education the student has achieved. These duties range from the provision of hygiene and comfort measures, and simple observations in the first year, through to more complex procedures in the third year.

There are various titles given to people fulfilling the AIN (or very similar) role, and these various titles are applied in various locations. Some of the other titles are nurse's aide, care worker or personal care assistant. AINs (and similar workers) are known as unregulated health workers, and they do not come under the auspices of nurse-registering authorities. Rather, the registered nurse under whose supervision they are working is accountable in the event of an adverse situation occurring.

Enrolled nurse

The enrolled nurse (EN) is one who has completed an approved educational course leading to enrolment with nurse-registering authorities. The EN course is shorter than courses leading to registration as a nurse, usually being of 12–18 months' duration. The model of education also differs, in that trainee ENs are employed by health facilities and work during their training. In New South Wales, trainee ENs experience much of their classroom teaching in the Technical and Further Education (TAFE) sector.

Unlike the registered nurse (whose names appear in a register), the names of ENs are entered onto a roll. Like the registered nurse, the EN is subject to the regulation and censure of nurse-registering authorities. ENs have responsibility for their actions and are accountable to registering authorities and also to the registered nurse under whose supervision they are working. Unlike the AIN, who must work under the direct supervision of a registered nurse, some registering authorities permit the EN to practise under the direct or indirect supervision of a registered nurse (www.nursesboard. sa.gov.au). Furthermore, some registering authorities authorise ENs who are able to meet certain requirements to practise without the supervision of a registered nurse (e.g. www.nursesboard.sa.gov.au). However, this practice is strictly monitored.

There are a number of career development opportunities available to ENs and these can include access to professional development courses that permit an extended role, such as medication administration. Some ENs wish to study further to complete qualifications to become registered nurses. Many universities and colleges give some recognition of prior learning to ENs, meaning that they may be able to undertake a shortened version of the Bachelor of Nursing degree.

Registered nurse

The term *registered nurse* (RN) refers to one who has undertaken and completed an approved program leading to nurse registration as a nurse, holds an appropriate qualification, has met all the requirements of registering authorities, and whose name appears on a register of nurses in accordance with the relevant state or territory Act. The RN is considered to be a first-level nurse and, as such, is permitted to practise without supervision and is accountable and responsible for actions taken and decisions made. Nurses who are registered include nurses or nurse practitioners. However, a change to national registration for nursing and a number of other health professions has been foreshadowed in Australia and this is expected to take effect from July 2010 (see www.nhwt.gov.au/natreg.asp for further information).

RNs have various career progression paths and various titles, depending on where they are located, so as you enter hospitals and community health settings you will encounter RNs with varying degrees of experience and status. These can include clinical nurse consultants (CNCs), clinical nurse specialists (CNSs), nurse managers, nurse educators, nurse researchers and other levels of nurse.

PROFESSIONAL CONDUCT

Nurses are expected to be people of integrity who conduct themselves with a high level of personal honour and veracity. It is important that members of the public feel safe in hospitals, and believe themselves to be in trustworthy and competent hands. If people do not feel safe, they would not be able to feel secure in leaving their loved ones in the care of nurses and healthcare facilities. Nursing authorities act to ensure the safety of the public by holding nurses accountable for their actions and making nurses answerable for their behaviour and any complaints that are made against them. In order to gain initial registration, nursing applicants need to demonstrate they are of good character.

Nurses are answerable to registering authorities that have the power to question nurses, and suspend or remove them from the register. These same authorities can also place conditions on registration, restricting practice or, in certain circumstances, requiring a nurse participate in educational programs. The conduct of nurses is also guided by various codes that inform professional conduct. In 1990, the Australasian Nurse Registering Authorities Conference (ANRAC) instigated the Code of Professional Conduct for Nurses in Australia in response to a perceived need for a clear statement to guide registered and enrolled nurses. Subsequently, the Australian Nursing Council (now the Australian Nursing and Midwifery Council or ANMC) continued to progress the Code to ensure its continued relevance to contemporary health environments. In order to maintain currency, the Code was reviewed in 1995 and 2003. It is the responsibility of every Australian nurse to be familiar with the Code and use it to guide their everyday practice (www.anmc.org.au). The ANMC Code of Professional Conduct for Nurses in Australia is available from the ANMC website at www.anmc.org.au. The International Council of Nurses (ICN) has a Code for nurses and this is considered to provide the basis for ethical international nursing practice. The ICN Code of Ethics for Nurses Australia can be downloaded from the ICN site at www.icn.ch/icncode.pdf.

REGULATION OF PRACTICE

In Australia, nurse registration in each state and territory is governed by registration Acts, and administered by state and territory registration authorities. These authorities are charged with regulating nursing practice. Although there has been a lot of discussion in Australia about national registration, the current situation is that nurse registration is obtained on a state-by-state basis. Thus, if nurses are registered in New South Wales and wish to work as nurses in South Australia, they first need to apply to the South Australian Nurses Board for registration. In New Zealand, nurses are registered by a central registering authority, the Nursing Council of New Zealand. However, if nurses are registered in New Zealand and wish to practise in Australia, they need to seek registration in the state or territory in which they wish to practise. Australian and New Zealand nurses have mutual recognition through the *Trans Tasman Mutual Recognition Act 1997*. For more information about this Act in relation to nurses, see www.nmb.nsw. gov.au.

When seeking to register in Australia, nurses from some countries receive recognition, while nurses from other countries need to sit exams or complete other education prior to gaining registration. More information about initial registration and registration from state-to-state and country-to-country can be found on relevant websites. A selection of these websites appears below and you may find it interesting to browse through some of these:

- Nurses and Midwives Board New South Wales: www.nmb.nsw.gov.au
- Nurses Board of South Australia: www.nursesboard.sa.gov.au/reg_cre.html
- Nursing Council of New Zealand: www.nursingcouncil.org.nz/reg.html
- Nursing Board of Tasmania: www.nursingboardtas.org.au/nbtonline.nsf/ $LookupDocName/FEES
- Nurses Board of Victoria: www.nbv.org.au/nbv/nbvonlinev1.nsf/ $LookupDocName/registration_&_practice_standards

CONCLUSION

Nursing attracts people from all walks of life. Many readers of this text will be entering nursing as school leavers, but others will be mature-aged students who come to nursing with a variety of life experiences. Welcome to nursing, and congratulations on making a choice that will open many doors for you and provide you with a career for life. You may find it challenging and, possibly, not quite what you expected. But, go with your passion, and believe in yourself—because you can create your life. The road you have chosen is not an easy one, but you need to believe in yourself, as we do, to succeed.

We may have had a more facilitative environment, so for that we are grateful, and we need to be. What a blessed life we have had, on behalf of nursing.

> **REFLECTIVE QUESTIONS**
>
> 1 What are the main reasons you have chosen a career in nursing?
>
> 2 Why do you think nursing has proved difficult to define?
>
> 3 What do you see as essential personal qualities for nurses?
>
> 4 Consider the popular stereotypes of nurses. How many can you identify? Did any of these stereotypes influence your decision to become a nurse?
>
> 5 Spouse (2000) suggests that many students come into nursing with strongly held images in their minds about how they will practise and what sort of a nurse they will be. What sort of nurse do you want to be?
>
> 6 What has been your experience of nursing? What motivated you to go there? What now sustains you?

RECOMMENDED READINGS

Fletcher K 2007 Image: changing how women nurses think about themselves. Literature review. Journal of Advanced Nursing 58(3):207–215

Jackson D, Daly J 2004 Current challenges and issues facing nursing in Australia. Nursing Science Quarterly 17(4):352–355

Jackson D, Mannix J, Daly J 2001 Retaining a viable workforce: a critical challenge for nursing. Contemporary Nurse 11(2/3):163–172

Scannell-Desch E 2005 Lessons learned and advice from Vietnam War nurses: a qualitative study. Journal of Advanced Nursing 49(6):600–607

Spouse J 2000 An impossible dream? Images of nursing held by pre-registration students and their effect on sustaining motivation to become nurses. Journal of Advanced Nursing 32(3):730–739

Tracey C, Nicholl H 2007 The multifaceted influence of gender in career progress in nursing. Journal of Nursing Management 15:677–682

REFERENCES

Anthony AS 2004 Gender bias and discrimination in nursing education: can we change it? Nurse Educator 29(3):121–125

Antrobus S 2004 Why does nursing need political leaders? Journal of Nursing Management 12(4):227–228

Baumgardner J, Richards A 2003 The number one question about feminism. Feminist Studies 29(2):448–454

Biedermann N 2004 Tears on my pillow: Australian nurses in Vietnam. Random House, Sydney

Bulter A, Garvey A 2003 Professional issues: the more things change … The Lamp 60(6):24–25

Ceci C 2004 Gender, power, nursing: a case analysis. Nursing Inquiry 11(2):72–81

David A 2000 Nursing's gender politics: reformulating the footnotes. Advances in Nursing Science 23(1):83–94

Darbyshire P 1995 Reclaiming 'Big Nurse': a feminist critique of Ken Kesey's portrayal of Nurse Ratched in *One Flew Over the Cuckoo's Nest*. Nursing Inquiry 2(4):198–202

Dendaas N 2004 The scholarship related to nursing work environments: where do we go from here? Advances in Nursing Science 27(1):12–21

De Vries S, Dunlop M, Goopy S, Moyle W, Sutherland-Lockhart D 1995 Discipline and passion: meaning, masochism and mythology in popular medical romances. Nursing Inquiry 2(4):203–210

Donnelly C 2003 Leadership: professional, inspirational or dysfunctional? Journal of Nursing Management 11(2):65–67

Fealy GM 2004 'The good nurse': visions and value in images of the nurse. Journal of Advanced Nursing 46(6):649–656

Fletcher K 2007 Image: changing how women nurses think about themselves. Literature review. Journal of Advanced Nursing 58(3):207–215

Hallett C 2007 The personal writings of First World War nurses: a study of the interplay of authorial intention and scholarly interpretation. Nursing Inquiry 14(4):320–329

Hunter K 1988 Nurses: the satiric image and the translocated ideal. In: Jones A (ed.) Images of nurses: perspectives from history, art and literature. University of Pennsylvania Press, Philadelphia

Hutchinson M, Jackson D, Wilkes L, Vickers MH 2008 A model of bullying in the nursing workplace: organizational characteristics as critical antecedents. Advances in Nursing Science 31(2):E60–E71

Jackson D 2003 Culture, health and social justice. Contemporary Nurse 15(3):347–348

Jackson D 2008 Servant leadership: a framework for developing sustainable research capacity in nursing. Collegian 15(1):27–33

Jackson D, Mannix J, Daly J 2001 Retaining a viable workforce: a critical challenge for nursing. Contemporary Nurse 11(2–3):163–172

Jones A 1988 *The White Angel* (1936): Hollywood's image of Florence Nightingale. In: Jones A (ed.) Images of nurses: perspectives from history, art and literature. University of Pennsylvania Press, Philadelphia

Kalisch P, Kalisch B, Scobey M 1983 Images of nurses on television. Springer Publishing, New York

Kitson A 2004 Drawing out leadership. Journal of Advanced Nursing 48(3):211

McQueen ACH 2004 Emotional intelligence in nursing work. Journal of Advanced Nursing 47(1):101–108

McVicar A 2003 Workplace stress in nursing: a literature review. Journal of Advanced Nursing 44(6):633–642

Muff J 1988 Of images and ideals: a look at socialization and sexism in nursing. In: Jones A (ed.) Images of nurses: perspectives from history, art and literature. University of Pennsylvania Press, Philadelphia

Peter E 2004 Nursing resistance as ethical action: literature review. Journal of Advanced Nursing 46(4):403–416

Reinhardt AC 2004 Discourse on the transformational leader metanarrative or finding the right person for the job. Advances in Nursing Science 27(1):21–32

Roberts SJ 2000 Development of a positive professional identity: liberating oneself from the oppressor within. Advances in Nursing Science 22(4):71–83

Robinson-Walker C 1999 Women in leadership and health care: the journey to authenticity and power. Jossey-Bass, San Francisco

Rudan V 2003 The best of both worlds: a consideration of gender in team building. Journal of Nursing Administration 33(3):179–186

Scannell-Desch E 2005 Lessons learned and advice from Vietnam War nurses: a qualitative study. Journal of Advanced Nursing 49(6):600–607

Speedy S 1999 The therapeutic alliance. In: Clinton M, Nelson S (eds) Advanced practice in mental health nursing. Blackwell Science, Oxford

Spouse J 2000 An impossible dream? Images of nursing held by pre-registration students and their effect on sustaining motivation to become nurses. Journal of Advanced Nursing 32(3):730–739

Tomey AM, Alligood MR 1998 Nursing theorists and their work. Mosby, St Louis

Tracey C, Nicholl H 2007 The multifaceted influence of gender in career progress in nursing. Journal of Nursing Management 15:677–682

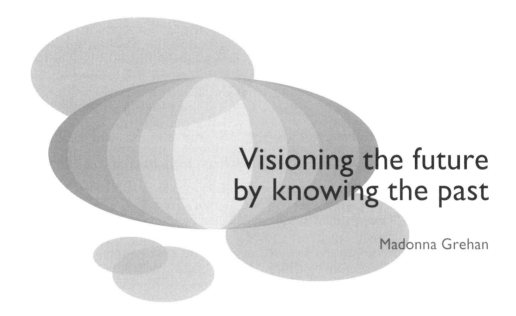

Visioning the future by knowing the past

Madonna Grehan

LEARNING OBJECTIVES

After reading this chapter, students should be able to:

- understand the benefits of having a knowledge of nursing's history
- develop a critical understanding of received accounts of nursing's history
- identify the lineage of nursing and its occupational relatives
- identify significant events which have influenced nursing's evolution in Australia, and
- describe aspects in nursing and midwifery that warrant historical research.

KEY WORDS

History, nursing, midwifery, regulation, education, hospitals

---

HISTORY AND ITS PURPOSE

History, heritage, tradition and the past are concepts that may be familiar to most of us, but what is their relevance to nursing? What is the relationship between knowing about the past and seeing into the future? This chapter is about nursing's history. It explains why knowing about nursing's history is useful for all nurses. For some people, history consists merely of important dates, events and celebrated individuals. These elements have a place in history's narrative, but history has so much more to offer than time lines and famous faces. Some people also think that history is about heritage and tradition, but an Australian historian, Graeme Davison (2000), argues that the concepts of 'heritage' and 'tradition' are concerned with sentimentality, not the accuracy and objectivity of history that is critical and self-aware. We will return to these concepts later in this chapter.

Why is history important for nurses to know about? Davison writes that, among other things:

> History … tells us who we are, gives us an imaginative and sympathetic insight into the lives of others, encourages a critical attitude to question social and political change, and equips us to participate in a political community (Davison 2000:263).

Furthermore, an understanding of history can help to explain how things have come to be the way that they are (Davison 2000). Applied to nursing, for example, we can use the tools of history to examine why nursing is a profession dominated by women. History can also help to explain why some issues in nursing seem complicated, such as Australia's plan to implement national nursing registration. An examination of social and political developments in the history of healthcare can help us to understand how nursing's identity as a profession has developed compared with other professions (Connolly 2004).

Sometimes, too, history offers valuable insights into what the future might bring, although clearly it is impossible to be certain what will happen in the future. We can use history to examine the background to current issues and problems. Taking one contemporary concern, the worldwide shortages of nurses and midwives, historical inquiry might explain if these shortages have occurred in the past, and how they were dealt with. Armed with a historical perspective of nursing shortages, it may be possible to shed light on the current situation and to plan future workforces differently. How, then, do we, as nurses, learn about history?

Traditional views of history

Each of us learns about history in different ways. We hear stories and read texts. Sometimes we might ask people about their experiences. A lot of what we have come to accept as nursing's history derives from popular culture, such as movies and television. Thinking about an 'image' representative of nursing's history, the Australian imagination might picture a neatly frocked Florence Nightingale, carrying a burning lamp in the military wards of Scutari in the Crimean War in the 1850s. We might see a nurse soothing the brow of an injured soldier in World War I, or picture Sister Kenny, the controversial Australian woman who applied novel treatment regimes to children affected by polio. What do these images say about nursing's history?

These are romantic impressions to say the least. It is likely that most of us have not questioned whether there is any accuracy or objectivity to these images of nursing's history. This is not surprising, as stories of Nightingale, Kenny and noble nurses have been told and retold. They have come to be accepted as how nursing 'was'.

Commonly accepted interpretations of history are also known as 'received' histories. Received histories of nursing summarise this complex history as follows. Before Miss Nightingale's influence and the later professionalisation of nursing, the care of the sick and childbearing women was unskilled work of low status. The installation of structured training schemes and, later, nursing's professionalising movement, transformed nursing into a profession for educated women. Received histories, lauding the transformation of nursing from old to new, from darkness to light, were recorded by nurse luminaries in the United States of America by Adelaide Nutting and Lavinia Dock (1907), and in Britain by Sarah Tooley (1906). Nurses in Australia (Webster 1942) and in New Zealand (Maclean 1932) reiterated this triumphal tale.

However, in recalling history as a narrative of progress, received histories inevitably have drawbacks. While they champion the achievements of individuals and celebrate progress, they leave out the more mundane, the contribution of everyday nurses, and those aspects of history which do not 'fit' the story of progress. In so doing, nursing becomes distanced from the society it serves. It becomes distanced from the political times in which nurses have lived and worked, from those in which nursing has evolved, from other professions, and from nursing as practice. Until very recently, received accounts of nursing's history were accepted as accurate. They are now being challenged.

An enlightened view of the past

Recent scholarship in nursing history has questioned the tale of nursing's triumphs over ignorant nurses through professionalisation and the Nightingale influence. This scholarship applies critical inquiry to history (Dean 1994). Critical history rejects assumptions such as the idea that history is about progress, or that complex events can be explained simply (Connolly 2004). Critical history throws a wide net to examine issues, events, processes and the people who received histories have ignored, so that nursing's history may be seen in a different light.

One example of groups whose contribution to nursing has not been noted in received histories of nursing is Aboriginal nurses like Sadie Corner (pictured) and Lowitja (Lois)

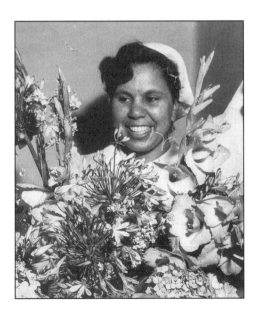

Sadie Corner. Reproduced with the permission of the Salvation Army Australia, Southern Territory Archives and Museum, Melbourne.

O'Donohue, who overcame considerable odds to train as nurses and work in Australia's white healthcare system. To explore this and other fascinating and instructive aspects of nursing history would entail a story of politics, race, social attitudes and geography. It is one of many in Australian nursing history waiting to be told, using the tools of critical history.

Here we can offer only a snapshot of nursing's history. To begin this overview, we look past received history to other explanations of nursing's evolution. We discuss contemporary nursing's antecedents and examine the formations of care, using the example of the Australian arena. We consider some historical influences on nursing and some of the events in nursing's evolution in Australia and New Zealand, and discuss the relationship between history and professional identity. The chapter concludes with remarks on nursing's future.

THE ROOTS OF MODERN NURSING

Given that the act of nursing is as old as the human race (Nelson 2000), it is difficult to identify nursing's so-called 'roots'. However, in the interests of advancing a discussion about nursing's history, it is useful to agree upon some point in history and work from there. If we agree that nursing in the twenty-first century is 'modern', we can attempt to visualise what its antecedents are. Much of contemporary healthcare in the twenty-first century is provided in what we call the 'modern' hospital.

The 'modern' hospital as a concept emerged in the late nineteenth century, a time when medicine was developing a sophisticated understanding of disease and illness, and experimenting with novel treatments (Rosenberg 1987). The modern hospital was hailed as a complete innovation with its ordered and hierarchical system of caregiving and the emergence of modern nursing, with its hierarchical structures, as parallel in this innovation (Nelson 2000). However, scholars of nursing and health history, including the Australian nursing historian Sioban Nelson (2000), have argued that the idea of the hospital as a place where a systematic care was provided was not 'new'. Rather, it constituted new ways of doing 'old' things in which structure and standards were replicated, but were evangelised as modern innovations. It is in these older ways of providing care that the roots of modern nursing can be found.

Pre-modern nursing

In the early Christian era and beyond, care in hospices (early forms of hospitals) was performed by religious communities to those on spiritual pilgrimages (Nelson 2000). Religious orders sought to emulate the work of Jesus Christ in tending to his flock by caring for strangers, the sick poor, providing them a place of refuge, giving nourishment, tending the infirm, and perhaps applying palliative treatments (Nelson 2000). One group of nurses who have sustained this care is the Catholic religious order, the Sisters of Charity of St Vincent de Paul, mentioned later in this chapter. However, the care of the sick poor was not the sole domain of Catholic organisations. Protestant female followers of Christianity, such as Elizabeth Fry, Jane Shaw Stewart, Agnes Jones and Sister Dora [Pattison], in the nineteenth century formed nursing 'sisterhoods' through which nursing care was provided to the sick poor in a similar way (Summers 1989). Thus, nursing's foundations can be found in care in the sick poor as strangers, provided by religious orders as 'an integral part of Christian practice' (Nelson 2000:3).

There is of course, another form of care that is not concerned with the Christian practice of caring for strangers. That care is familial care, undertaken conventionally by women as extensions of their roles as wives and mothers (Summers 1988). In the following discussion, familial care is considered within the context of the nineteenth century, a period when Britain was expanding its empire, establishing colonies around the world. With colonial expansion, the customs, conventions and system of government of Britain were carried to new horizons. What was happening in Britain, therefore, impacted on its colonies, including Australia and New Zealand.

The old style nurse

For those with family to attend them, for centuries the person's home or 'domicile' had been the primary domain for the care of the sick, the dying and the place for birth (Summers 1989). This caring work was undertaken as part of familial duties, usually by women; by the nineteenth century and for those who could afford to pay, it was possible to engage a secular (non-religious) nurse to watch over the patient (Summers 1989). These nurses had varying backgrounds, with some relying on their experience of childbearing and rearing, while others, particularly those practising midwifery, were educated by apprenticeship (Evenden 2000). In mid-nineteenth century Britain, popular culture opened a window on the world of the domiciliary nurse via the writings of the social commentator, Charles Dickens. Through one of his serialised novels, *The Life and Adventures of Martin Chuzzlewit*, published in 1843, Dickens brought to the imagination of the reading public two memorable characters who symbolised all that was perceived to be wrong with nurses and nursing (Grehan 2004).

The Life and Adventures of Martin Chuzzlewit introduced Mrs Sarah Gamp and her friend Betsy Prig. Gamp was a domiciliary nurse and midwife in London attending births, the sick and the deceased; Prig was a hospital nurse who moonlighted as a 'private' nurse in people's homes. Gamp and Prig were depicted as middle-aged, fat, uncouth, drunken, ignorant, unrefined and untrustworthy attendants. Accompanying Dickens' text were graphic pen and ink sketches of Mrs Gamp and Betsy Prig, leaving little to readers' imaginations. Dickens' narratives helped to build perceptions that many nurses were unsuited to the important duty of caring for the sick and for childbearing women, adding to calls for reforms in hospital and private nursing (Grehan 2004).

The 'modern' nurse

Calls for a new style of nurse must be considered, not as a result of, but within the context of other developments in society in the nineteenth century. For example, in the Western world at this time, medicine was developing new understandings of diseases and ways to treat them. The modern hospital was the place where medicine's innovations were carried out; innovations in surgery called for a team of people to guarantee their success (Rosenberg 1987). Nurses providing after care for operation cases needed to be cooperative, literate and diligent, and they needed to be able to observe changes in the patient's state, using new technologies such as the thermometer (Grehan 2004). Nurses who could perform the new skills required of them were not always easy to find, particularly in the colonies. To understand the development of what is considered in received history to be the era of modern nursing, our discussion continues in the geographic location of colonial Australia and New Zealand.

HEALTHCARE IN EARLY AUSTRALIA AND OTHER COLONIES

As we have noted, colonies transplanted the conventions of their homelands to their new surroundings, so that people who required nursing in childbirth, or as a result of some injury or ailment, were tended at home by the most able member of the family (Grehan 2004). Few records have survived that might explain precisely what nursing constituted in the newly settled British colonial world. It is sobering to consider, however, that care was performed in the absence of modern-day sanitation, where access to running water meant the existence of a nearby stream or perhaps a stagnant pond, where 'watching' the patient at night was done by candlelight, and where help in the form of a doctor or nurse might be several days ride away on horseback.

Care provided in the community

As was the case in Britain, governments in Australia tended to leave the responsibility of healthcare to individuals (Grehan 2004). We know from private diaries, letters and administrative documents, including birth registers and coronial inquests, that a variety of people were available to attend the infirm and childbearing women. For example, doctors, nurses, midwives, herbalists, oculists, druggists and dentists were just some of those advertising in the town of Melbourne in 1847 (*Port Phillip Almanac and Business Directory*). Who the patient chose depended on who was available, what the purchaser expected of his or her care, and what he or she was willing to pay (Martyr 2002).

Birth, for example, was a time when women needed help. Doctors and experienced attendants were not always available, especially in isolated rural areas. Local women often filled this gap, attending births as a neighbourly gesture, or sometimes as paid employment (Grehan & Nelson 2005). A study of births registered in an isolated rural district of New South Wales found that, in the period 1856 to 1896, women were recorded as the primary birth attendant in almost half of the births (Strachan 2001). In some ways, this array of persons was the ultimate in consumer 'choice'. In reality, however, obtaining an attendant at birth or at times of sickness was a risky business, because there was no real way to measure the qualifications or skills of an attendant. Some nurses were known to have undertaken formal education in midwifery; others had the experience of having their family to rely on (Grehan 2003). Others had no experience whatsoever (Peel 2006).

In the colonial world, where employment for women was hard to find, nursing and midwifery was easily adopted when family circumstances changed. For instance, the Australian nurse historian, Joan Durdin, writes that Mrs Elizabeth Knight, a well-respected midwife in the Mount Gambier region of South Australia, began work at the age of 70 after the death of her husband (Durdin 1991). Women attending others as paid work were known as 'handywomen', in the same way that a handyman performs a multitude of tasks around a house (Grehan 2004). These women combined the roles of tending the sick, preparing the dead for burial, acting as midwife, and sometimes running the local postal service too (Forth et al 1998).

Institutional care

As it was in Britain, institutional healthcare in the colonies was a product of the charity sector; some hospitals and asylums in the colonial world were part of the government's management of prisoners and those deemed to be lunatics (Martyr 2002). Where colonists expanded the white frontier, voluntary hospitals were established in response to industrial catastrophes, such as mining disasters (Collins 1999), but what institutional care was available depended on the geographic locality, the size of the population and its perceived need. The Melbourne Lying-in Hospital and Infirmary for Diseases Peculiar to Women and Children, for example, was established in 1856 for the indigent in the colony of Victoria, mirroring similar institutions in Britain, Scotland and Ireland (McCalman 1998).

The voluntary hospitals, also called 'charitable institutions', were established by philanthropically minded people and funded by subscription, so that, in return for their financial support, subscribers were able to recommend people for the institution's charity (McCalman 1998). However, hospitals were thought to harbour miasmas, noxious vapours said to emanate from suppurating wounds, ill-ventilated rooms, cesspits and cemeteries (Nelson 1998). According to mid-nineteenth century medical orthodoxy, diseases were a result of absorption of miasmas; the practice of 'sanitary' science was the method to minimise them (Nelson 1998). Sanitary science and miasmatic theory demanded an extensive regime of cleanliness and ventilation practices for this purpose, and the exclusion of certain conditions from hospital admission. Among them were smallpox and forms of cancer (Bashford 1998). Pregnant women were excluded from hospital admission, too, because healthy people were thought to be at risk from miasmas.

Institutional nurses

Just as in Britain, hospitals in the colonial world were hierarchical places. What a nurse was expected to do depended on the type of establishment in which she was employed, and on what basis she was employed—that is, as head nurse, assistant nurse or pupil nurse. In the colony of Victoria, for example, hospitals might be operated by a married couple as attendants who provided food, did the laundry and attended to the patients; other establishments employed men as nurses (Collins & Kippen 2003). According to the dictates of sanitary science, the nurse's role in maintaining the cleanest possible environment, through promoting fresh air and cleanliness, was of paramount importance (Nelson 2000).

Given that hospitals were not sewered until the late nineteenth century, it was also the nurses' job under this regime to dispose of bodily wastes such as blood, faeces and urine. Excreta were placed in buckets stored at the end of wards and later thrown out into a cesspit within hospital grounds (Templeton 1969). Institutional nurses' work also included scrubbing floors, brushing carpets, dusting, polishing brassware and furniture, washing the patients and providing nourishments for those who could not do it for themselves. Nurses had to clean and fumigate straw mattresses, known as palliasses, in special airing rooms (McCalman 1998). They carried soiled linen to the laundry for washing. In some hospitals they slept at the end of wards so that they could attend people when required.

Mid-nineteenth century nursing consisted of a mixture of bedside attendance and lots of domestic work. It was extremely hard work for little reward. Little wonder, then, that few people were attracted to the position of 'hospital nurse' and the descriptor of 'Sarah Gamp' was applied to many of them (Grehan 2004). Those who applied for positions at Melbourne's Lying-in Hospital in the nineteenth century, for example, either as nurses or pupils, had to provide a testimonial or letter from a minister of religion or medical practitioner as a recommendation that the hospital employ them. This was designed to weed out potential troublemakers (McCalman 1998). However, even with these attempts at control, nurses were found wanting in their behaviour, had bad language, were drunk on duty and were cruel to patients (Grehan 2004). What is clear is that we hear only about those nurses who did not comply with institutional expectations. This quirk in nursing's history is not so surprising. As the American historian Laurel Ulrich has noted in the title of her recent (2007) book, 'Well behaved women seldom make history'!

Institutional training schemes

In the last quarter of the twentieth century, as the expansion of the modern hospital created a demand for more staff, hospitals introduced their own training schemes for nurses. Training, it has to be said, was far less sophisticated than the term suggests. It involved on-the-job learning, combined with lectures by medical practitioners, which pupil nurses attended only if they could be freed from their ward work (Mitchell 1977). Hospitals, always starved of funds, sometimes hired out pupil nurses to nurse private paying patients in their own homes, meaning that pupil nurses could spend a substantial portion of their training time away from the hospital, learning very little (Templeton 1969).

Another issue was that training tended to be organised around the institution's associated medical speciality, so that wildly varying schemes proliferated and a lack of uniformity in training was the outcome. For example, a training scheme in a hospital established for people with eye and ear conditions produced eye and ear nurses. Training was so specific to the hospital's needs that the 'trained' nurses' skills were not always transferable to another environment (Trembath & Hellier 1987).

Nightingale trained nurses

Given the reported variability in nurses, their care, and the low status of nursing, it is not surprising that Miss Florence Nightingale's ideas about training nurses were seen as necessary solutions to the various ills pervading colonial healthcare. When news emerged that Nightingale was to establish a training school where nurses could be trained 'properly', the Australian public embraced the idea (*Argus*, 10 July 1856).

In Britain, a charitable organisation known as the 'Nightingale Fund for Nursing' was founded in 1856, to commemorate Nightingale's work with the Crimean War wounded. Headed by a group of social reformers, not Nightingale herself, the Nightingale Fund wanted to support nurse training in institutions all around the colonial world. The Nightingale Fund's enduring message was that nursing needed educated 'ladies' of good character who could act as role models for the less educated nurses around them (Baly 1987). Under the auspices of the Nightingale Fund, two training schools in London were established. One was for general nursing at St Thomas's Hospital; the other was for midwifery nursing at King's College Hospital, although it lasted only for five years (Baly 1987). The so-called 'model' of Nightingale nurse training spread to hospitals throughout the English-speaking world.

Nightingale nursing was introduced into New South Wales with much fanfare in 1868 after Sir Henry Parkes, then Colonial Secretary of New South Wales, requested the Fund's help to improve conditions at the Sydney Hospital (Godden 2006). Miss Lucy Osburn arrived in Sydney in 1868, ready for reform with the help of five Nightingale nurses. This episode in Australian nursing has been much celebrated (Godden 2006). But recent research by Judith Godden, an Australian historian, shows that reports of the Sydney Hospital's condition were greatly exaggerated, and that Osburn's capabilities as a nurse were of similar, mythical proportion (Godden 2006). Nevertheless, the idea caught on that colonial nursing desperately needed cleaning up and that Nightingale nursing was the prescribed method to effect it. In 1885, the Australian colony of Tasmania welcomed three Nightingale nurses to institute reforms in that colony (Grehan 2004). The Nightingale Fund's two-tiered model of pupil nurses being 'lady nurses' and 'regular probationers' was subsequently adopted throughout Australia (Grehan 2004) and in New Zealand (Hill 1982) to much acclaim.

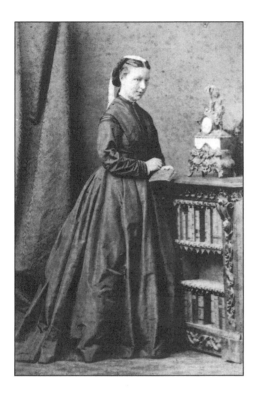

Lucy Osburn. Reproduced with the permission of the Sydney Hospital.

The story of modern nursing as having emerged through the reform of hospitals, as well as private and institutional nursing, with systematised training and professionalisation, is the received version of nursing's history. However, nursing and hospital reforms came very, very slowly in the colonies, just as they did elsewhere. There was little agreement on how to run hospitals, on how to teach nurses, what to teach nurses, and even on whether training was beneficial (Grehan 2004). Reforms in nursing and hospitals were just one small element in a wave of rapid and lasting social change in the mid-nineteenth century (Nelson 2000). In the early years of the twentieth century, a degree of uniformity in nurse training schemes was achieved, although this was a lengthy and complicated process, discussed later in this chapter.

Religious nurses

Earlier in our discussion about the deficits of received histories of nursing, we noted that these accounts tended to celebrate milestones and ignore other aspects of nursing and healthcare. Given the profile of 'Nightingales' in received histories of nursing, one can be forgiven for imagining that there were no skilled nurses in Australia and very low standards in healthcare until 1868. However, as early as 1838, five religious nurses from Dublin were providing care in Sydney, 30 years before Miss Osburn set foot in the colony. Of these five Catholic Sisters of Charity, one had trained as a nurse; another had been sent to Paris to gain nursing experience (MacGinley 2002). The Sisters visited Parramatta's female factory, the women's jail and 'the sick poor in their own homes' (MacGinley 2002:72). In 1857, the Sisters of Charity opened the first St Vincent's Hospital at Sydney's Pott's Point. Today, the St Vincent's hospitals provide a considerable proportion of public health services.

The Australian Inland Mission

Another charitable religious organisation, which pioneered the provision of nursing care in remote regions of Australia, is the Australian Inland Mission (AIM), an offshoot of the Presbyterian Church. In the early twentieth century, the Reverend John Flynn, of the Flying Doctor fame, established a network of health centres staffed by trained nurses in extremely isolated territory (Cockrill 1999). The nurses were trained general nurses and also deaconesses of the Presbyterian Church, which enabled them to provide the dual roles of nursing care and spiritual support to the people they attended (Cockrill 1999).

AIM nurses faced all kinds of challenges because of the isolation in which they worked. For instance, they were often called upon to attend births. To prepare them for this work, deaconess nurses were allowed to undertake brief terms of midwifery training at the Women's Hospital in Melbourne. Nurse Bett completed a short stint of training prior to taking up her position at Oodnadatta in South Australia in 1909 (Women's Hospital Board of Management Meeting Minutes 1909). Sister Jean Finlayson also worked at the AIM's Oodnadatta centre. Jean, pictured below on a mode of desert transport, was the inaugural trained nurse at the Northern Territory's Alice Springs AIM Centre in 1915. It later became the Alice Springs Hospital (Cockrill 1999).

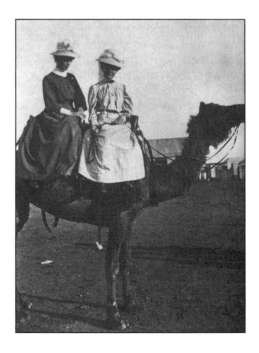

Jean Finlayson (right) and fellow deaconess at Alice Springs c1915. Reproduced with the permission of Adelaide House Museum, Alice Springs.

Aboriginal nurses

One religious organisation, the Salvation Army (SA), had a significant role in the training of nurses and in the provision of healthcare. Like the Catholic hospitals, the SA formed their own district nursing services in cities, building a network of hospitals around Australia that were big enough to become training schools for nurses. They also offered opportunities where few existed. For example, according to SA records, mainstream hospitals would not accept Aboriginal women as pupil nurses (Salvation Army Archives). One SA hospital in the state of Victoria, Bethesda, in the 1950s was a training ground for several young women from the Aboriginal missions at Mount Margaret in Western Australia and Colebrook in South Australia.

Miss Sadie Corner, pictured earlier in this chapter, graduated from Bethesda in the 1950s, first as a nurses' aide, then as a general nurse, and then as a midwifery nurse. She was the first Aboriginal woman to work as a trained nurse and hospital matron in Western Australia. Miss Corner was later awarded an MBE and Queen's Jubilee Medal for her contribution to the health needs of the community of Leonora and surrounding district (Australian Legal Information Institute 2000). Another Aboriginal woman, Lowitja (Lois) O'Donohue CBE, AM, initially was rejected as a nursing trainee simply because she was of Aboriginal descent. Subsequently, Ms O'Donohue graduated from the Royal Adelaide Hospital in 1954 as a trained general nurse and later worked in Adelaide as a charge sister. She then spent time in India with a missionary society before taking up positions in national Aboriginal affairs (State Library of South Australia 2001).

Summary

The brief discussion of nursing's evolution presented here has offered only a glimpse of the colonial health landscape since the arrival of Europeans and of nursing's antecedents. Clearly, there are many aspects of nursing's history which will make fascinating subjects of critical historical inquiry in the future. In the second half of this chapter, we touch on some examples of external pressures which have shaped the profession in Australia and New Zealand, and consider some of the milestones in nursing's historical narrative.

HISTORICAL INFLUENCES ON NURSING

No profession or occupation can escape outside influences. The profession or occupation exists as part of the society it serves. The external influences on nursing might also be described as 'accidents of history', such as natural disasters, epidemics and war. We are not always conscious of the broad effects of these dramatic influences on our history, particularly if we happen to be living through them. We are even less aware of the influences that are far less dramatic, such as the political and social climate. With a critical examination of nursing's history, however, we can reflect on the way that events and trends, momentous and less momentous, have shaped nursing as we know it today. Here, we mention two intricately interconnected issues which have undoubtedly influenced nursing's development in Australia and New Zealand. These are: the consequences of a lack of government interest in healthcare in the nineteenth century, and the development of responsible government, respectively in New Zealand as a national government, and in Australia initially as colonies and from 1901 as a federation of states and territories.

The effect of the unregulated marketplace and subsequent regulation

One of the consistencies between the British arena and those of Australia and New Zealand is the initial lack of government interest in matters of nursing and midwifery in the nineteenth century. This set a pattern that was difficult to change, at least in Australia. With no real restrictions on individuals or their practices as nurses, midwives or healers in Australia or New Zealand or Britain until the early twentieth century, anyone could claim to have skills learnt through personal experience, by working as an apprentice, or by attending public lectures given by doctors on nursing (Grehan 2004). The problem was that the unfortunate public had no way of knowing if a nurse or midwife who claimed qualifications or skills actually possessed them.

In the previous section, we referred to the movement to reform nursing and hospitals towards the end of the nineteenth century. Up to this point in time, Australian and New Zealand nursing had developed in tandem, mostly haphazardly and taking cues from the trends in Britain. However, in the last decade of the nineteenth century, New Zealand's government took an entirely different direction from governments in Australia. New Zealand introduced statutory regulation for nursing in 1901 (French 2001) and a *Midwives Registration Act* in 1904 (Neill 1961). In Australia, where colonial governments were disinclined to interfere in the private matter of healthcare, Australia's nurses had no option but to pursue a voluntary, professional, self-regulation of nursing.

Voluntary regulation

Efforts to introduce voluntary professional regulation for nurses and midwives in Australia mirrored those in Britain where a British Nurses Association was established in late 1887 (Grehan 2004). Voluntary professional regulation was designed to differentiate trained nurses from untrained people by setting standards in education and training, and by maintaining registers of trained nurses so that the public could engage a nurse whose qualifications had been assessed as adequate (Grehan 2004). There was an expectation that the public would choose trained nurses, even if their fees were higher than those of untrained nurses.

A Nurses Association of Australasia, founded in Melbourne in 1892, was spectacularly unsuccessful (Grehan 2004). An ongoing professional organisation for nurses was formed in the colony of New South Wales in 1899; it became the Australasian Trained Nurses Association (ATNA) (Grehan 2004). Victoria founded its own association in 1901, the Victorian Trained Nurses Association (VTNA). After being awarded Royal Charter in 1904, the VTNA became the Royal Victorian Trained Nurses Association (RVTNA) (Trembath & Hellier 1987).

The professional associations for nurses in Australia attempted to force hospitals to accept uniform curricula and registration categories. The idea was that uniform standards would make the term 'trained nurse' mean something recognisable to the public and to the medical profession (Grehan 2004). The success of voluntary regulation was marginal because their voluntary nature was their greatest flaw (Trembath & Hellier 1987). For nurses and midwives in many parts of Australia, and in private hospitals, voluntary regulation made little difference (Grehan & Nelson 2005). Eventually, however, legislation came to be introduced for nursing and midwifery across Australia. The categories of nurse and curricula laid down by the ATNA and the VTNA formed the basis of many statutes.

Thus, in Australia, voluntary regulation preceded statutory regulation of nursing and midwifery. In New Zealand it was the reverse. National regulation had set the tone for the whole country with uniform curricula and restrictions on training centres, but New Zealand formed a voluntary professional association for 'private' nurses in any case (Maclean 1932). This happened because of movements in the international nursing arena. In 1899, an International Council of Nurses (ICN), a professional organisation, was formed to provide a voice for nurses worldwide (Nelson 1999). To belong to the ICN, a country was expected to have a national nurses association, governed by nurses, which made ICN affiliation difficult in Australia given the existence of two separate professional associations for nurses (Trembath & Hellier 1987). New Zealand, however, was able to take advantage of membership of this international organisation by forming the New Zealand Trained Nurses Association in 1909 (Maclean 1932).

Statutory regulation

Australia's pathway to statutory regulation was different because of its history of responsible government of several colonies, compared to New Zealand's national government. Each Australian colony was established at a different time, and developed unique regulatory requirements for aspects of commerce, trade and legal matters conducted under its own constitution (Macintyre 1986). The colonies were protective of their own borders and interests, but, in 1901, overcame their territorial differences to form a federation of states with a national government (Macintyre 1986). Under the 1901 Australian Constitution, the states' capacity to make their own regulations was protected. This included those pertaining to nursing and midwifery, with the result that nursing and midwifery regulations across Australia have varied considerably.

National registration

With different registration systems and regulations in each Australian state, nurses who want to work in a variety of jurisdictions need to hold multiple registrations. It has also been difficult to accommodate nurses and midwives trained in places other than Australia. The globalisation of workforces, worldwide shortages of nurses and development of trade agreements, however, have forced change in the way that nurses and midwives in Australia are registered as healthcare practitioners.

In 1992, the Australian and New Zealand national governments signed a *Mutual Recognition Agreement*, which was extended more recently to include the Australian state governments under the *Trans-Tasman Mutual Recognition Arrangement* (Council of Australian Governments undated). Designed to 'promote economic integration and increased trade', these agreements also were expected to enable the equal recognition of occupational qualifications in both jurisdictions. More recently, the problem of nurse and midwife shortages all over Australia, rather than free trade requirements, has provided the impetus to ease regulatory restrictions on nurses and midwives. A national registration system for all nurses and midwives is expected to come into force in Australia in July 2010 (Australian Nursing and Midwifery Council 2008).

The political landscape, the unregulated healthcare arena and the consequent challenge of regulation are just some examples of the historical influences which deserve consideration when developing a vision of nursing's history in Australia and in New Zealand. Tumultuous events, also, have had an influence on nursing as a profession. Some of these are explored in the next section.

MILESTONES IN AUSTRALIAN AND NEW ZEALAND NURSING

Even in the relatively short history of Australian and New Zealand nursing, there have been notable events and momentous occasions which can be seen as milestones. In the next section, we concentrate on two milestones in Australian nursing history. These are simply events or stages when seen in isolation, as is often the case in received histories. However, it is their context and their sequelae that are of interest to us in historical terms. The first milestone is the role of war; the second is the transition of nursing and midwifery education from the apprentice system into tertiary education.

War

Conflicts have been a significant theme in nursing history in Australia and New Zealand and elsewhere. The work of Florence Nightingale with the war wounded of the Crimea and that of women in the American Civil War attracted the admiration of the public worldwide. Nelson writes that 'the successes of the war nurses stimulated a shift in public perceptions of the role of the nurse' because, in the organised arena of tending the war wounded, 'nursing came to be seen as a useful profession' and a rather more lofty exercise than nursing the poor (Nelson 2000:148). In Australia, New South Wales was the first colony to have a military nursing 'reserve' (Smith 1999). Australian nurses have since served in Korea, Vietnam and in the Pacific (Reid et al 1999).

The Boer War, World Wars I and II

During the 1899–1902 South African (Boer) War, nurses from each state in Australia joined volunteer troops, serving as private citizens or with the British nursing forces. A small collection of photographs and letters held at the Australian War Memorial in Canberra tells a little of their experiences in South Africa. We know more about nursing in World War I between 1914 and 1918, as many nurses kept diaries of their experiences. Recent research by Harris (2007) estimates that 2500 nurses served with the Australian Army Nursing Service (AANS). Among other places, they served in the Middle East, in the south of Europe, France, England and India. It is estimated that 23 nurses died on military duty in World War I.

Around the same number of Australian nurses volunteered for service during World War II (Harris 2007). Among other places, nurses served in North Africa, the Middle East, the south of Europe, and across the Pacific, as members of the three areas of the Australian military forces: the AANS, the Royal Australian Air Force Nursing Service and the Royal Australian Naval Nursing Service (Reid et al 1999). A significant event in 1943 was the awarding of military rankings to nurses in the Australian forces, formally placing women in charge of men at a time when no comparable positions were open to women in civilian life (Milligan & Foley 1993). Two other events, judged as war crimes, encapsulated the inhumanity of World War II, and drew the attention of the public to the roles of ordinary women who risked their lives in their work as military nurses.

The sinking of the *Vyner Brooke* and the Bangka Island massacre

Vivian Bullwinkel was 26 years of age when she enlisted in the AANS. In 1942, Bullwinkel and 64 other AANS sisters were serving in an army general hospital in Singapore when they were forced to evacuate (Jeffrey 1954). Just before the city fell to the Japanese army in February 1942, the nurses left Singapore with more than 200 passengers on a small coastal steamer, the *Vyner Brooke* (Jeffrey 1954). The *Vyner Brooke* was one of several vessels attacked by Japanese bombers at sea.

A number of passengers on board the *Vyner Brooke* died when it sank, but others managed to swim ashore to Radji Beach on Bangka Island in the Malacca Straits, landing in two parties on different parts of the coast. One party was taken as prisoners of war. A second party was discovered by Japanese soldiers two days after their landing on Bangka Island. The soldiers ordered this group of 22 nurses to march into the sea, where they were shot. Twenty-one were killed. Vivian Bullwinkel was the only survivor of what is known as the Bangka Island massacre. After hiding for 12 days in the jungle with a wounded British soldier, Bullwinkel surrendered to the Japanese army, and was reunited with the other party of 31 nurses. These women spent the next three and a half years as Japanese prisoners of war (Jeffrey 1954). News of the Bangka Island massacre did not reach Australia until the war ended in 1945.

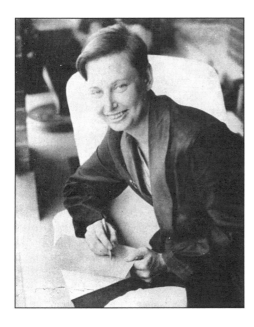

Vivian Bullwinkel.

The sinking of the *MV Centaur*

A second shocking incident occurred in May 1943, not 80 kilometres from Australia's shores. Just off the coast of Brisbane, the Merchant Vessel *Centaur*, a converted hospital ship, was on its way from Sydney to Papua New Guinea with 332 personnel on board: doctors, field ambulance officers, ship's crew and 12 army nurses (Milligan & Foley 1993). At 4.10 a.m. and without warning, the *Centaur* was torpedoed by a Japanese submarine. Of the 12 nurses on board, only one survived. During the 36 hours which passed until the *Centaur's* survivors were rescued, this remarkable nurse, Ellen Savage, took charge of rationing food and attended to some of the 63 injured survivors. Her nursing work took place on a raft in the Pacific Ocean and despite her own severe injuries: a fractured palate, nose and ribs, as well as perforated ear drums and severe bruising (Milligan & Foley 1993). Given that this assault was committed on a well-lit and clearly marked hospital ship, which had previously completed this same journey unhindered, the sinking of the *Centaur* was judged to be a war crime (Milligan & Foley 1993).

On the home front

The war had effects away from the battlefront. Four thousand nurses in Australia volunteered out of an estimated workforce of 13,000 (Nelson & Rabach 2002), creating deficits in every area of nursing across the nation (Harris 2007). Some hospitals attempted to overcome this shortage by extending nursing training from three to four years in some cases, but this had an unintended effect of discouraging young women from applying for training places. 'War emergency nurses' were introduced when there were no trained nurses (Trembath & Hellier 1987). These were members of the Australian Red Cross or Voluntary Aid Detachments (VADs) and members of the Order of St John, who usually worked without pay in medical support roles (Reid et al 1999).

The shortages of trained nurses were so dire that the national government recognised that nursing was one of many occupations important for national stability (Nelson & Rabach 2002). For the duration of the war, nursing was a protected industry under the control of a federal authority, the Manpower Directorate (Nelson & Rabach 2002). Because the Directorate controlled the movement of nurses all over the nation, nurses who wished to work interstate had to obtain the permission of this organisation to do so.

Postwar

Following the war, serving nurses were repatriated. Adjustment to civilian life must have been difficult for service nurses, but particularly so for those who had occupied positions of authority in the military. For them, positions offering equal status, authority and respect, as their officer ranks had done, were few and far between. In Australian civilian workplaces, women like Miss Annie Sage, Matron-in-chief of the AANS, were unable to reach the heights of leadership tacit in the military arena. Sage's aspirations to lift nursing out of the realm of women's work into an even more professional sphere were dashed as she was devolved of the level of responsibility and authority to which she had been accustomed in her role as commander of army nursing services (Nelson & Rabach 2002).

Another tier of nurses disappointed with their status postwar were members of the VADs who had assumed considerable responsibility during the war under the direction of the Army Medical Service. On demobilisation, they found themselves unable to join the ranks of civilian nursing because VADs were not considered qualified enough to register as 'trained nurses' (Reid et al 1999). Without a career structure and system for postgraduate education, and without recognition or recompense for experience, the situation for a range of aspirational nurses remained as difficult as it had before the war.

The transfer of nursing education to the tertiary sector

A second milestone in nursing's history in Australia is the transfer of nursing education to the tertiary sector. The apprentice mode of training nurses on-the-job in hospitals was the mainstay of nursing education throughout the twentieth century. Education of nurses was part education, part service provision, with a greater weighting on service provision (Trembath & Hellier 1987). Australian nurses, since the 1930s, had recognised that nursing lacked the postgraduate education opportunities available to nurses in England and America. Their aspirations to have postgraduate education available locally came to fruition after World War II, albeit in two different forms. In the state of Victoria, postgraduate courses in teaching, administration and industrial (now occupational health) nursing were offered by the Royal Victorian College of Nursing (RVCN), which had metamorphosed out of the Royal Victorian Trained Nurses Association. This organisation, now known as the Royal College of Nursing Australia (RCNA), secured funding to lay the foundations for a national college of nursing, but state rivalries between Victoria and New South Wales guaranteed that a national college did not eventuate (McCoppin & Gardner 1994).

In the meantime, New Zealand nurses were accepted into the ICN where international exchanges between nurses flourished (Maclean 1932). In 1949, the state of New South Wales formed its own college and commenced postgraduate education programs with support from the New South Wales Nurses Association, the Australian Trained Nurses Association and the Institute of Hospital Matrons. The RCNA and the College of Nursing, the latter incorporating the New South Wales College of Nursing, coexist.

By the 1960s and 1970s, nursing and midwifery education began to be seen as more about education than service provision while learning. In 1977, the state government in New South Wales moved nursing education from the health portfolio to education so that the state's colleges of advanced education assumed responsibility for nurse education. In 1984, under an Australian federal government plan, tertiary education for all nurses was formally adopted (McCoppin & Gardner 1994). Midwifery education followed in the 1990s. This transition in Australia ended 140 years of nursing by apprenticeship.

Emerging streams of specialisation

Just as the transfer of education to the tertiary sector signalled a new way of thinking about nurses and their preparation for practice, opportunities for nurses have opened up in tandem with twentieth century developments in the treatment of disease and new ways of understanding health and illness. Rapid developments in medical science opened opportunities to nurses in specialised areas of practice (Fairman & Lynaugh 1998). For example, improved anaesthetic methods in the 1960s allowed previously haemodynamically unstable cases to survive life-threatening injuries with skilled nursing and medical care. Out of such developments, including a specific body of knowledge particular to an area of care, specialisms within nursing have emerged, one being the intensive care nursing units in the 1960s (Fairman & Lynaugh 1998).

Neonatal intensive care units, coronary care units, burns units and myriad others are now accepted as requisite by modern healthcare standards in the Western world. Stomal therapy, diabetes education, mental health, women's health, cancer nursing, tissue transplant nursing, health promotion and palliative care are just some examples of the speciality practice areas offering nurses the opportunity to expand their skills. These fields tend to be seen as specialisations of 'nursing'. The status of midwifery as a branch of nursing, as it has been throughout the twentieth century, however, is a little more contentious. Let us turn to the arena of midwifery and nursing and to the issue of history and identity.

HISTORY AND IDENTITY

Earlier in this chapter, we noted that history can tell us a lot about who we are, about our identity as part of the broader nursing profession, and about our identity as individuals. We have seen that nursing's identity in received histories is linked to a sense of itself as a modern profession with many branches, one of which was midwifery. In the last quarter of the twentieth century and continuing into the twenty-first century, midwifery's identity as a branch of nursing has been questioned, as part of a worldwide movement in professionalising midwifery. This movement seeks to have midwifery in Australia recognised as a profession, separate and distinct from nursing, as it is in the Netherlands, New Zealand and other parts of the Western world (Australian College of Midwives Incorporated Victorian Branch 1999). To this end, a freestanding educational pathway leading to registration as a midwife, the Bachelor of Midwifery, has been underway since 2001 in Australia. The Bachelor of Midwifery has been underway in New Zealand since the early 1990s, following the government's recognition that midwifery was different from nursing. This brings to the fore the relationship between a profession, its identity and its history.

Midwifery's identity, not 'nursing'

Midwifery is said to be different from nursing for several reasons. One central point of difference is said to be that midwifery concerns care in a natural episode in the female life cycle, while nursing concerns the care of the sick (Fahy 1998). Midwifery is also said to have a history that is different from nursing's (Australian College of Midwives Incorporated Victorian Branch 1999). So what is the relationship between profession, history and identity? 'Identity' histories, sometimes referred to under the banner of 'revisionist' histories, have been popular since the 1960s when second wave feminism and the broader movement in social change at that time critiqued received historical narratives as a march of progress (Davison 2000). Revisionist history aimed to give 'voice' to groups whose contributions had been ignored in conventional interpretations of history, such as women, African Americans and other ethnic groups (Davison 2000).

In some ways, however, this type of history is no less problematic than received history. While it can give voice to those whose voices have been ignored previously, one of the main concerns with identity history is its purpose—that is, righting wrongs or locating origins that resonate with the present (Davison 2000). When the aim of history becomes a search for roots, or righting history's wrongs, history can be crafted so that it 'fits' with the author's view of the world (Davison 2000). In other words, this kind of history is not critical, does not question its assumptions, is not objective and is not self-conscious. The outcome can be that the past is invested with nostalgia (Ulrich 2002).

Two examples of the effects of an uncritical approach to examining identity are histories of midwifery, produced during midwifery's revival in the 1990s. One is an oral history of midwifery in England; the second is a study of South Australian midwifery. Leap and Hunter, the authors of the English text, declare in their introduction that: 'We expected to uncover a treasure chest of forgotten skills: experience that would enhance midwifery practice and inspire the midwives of today' (Leap & Hunter 1993:xi). In the Australian text, Annette Summers aims to examine the 'historical terrain which led to the demise of the community midwife, whose lost autonomy is lamented by the midwife of the 1990s' (Summers 1995:1).

We can see that both texts are searching for forgotten skills and lost autonomy. These concepts certainly resonate with contemporary midwifery's professional aspirations to make itself distinct from nursing and regain what it believes to be its lost independence (Summers 1995). This search for a preconceived kind of history, however, is no different from received nursing's history's search for Nightingale-style nurses, who we now know were largely mythical. It is no surprise that Leap and Hunter, and Summers, for the most part find the history they were looking for.

Leap and Hunter, for example, having interviewed some handywomen, found no evidence to suggest that handywomen were in any way dealing out 'death and destruction' or that handywomen midwives were involved in providing abortions (Leap & Hunter 1993:22). This assessment is despite ample documentary evidence in Britain confirming that some untrained women and trained midwives were ill-equipped for even the most common of complications in labour, such as haemorrhage (as were many doctors ill-equipped), and that female midwives' facilitated the crimes of abortion and infanticide (Grehan & Nelson 2005). Summers locates midwifery's 'lost' autonomy in South Australian midwifery at a time before the profession of nursing eclipsed this 'ancient' form. In adhering to a preconceived view that independent midwifery was unjustifiably subsumed by nursing with the help of medicine, Summers does not pay any attention to Australian documentary evidence which shows that midwives played a role in abortion and infanticide and that they lacked basic skills.

Our criticism of these revisionist histories is not to suggest that midwifery was not extinguished. Nor is it to suggest that medicine and nursing were somehow innocent bystanders in this process. What we are suggesting is that nurses should question the way that both received and revisionist histories have approached their subject. When accounts of history inform a professional identity and make special claims on that basis, it is important for nurses to understand how those histories have been assembled.

THE FUTURE

At the beginning of this chapter, we stated that sometimes history can offer insights that might be applied to the future. Of course, it is impossible to tell what the future will bring, but Graeme Davison, the Australian historian, suggests that history can tell us what is *unlikely* to happen, rather than what will happen, simply because history never repeats itself, although over a sweep of time it may show patterns. In this sense, then, the trends that have featured consistently in nursing's history emphasise the perennial nature of some issues in nursing and healthcare. For example, arguments about professional identities are unlikely to dissipate and may even strengthen. Given the recent separation of midwifery from nursing, it is possible that in the future other branches of nursing might pursue a similar path. One branch might be psychiatric nursing, which, formerly known as mental nursing, had its foundations in asylums which were geographically and philosophically far away from general hospitals and general nurse training schemes. Just as contemporary midwifery argues its difference from nursing, so may psychiatric nursing.

The role of nurses in war service has been a consistent element in nursing's narrative, indicating that this is likely to remain so. Nursing, we have seen, has been affected by acute and chronic shortages of personnel, necessitating novel ways of education and even government intervention in wartime to control supply of nurses. There is no guarantee that government will not institute similar controls if it sees the need. Such controls would be infinitely more achievable once national registration comes into force in Australia in 2010. Over the sweep of nursing's history, we have seen the primary domain for care shift from the home, to the modern hospital, and recently back to the home. A continuation of this cycle cannot be ruled out.

Technology has impacted greatly on nursing's development. Technological advances, coupled with sophisticated understandings of trauma and illness, have transformed the way in which care in hospitals and homes is provided. Technical demands call for a different style of education than was required in the 1960s for example. Technological advances are part and parcel of modern healthcare. They are likely to remain so in the future.

CONCLUSION

In this brief survey of nursing's history in Australia and New Zealand, there are many aspects of nursing history that have not been raised but are worthy of examination using the tools of critical history. Some areas for future research might include the contribution of women combining nursing with their evangelical missionary work, the impact on nursing of world events and globalisation, the role of Aboriginal women as nurses, migrant nurses and aspects of nursing practice— that is, doing, organising, planning and implementing the care of others. More research in the form of critical history will illuminate the most contentious areas in nursing's history, such as nursing's relationship with midwifery and the care of women. What is important for nursing is to accept its past 'warts and all' (Nelson 1997:234). Only this pursuit, using the tools of critical history, will provide a realistic vision of nursing's and midwifery's history in the Australian and New Zealand context.

REFLECTIVE QUESTIONS
1 How does knowing about nursing's past help nurses to understand the present and the future?
2 What have been the major historical influences on nursing and midwifery?
3 What new questions could be asked about aspects of nursing history?

RECOMMENDED READINGS

Bashford A 1998 Purity and pollution: gender, embodiment and Victorian medicine. St Martin's Press, New York

Fairman J, Lynaugh JE 1998 Critical care nursing: a history. University of Pennsylvania Press, Pennsylvania

Nelson S 2001 Say little, do much: nurses, nuns, and hospitals in the nineteenth century. University of Pennsylvania Press, Pennsylvania

Reverby S 1988 Ordered to care: the dilemma of American nursing, 1885–1945. Cambridge University Press, Boston

Rosenberg C 1987 The care of strangers: the rise of America's hospital system. John Hopkins University Press, Baltimore

REFERENCES

Argus, 10 July 1956, Melbourne

Australian College of Midwives Incorporated (ACMI) Victorian Branch 1999 Reforming midwifery: a discussion paper on the introduction of Bachelor of Midwifery Programs into Victoria. ACMI Victorian Branch, Melbourne

Australian Legal Information Institute 2000 Council for Aboriginal Reconciliation archives, Members of Council 1991–2000. Online. Available: www.austlii.edu.au/au/other/IndigLRes/car/2000/16/appendices04.htm 20 Feb 2006

Australian Nursing and Midwifery Council (ANMC) 2008 Media release. Online. Available: www.anmc.gov.au/docs/media_releases 16 May 2008

Baly M 1987 The Nightingale nurses: the myth and reality. In: Maggs C (ed.) Nursing history: the state-of-the-art. Croom Helm, New Hampshire, pp 33–59

Bashford A 1998 Purity and pollution: gender, embodiment and Victorian medicine. St Martin's Press, New York

Cockrill P 1999 Healing the heart: 60 years of Alice Springs Hospital 1939–1999. Alice Springs Hospital's 60th anniversary reunion organising committee. Alice Springs

Collins Y 1999 The provision of hospital care in country Victoria 1840s to 1940s. Unpublished PhD thesis. Department of History of Philosophy and Science, University of Melbourne, Melbourne

Collins Y, Kippen S 2003 The 'Sairey Gamps' of Victorian nursing? Tales of drunk and disorderly wardsmen in Victorian hospitals between the 1850s and the 1880s. Health and History 5(1):42–64

Connolly C 2004 Beyond social history: new approaches to understanding the state of and the state in nursing history. Nursing History Review 12(3):5–24

Council of Australian Governments (undated) Trans-Tasman Mutual Recognition Arrangement. Online. Available: www.coag.gov.au/recongition.htm#ttmra 20 Feb 2006

Davison G 2000 The use and abuse of Australian history. Allen & Unwin, Sydney

Dean M 1994 Critical and effective histories: Foucault's methods and historical sociology. Routledge, London

Dickens C 1843 The life and adventures of Martin Chuzzlewit. Chapman and Hall, London

Durdin J 1991 They became nurses: a history of nursing in South Australia 1836–1980. Allen & Unwin, Sydney

Evenden D 2000 The midwives of seventeenth century London. Cambridge University Press, Cambridge

Fahy K 1998 Being a midwife or doing midwifery? Australian College of Midwives Incorporated Journal 11(2):11–16

Fairman J, Lynaugh JE 1998 Critical care nursing: a history. University of Pennsylvania Press, Pennsylvania

Forth G, Critchett J, Yule P (eds) 1998 The biographical dictionary of the Western District of Victoria. Hyland House, Melbourne

French P 2001 A study of the regulation of nursing in New Zealand. Victoria University of Wellington Graduate School of Nursing and Midwifery Monograph Series 2/2001, Wellington

Godden J 2006 Lucy Osburn, a lady displaced: Florence Nightingale's envoy to Australia. University of Sydney Press, Sydney

Grehan M 2003 Midwives and nurses in colonial Victoria: Sarah Barfoot and her contemporaries. Genealogist 10(11):496–498

Grehan M 2004 From the sphere of Sarah Gampism: the professionalisation of nursing and midwifery in the colony of Victoria. Nursing Inquiry 11(3):192–201

Grehan M, Nelson S 2005 Not fit persons: Sarah Gamp, midwives and nationhood in Australia 1890–1919. 27th Congress of the International Confederation of Midwives. Pathways to Healthy Nations, Brisbane, 25–29 July 2005

Harris K 2007 Not just 'routine nursing': the roles and skills of the Australian Army Nursing Service during World War I. Unpublished PhD thesis, History Department, University of Melbourne

Hill A 1982 The history of midwifery from 1840–1979: with specific reference to the training and education of student midwives. Unpublished MA thesis, Department of Education, University of Auckland

Jeffrey B 1954 White Coolies: a graphic record of survival in World War Two. Angus & Robertson, Sydney

Leap N, Hunter B 1993 The midwife's tale: an oral history from handywoman to professional midwife. Scarlett Press, London

McCalman J 1998 Sex and suffering: women's health and a women's hospital. Melbourne University Press, Melbourne

McCoppin B, Gardner H 1994 Tradition and reality: nursing and politics in Australia. Churchill Livingstone, Melbourne

MacGinley MR 2002 A dynamic of hope: institutes of women religious in Australia, 2nd edn. Crossing Press for the Institute of Religious Studies, Sydney

Macintyre S 1986 A concise history of Australia: Vol. 4, 1901–41. The succeeding age. Cambridge University Press, Cambridge

Maclean H 1932 Nursing in New Zealand: history and reminiscences. Tolan Printing, Wellington

Martyr P 2002 Paradise of quacks: an alternative history of medicine in Australia. Macleay Press, Sydney

Milligan CS, Foley JCH 1993 Australian hospital ship *Centaur*: the myth of immunity. Nairana Publications, Brisbane

Mitchell A 1977 The hospital south of the Yarra: a history of the Alfred Hospital Melbourne from foundation to the nineteen-forties. Alfred Hospital, Melbourne

Neill J 1961 Grace Neill: the story of a noble woman. NM Peryer, Christchurch

Nelson S 1997 Reading nursing history. Nursing Inquiry 4:229–236

Nelson S 1998 How do we write a nursing history of disease? Health and History 1(1):43–47

Nelson S 1999 Deja vu and the regulation of nursing in Victoria. Australian Journal of Advanced Nursing 16(4):29–35

Nelson S 2000 A genealogy of the care of the sick: nursing, holism and pious practice. Nursing Praxis International, Hants, England

Nelson S, Rabach J 2002 Military experience: the new age of Australian nursing and other failures. Health and History 4(1):79–87

Nutting MA, Dock LL 1907 A history of nursing, Vol. 1. Putnam, New York

Peel D 2006 Year of hope: 1857 in the Colac district. Published privately

Reid R, Page C, Pounds R 1999 Just wanted to be there: Australian service nurses 1899–1999. Commonwealth Department of Veteran's Affairs, Canberra

Rosenberg CE 1987 The care of strangers: the rise of America's hospital system. John Hopkins University Press, Baltimore

Salvation Army Archives, Melbourne, Appendix 1, unpublished SOC BEV BK000825.2

Smith R 1999 In pursuit of excellence: a history of the Royal College of Nursing, Australia. Oxford University Press, Melbourne

State Library of South Australia 2001 Lowitja O'Donohue: Elder of our nation. In: Women and politics in South Australia: the Aboriginal voice. Online. Available: www.slsa.sa.gov.au/women_and_politics/abor1.htm 20 Feb 2006

Strachan G 2001 Present at the birth: 'handywomen' and neighbours in rural New South Wales 1850–1900. Labour History 81:13–27

Summers A 1988 Angels and citizens: British women as military nurses, 1854–1914. Keegan Paul, London

Summers A 1989 The mysterious demise of Sarah Gamp: the domiciliary nurse and her detractors c. 1830–1860. Victorian Studies 32(2):365–386

Summers AD 1995 For I have ever so much more faith in her ability as a nurse: the eclipse of the community midwife in South Australia, 1836–1942. Unpublished PhD thesis, History Department, Flinders University

Templeton J 1969 Prince Henry's: the evolution of a Melbourne hospital. Robertson and Mullens, Melbourne

Tooley S 1906 A history of nursing in the British Empire. SH Bousfield, London

Trembath R, Hellier D 1987 All care and responsibility: a history of nursing in Victoria 1850–1934. Florence Nightingale Committee, Australia, Victorian Branch, Melbourne

Ulrich LT 2002 The age of homespun: objects and stories in the creation of an American myth. Random House, New York

Ulrich LT 2007 Well behaved women seldom make history. Alfred J Knopf, New York

Webster ME 1942 The history of trained nursing in Victoria. Typescript copy. Royal Women's Hospital Archives, Melbourne, unaccessioned

Women's Hospital Board of Management Meeting Minutes 1909 Royal Women's Hospital Archives Melbourne, unpublished, Accession No. RWHA 1991/6/26

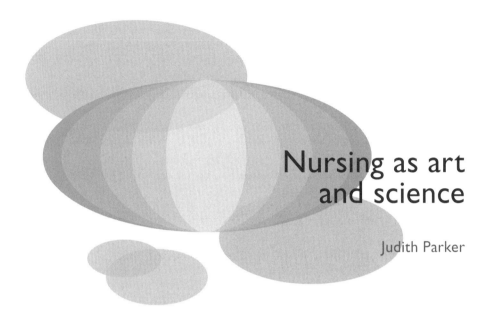

CHAPTER 3

Nursing as art and science

Judith Parker

LEARNING OBJECTIVES

Upon completion of this chapter, the reader should have gained:

- an understanding of the development of ideas about nursing as an art and a science within an historical context
- an appreciation of the meaning of the art of nursing within the Florence Nightingale school of thought
- an appreciation of debates about the art and science of nursing in the US context
- an appreciation of emerging ideas about art and science and the relationships between them in the current context of healthcare, and
- insight into the implications of these ideas for current nursing education, practice and research.

KEY WORDS

Art, science, nursing, gender, aesthetics, enlightenment, contemporary

NURSING: AN ART AND SCIENCE?

What is nursing? Is nursing an art? Is nursing a science? Is nursing both an art and a science? Is nursing neither an art nor a science? Over the years there has been extensive debate in the nursing literature about the art and science of nursing. Why are questions about the nature of nursing posed in these terms? What is it about how knowledge and practices are understood in our society that invites us to ask these questions about nursing? What are the implications of these perceptions for education, practice and research in nursing?

This chapter seeks to explore a number of these questions. It considers some of the history of the development of ideas about modern nursing as an art and a science. More specifically, it examines the division between art and science, and explores the impact that this separation has had upon ideas about nursing.

Two particular developments in the history of nursing ideas are discussed, one stemming from the United Kingdom, and the other from the United States. One of these, often described as the Florence Nightingale school of thought, represents the first expression of nursing as an art in modern times. In this development, nursing as an art is conceived of in relation to the character of the nurse and the importance of character training in nursing education programs. The other concerns the development of nursing ideas within the university context of the United States. Of particular note in this discussion are the attempts to construct closed systems of thought through nursing theory development and the production of nursing science. It was in this context that contradictions between nursing as an art and as a science began to be recognised and attempts made to reconcile the two.

The chapter then examines some of the implications of these ideas for nursing in the contemporary context where many of the binary divisions that occurred historically, including those between art and science, are collapsing. It concludes with a discussion of the art and science of nursing within the emerging milieus of healthcare delivery.

WHAT IS AN ART? WHAT IS A SCIENCE?

Many modern ideas about art and science have their origins in the scientific revolution of the seventeenth century and the eighteenth century 'age of reason' that was generated by the philosophical movement known as the French Enlightenment.

The scientific revolution was a quest to understand, control and manipulate nature through rational, empirical means. As Capra pointed out in 1982:

> This development was brought about by revolutionary changes in physics and astronomy, culminating in the achievements of Copernicus, Galileo and Newton. The science of the seventeenth century was based on a new method of inquiry, advocated forcefully by Francis Bacon, which involved the mathematical description of nature and the analytical method of reasoning conceived by the genius of Descartes (Capra 1982:54).

The Enlightenment project had the aim of civilising all—of implementing its ideal of social betterment through the power of reason. It was based on beliefs in the universal superiority of the knowledge and values produced by Western science and culture. Those who believed in the democratic ideals of the Enlightenment sought to perfect humankind through reason and create a better world—a civilised and cultured one aided by the new knowledge produced by science (Parker & Gibbs 1998). Two ways of thinking about art can be linked to the Enlightenment, one concerning the cultural production of knowledge and the other the art of living.

A separation of the arts and the sciences occurred in the educational structures and processes that emerged in the wake of the Enlightenment period and with the rise of modern professions. Knowledge came to be packaged into the two domains of sciences and arts within university faculties, and a division emerged between those who were educated in the sciences and those who were educated in the arts (humanities). Each of these produced different ways of thinking and acting, and different types of knowledge. According to CP Snow (1964), writing of the United Kingdom, scientific training produces 'doers' and training in the arts produces 'thinkers' (intellectuals). He argued that by the 1950s, the science/art professional rift was so deep that the two groups worked completely independently of each other, a trend he saw as potentially dangerous for society.

Another way of thinking about art that emerged out of the Enlightenment concerns the art of living. The search for human perfectibility, which was a major plank of the Enlightenment, became linked to a philosophy of humanism, which, as Nelson (1995:37) points out, 'stresses the centrality of the human subject and sets freedom as the subject's destiny'. The human subject, however, was male, and rationality was understood to be a masculine attribute. The art of living for men was linked to the pursuit of freedom through rationality, as 'doers' and 'thinkers'.

Women were seen as neither free nor rational. They were understood 'as an essential nature defined by purposeful organic functions' (Berriot-Salvadore 1993:387). Medical discourse defined the feminine ideal in terms of natural determinism as 'the mother, the guardian of virtues and eternal values' (Berriot-Salvadore 1993:388). Thus, while men, defined as human subjects, were separated and freed from the constraints of nature via reason and culture, women, defined in relation to nature and the feminine, were not. Nature and culture merged in this understanding of the feminine, and women were defined on natural and moral grounds. Good women exercised their womanly arts and civilised others through the practice of these arts. By and large, women were excluded from education into the professions.

ART, SCIENCE AND MODERN NURSING

The constitution of modern secular professional nursing as it has evolved since the days of Florence Nightingale has been influenced by some of these ideas. Of particular importance to this discussion is how the divisions that occurred between art and science were managed in nursing. These will be considered first in relation to the Florence Nightingale school of thought stemming from Britain and then in relation to university-based nursing in the United States.

The Florence Nightingale school of thought

The Florence Nightingale school of thought developed and was sustained within the nurse training schools that sprang up in hospitals, not only in Britain, but also in Australia, New Zealand and other countries. I argue that within nursing education and practice, nursing as an art was seen to involve the character of the nurse in the exercise of feminine virtues, and the importance of character training in the development of nursing as a female profession/occupation. In this context, science was out of place: the scientific enterprise was a male one and, in the hospital and medical context, belonged to the doctor.

Nursing in nineteenth century industrial England was regarded as an inferior, undesirable occupation practised by morally suspect women. In *Martin Chuzzlewit*, Dickens epitomised the nineteenth century English nurse in the character of Mrs Gamp, writing that 'it was difficult to enjoy her company without being conscious of a smell of spirits' (Dickens 1910:312–313). The contrast of Florence Nightingale's work in the Crimea, and the subsequent publicity, brought about her identification in the public mind as a 'ministering angel' (*The Times*, London, 20 November 1854). This image was instrumental in elevating secular nursing to a female vocation based on Enlightenment ideals of the womanly virtues and the exercise of the womanly arts through the care of the sick. Indeed, Florence Nightingale described nursing as 'the finest of the fine arts' (Donahue 1996).

Enormous effort went into the attempts to position nursing as epitomising feminine ideals of the good woman. Nursing transgressed many prevailing ideas about the role of women in society and it was extremely difficult for nursing to gain acceptance as a legitimate and respectable occupation. Mrs Gamp and the 'bad woman' were never far beneath the surface; it is therefore not surprising that Florence Nightingale and her followers placed so much emphasis upon ensuring appropriate character formation among nurses in training (Parker 1990).

The first Florence Nightingale training school began at St Thomas' Hospital in London in 1860 and became the model for many training schools in Britain and its overseas territories in the latter half of the nineteenth century (Trembath & Hellier 1987). Student nurses were judged on their qualities of trustworthiness, neatness, quietness, sobriety, honesty and truthfulness (Smith 1982). Additionally, nurses were trained to ensure they did not wish to usurp any of the doctor's functions. Isabella Rathie, the first trained Matron of the Melbourne Hospital, noted, 'we are in a great measure the handmaid of the medical man and our function in this particular is to be obedient in every detail' (Rathie, cited in Trembath & Hellier 1987:19).

Thus, the division between art and science as it was manifest within modern secular professional nursing of the Nightingale school of thought can be described as a gendered division. Nursing as a feminine art was developed through character training that resulted in non-assertiveness, obedience and compliance with medical directives. Specific nursing arts comprised nursing procedures such as bathing, bed-making, positioning patients and comforting techniques. While some science content was included in nursing courses, '[t]here was minimal, if any, application of science content in nursing practice' (Peplau 1988:8). Nor were nurses educated in arts subjects of the university, which produced the thinkers of society, for that was primarily the sphere of men. Rather, they were instilled with womanly virtues.

Nursing education was a process of systematically inculcating a task orientation and the moulding of a set of appropriate attitudes within hospital training schools to produce nurses who exemplified the feminine ideal. Science belonged to the rational and objective world of men, of which medicine was one domain. Men were subjects (minds), while women were objects (bodies); nurses were therefore not positioned as rational subjects shaping the Enlightenment project and their own destinies, but rather as passive and compliant objects, subservient to medicine.

Hospital-based nurse training lasted for more than 100 years in Australia and much longer in Britain. Many changes occurred over that time, including considerable strengthening of the science content, particularly from the 1950s onwards. However, the gendering of nursing as a feminine art, developed in the restrictive environment of the hospital, placed limitations upon the possibilities for nursing to develop as a modern profession. It also limited the possibilities for nurses to develop knowledge, skills and attitudes in ways that would enable them to act as autonomous subjects. Nevertheless, it equipped them powerfully to work as moral agents engaged in socially significant work and to develop in-depth knowledge of the human condition in sickness and in suffering, albeit in an unarticulated, scientifically untested form.

Nursing in the university

In the United States, a 4-year entry-to-practice program had been established within a university by 1919. Within this system, it was possible to ensure the development of knowledge in a systematic and orderly way. By the late 1950s, programs for training nurse scientists had developed in a number of major universities, which stimulated interest in theoretical and scientific bases of practice. These were supported by a huge federal investment in nursing education during the 1960s and early 1970s (Gortner 1983). In the period from the late 1950s to the early 1980s, theories of nursing proliferated as nurse scholars sought to include in the concept of nursing an understanding of biological, behavioural, social and cultural factors in health and illness. Of particular note in this discussion were the attempts made to produce closed systems of thought through nursing theory development and the creation of nursing science.

This scientific orientation in nursing, however, came into conflict with ideas about the art of nursing. These stemmed not only from the Nightingale school of thought, but also from consideration of the art of nursing in relation to humanism and the nature of the human subject, by this time conceived of as including women. It is in this context that most of the debates about the art and science of nursing have occurred.

Nursing as a science

As has already been noted, a significant feature of the modern era has been the rise of professions, each clearly delineated by a separate body of knowledge. In the early modern era, nursing could not be regarded as a profession because it was seen to be subservient to and complicit in the medical tasks of diagnosis and treatment. With the location of nursing education within universities, and with the goal of securing professional status for nurses, a major task was to establish its own scientific base, separate from that of medicine.

One early nursing theorist, Johnson (1961), distinguished medicine from nursing by arguing that while the scientific basis of medical knowledge was biological systems, the scientific basis of nursing was behavioural systems. She proposed a behavioural subsystem model of the person 'with behaviour understood as the sum total of physical, biological and social factors/behaviours' (Parker 1995:334). These ideas were further developed by Roy (1980), who conceived of the person as an open, adaptive system, and nursing as the science and practice of promoting adaptation.

Other theorists, however, argued that these approaches did not sufficiently distinguish nursing from medicine. Like medical knowledge, the knowledge produced through study of systems was overly simplistic and mechanistic. Nursing, by contrast, needed to be conceptualised in broader, more encompassing, terms (e.g. Levine 1971). Ideas about nursing as a holistic science were developed by writers such as Rogers (1970) who conceived of the person as an energy field, coextensive with the environment, identified in terms of unified wholeness, openness, pattern, organisation and sentience.

Other writers further differentiated nursing science from medical science by emphasising nursing's caring function in opposition to medicine's curative function. Watson (1985), for example, pulled together two of the central ideas of the modern era by describing nursing as a humanistic science, with caring the central unifying dimension of nursing (Cohen 1991).

Thus, with the shift of nursing education to universities in the United States, strong schools of nursing thought emerged. Each was developed in opposition to medicine, and understood nursing as a behavioural science, a holistic science or a caring science. These conceptual models for nursing practice were the work of a number of nursing intellectuals who had undertaken higher degree work in a range of disciplines, particularly in social sciences and education. Each model was designed to capture the complex dimensions of nursing, although, naturally enough, each one tended to reflect the disciplinary base of its author.

Following the establishment of the basis for nursing science through these models, there were calls to test the models against practical experience and refine them. However, progress was slow, as Flaskerud and Halloran pointed out in 1980, and Fawcett in 1984. There was also concern that the proliferation of models would weaken nursing's claims to be seen as a profession based in a single unique body of knowledge. Fawcett made the point that '[t]he discipline of nursing will advance only through continuous and systematic development and testing of nursing knowledge' (Fawcett 1984:84). Nursing authors sought to concentrate on the common ground in nursing conceptual models. Fawcett, for example, proposed a 'metaparadigm' (an explanatory framework) for nursing built on the central concepts of the discipline—person, environment, health and nursing—and attempts were made to further unify nursing knowledge around these concepts.

Many nurses, however, rejected nursing theories altogether as a means of establishing a science base for nursing. Nursing administrators and clinicians were particularly vocal in their rejection following frustrating experiences of trying to implement them in practice. Nursing theories were seen to reinforce the splits between the theory and practice of nursing, between the education students received and the realities of healthcare service provision, and between nursing thinkers (academics in universities) and nursing doers (nursing administrators and clinicians). In their attempts to develop nursing science through the advancement of nursing theory, nursing theorists, not surprisingly, replicated the binary modes of thought and the dividing practices of the general society.

While nursing theory was being developed, attempts were also being made to construct nursing science knowledge in ways that were linked more closely to practice. The nursing diagnosis movement attracted strong support following the first national conference on the classification of nursing diagnosis held in Missouri in 1973. Nursing diagnosis was developed to identify and classify the phenomena of nursing, to develop a common language for nursing and to facilitate the development and testing of nursing concepts and techniques. However, by 1983, the first broad-scoped critical rejection of nursing diagnosis emerged (Kritek 1985).

This more practice-focused approach to developing nursing science suffered from the same fundamental problem as the theory-based approach. Once again, nursing was attempting to develop its science in opposition to medicine by identifying a discipline-specific scientific knowledge base that would legitimate nursing's claims as a separate profession. In doing this, nursing opened itself to some of the same type of critiques that were made of medicine. The creation of a dedicated nursing language separated nursing not only from medicine but also, more importantly, from patients. When viewed through the nursing diagnosis lens, the patients were reduced to objects of nursing diagnoses and treatments, a positioning that was in opposition to nursing's understanding of the patient as a holistic subject.

Two broad approaches to the development of nursing science have been identified: one that focused on defining the domain of nursing theoretically and then testing propositions empirically; and another that focused on the phenomenon of nursing practice and on developing ways of defining and classifying them. Both approaches were consistent with prevailing philosophies of science. Neither appears to have been successful in providing a discipline-specific body of knowledge that would justify nursing's claims to professional autonomy and power.

Nursing as an art

Nursing's power seems to rest more in its moral claims than in its science base. Ideas that stem from the Nightingale school about the nature of nursing art as an expression of the essential goodness of feminine virtues persist in contemporary nursing practice. Peplau (1988), writing about the United States but presenting a view widely held internationally, points out that nursing has been called the conscience of the healthcare system, which 'suggests that nurses are major keepers of the morality, goodness, honesty, and ethics of client care' (Peplau 1988:9).

This positioning of nurses on the moral high ground in the battlefield of healthcare provision has been sustained by beliefs that nurses exemplify feminine ideals, and appears to have wide community support. It points to an ongoing belief in the Nightingale legacy that presents nurses as good women. It also suggests that nurses and nursing organisations recognise and exploit the ways in which this characterisation of nursing serves wider political agendas and social functions. Additionally, it supports the idea of nursing as a caring and holistic art that sets itself in opposition to the rationality and reductive practices of scientific medicine and healthcare organisation. As Tanya Buchanan (1999) noted: the 'Nightingale discourse generates myths about nursing that … appear to be eternal truths. We need to see past it' (Buchanan 1999:30).

And indeed, ideas that the art of nursing stems from essential female virtues have been challenged within the university setting. The essence of nursing has been claimed to lie in its humanistic philosophy and the artistic practice that flows from this philosophy. In a much-quoted paper, Munhall (1982) argued that nursing has identified itself as a humanistic discipline, adhering to a basic philosophy 'that focuses on individuality and the belief that the actions of men [sic] are in some sense free' (Munhall 1982:176).

Munhall focused attention on the extent to which university-based nursing education in the United States moved away from the Nightingale school of nursing thought based on female character training, and drew more upon a precisely set out philosophy of the discipline to provide the basis for artistic practice. However, this placed nursing philosophy in opposition to prevailing notions of nursing science. As Munhall pointed out, because nursing subscribed to a humanistic philosophy as well as a scientific research orientation, 'incongruities, paradoxes, and conflicting ideologies' (Munhall 1982:176) resulted between philosophy and research.

Munhall also drew attention to the attempts made within nursing education to accommodate both a scientific and humanistic (arts) orientation. This suggests that professional university-based nursing education in the United States attempted to bridge the divide between the sciences and the arts that had been identified by CP Snow (1964) in the British higher education context. Nursing in the university aimed to produce practitioners who were both scientists in orientation and humanists in practice.

However, in educational preparation, the aims and scope of scientific and arts training differ significantly, and the transfer of both scientific and humanistic orientations to the realities of practice is a complex process.

Many writers have noted that the differing orientations of art and science have resulted in problems for nursing practice. Peplau (1988), for example, pointed out that science and art are both essential for excellence in the performance of nursing's mission, but indicates the difficulty for a discipline of accommodating these two forms of professional behaviour:

> Combining both the art and science of nursing, seeing and bringing to bear the distinctive characteristics of each form and of the relation between them, imposes a complexity in professional nursing that virtually defies description (Peplau 1988:9).

Holden (1991), an Australian nurse, argued that the split between the arts and the sciences seriously complicates the notion of nursing. She pointed out that the caring role in nursing constrains nursing into the domain of the arts, while nursing that embraces high technology pushes into the domain of science. Jennings (1986) suggested that it is not a matter of choosing *either* art *or* science, but rather skilfully blending both for the betterment of nursing.

Peplau (1988) supported Jenning's view, pointing out that both science and art come together in practice, so that:

> There is surely a seamless quality, a graceful and delicately balanced movement, between art and science portrayed by experienced expert nurses that transcends as it uses the differences between these forms (Peplau 1988:14).

She suggested further that this transcending of the differing forms of art and science enables nursing to be practised not only as a helping art, but also as 'an enabling, empowering or transforming art'. People she noted 'are touched (literally and figuratively) and sometimes changed at a very personal level by the art nurses practice' (Peplau 1988:9).

The aesthetic dimension—the creative expression—of nursing has received increasing attention over the last few decades. It has built particularly upon the work of Carper who noted in 1978 that the primary emphasis in the professional literature of the time was being placed on the development of the science of nursing. She pointed out:

> There is, nonetheless, what might be described as a tacit admission that nursing is, at least in part, an art. Not much effort is made to elaborate or to make explicit this aesthetic pattern of knowing in nursing—other than to vaguely associate the 'art' with the general category of manual and/or technical skills involved in nursing practice (Carper 1978:16).

Chinn and Watson (1994) have been very influential in further developing ideas about aesthetics and nursing, drawing upon notions of nursing as a caring science. Subsequently, Chinn et al (1997) described the development of aesthetic enquiry in nursing and the conceptualisation that has emerged is of nursing as an art form. Further work along these lines was undertaken by Johnson who conducted a philosophical analysis of conceptualisations of nursing art as a means of contributing to debate on the specific abilities required for artistic creation in nursing (Johnson 1993, 1994, 1996).

Despite these developments, other writers (e.g. Darbyshire 1994a, 1994b, Lafferty 1997) have suggested that science content is still emphasised in nursing curricula at the expense of humanities content, and, as a result, humanistic aspects of care believed to be essential to the artistic component of nursing are not being addressed sufficiently. Lafferty argued that nursing's dual identity as an art and a science requires a balance and calls for the promotion and acquisition of aesthetic knowledge by nursing students. She suggests that studying literature is a way of fostering this. Darbyshire makes a similar point, arguing that nursing as an art and a science is in danger of becoming a cliché unless attempts are made to reverse the marginalisation of arts and humanities within nursing curricula.

It can be seen that nursing as a contemporary secular profession has developed out of ideas about the essential nature of women, wherein nursing has been regarded as an art practised by virtuous women. This essentialist notion of nursing as a gender-based art may help account for the continuing failure to attract equal numbers of men into nursing. This view has also resulted in nurses sometimes regarding themselves, and being regarded by others, as the conscience of the healthcare system. Nursing as a gendered art is a continuing thread in professional nursing.

However, this notion was challenged significantly by the shift of nursing education into universities in the United States and by the attempts that have been made to discuss nursing as a science and a humanistic art. The literature explored indicates that nursing lies somewhat uneasily in the domains of both science and art, a division that stemmed from dividing practices in the cultural production of knowledge. Nursing developments, too, have replicated many of these dividing practices.

NURSING AND CONTEMPORARY HEALTHCARE

Many of the old divisions of the modern era are collapsing in both contemporary higher education and the health sector. This is certainly true in Australia, with implications for practices that sustained the conceptual, methodological and practical separations between art and science in nursing. The clear division between arts and sciences in higher education that reinforced the arts/sciences divide in knowledge development and the professions is clearly breaking down. It is becoming less possible for professions to define themselves in relation to discrete bodies of discipline-specific knowledge. The continuing knowledge explosion, together with the information technologies now available, are resulting in new fields of scientific enquiry and the proliferation of new professions that draw upon knowledge from a range of sources.

The nexus between professional knowledge and power is being subverted in a number of ways, not least through the processes of mass higher education and the access consumers now have to information that enables them to make their own decisions, independently of professional advice. These changes are taking place in a wider context in which global market influences are strengthening and humanist principles are weakening. This is an era of market contestability, privatisation, accountability and competition. It is an era in which performance is measured and evaluated on the basis of outcomes.

The 'reinvention' of nursing

The healthcare sector has been rapidly transforming in response to demands for identifiable, quantifiable indicators of cost-effective quality outcomes. Clinical areas have been responding to the changes wrought in diagnosis and treatment through the use of new investigative and surgical technologies. Nursing, like many other professions, has been seeking to 'reinvent' itself to meet emerging challenges (Parker & Rickard 1999).

The reinvention of nursing, I would suggest, has been occurring on several fronts, all of which have implications for the art and science of nursing. Measures undertaken in nursing education, research and practice are ensuring that nurses have the necessary repertoire of knowledge and skills to play a part in the transformations aimed at cost-effective quality outcomes of healthcare (Parker 2001). Efforts are being made to identify the nursing practices that positively influence health outcomes (Hinshaw 2000) and to develop, test and apply new practice interventions (Aranda 2008). Nurses are investigating traditional nursing practices to determine both their continuing appropriateness and the skill level necessary for their implementation.

Competencies for general, specialist and advanced practice are being refined to ensure greater accountability in relation to consumers, within the profession, in relation to other health professionals, and with regard to various contexts of practice (Australian Nursing and Midwifery Council 2006). Nurses, in collaboration with other health professionals, are also contributing to the development, testing, implementation and evaluation of standardised clinical pathways. They are developing evidence-based nursing practices and contributing to developments in evidence-based healthcare (Fineout-Overholt & Johnston 2007, Pape 2003, Parker 2002, Parker et al 2000). They are working with consumers of health services to satisfy their learning needs.

What is becoming clear in this aspect of its reinvention is that nursing is shifting away from attempts to define itself as an autonomous profession with its own discipline-specific body of nursing science knowledge. As it moves into an interdisciplinary, team-based and consumer-oriented approach to practice and research, it is drawing upon current science/technology and information systems, and focusing upon nursing contributions to health outcomes and accountability for practices.

Nurses today need to draw substantially upon scientific knowledge to inform their practice, and scientific training needs to be a significant component of nursing education programs. At the same time, nurses can contribute to the development of scientific knowledge in interdisciplinary and nursing-specific research projects. Questions for—and about—nursing emerge out of what nurses ask about their practices and the people and communities that they serve.

But how is the art of nursing manifest in this reinvention of the discipline? In a multitude of ways, I would suggest. We live today in an era of diversity, multiplicity and hybrid practices. Nursing can be practised as a gendered art; as a humanistic, aesthetic endeavour; and it can take fragments from both of these traditions and draw upon others as well. It can take up aspects of traditional art forms such as music, movement and touch, and incorporate them in diverse ways into repertoires of skilful practice.

In all of the multiplicity that is the art of nursing there is, however, a continuing thread, expressed as support of the sense of wholeness and integrity of individuals and communities rendered vulnerable through sickness and suffering.

CONCLUSION

In the current climate, many nurses are expressing reservations about the market-driven approach and the economic ethic that underlie contemporary health reforms. They are worried that standardised approaches to care will compromise their ability to meet the demands of particular and unique situations. They are troubled that the increasing rationalisation of health services is causing fragmentation of services, despite the rhetoric of continuity of care. They are concerned that greater reliance upon advanced technologies is resulting in delivery of dehumanised services.

It is important that compliance with current healthcare reforms and resistance to them are not seen to be mutually exclusive endeavours. We can no longer think about the art and science of nursing as mutually exclusive endeavours. We can no longer claim that nursing is a holistic and artistic enterprise with humanistic and expressive concerns developed in opposition to the scientific, technical and instrumental dimensions of care (Parker 1995). The therapeutic tools and technologies of care we use are not separate from us: they are part of us and we are part of them. As they change, so we change. As we change, they change too. They are integral to our self-expression as nurses. The art of nursing, then, involves the perception and understanding of the inseparability of expression and technology.

Working within the framework of a standardised pathway does not prevent a nurse from recognising the individual and unique needs of particular patients. An aesthetic sensibility recognises the extent to which there is congruence between the standard (form) and the individual (content). Aesthetic integrity is responsive nursing in which standard and individual, form and content, become shaped into wholeness. An aesthetic sensibility facilitates expression of the art of nursing as part of the complex, ambiguous and technologically expressive milieus in which nurses work. An aesthetic sensibility is responsive to unified experiences both for recipients and providers of healthcare. It resists fragmented experience and can also 'empower people who are … sick, weak, vulnerable or disturbed to demand that attention is given to the particularities, complexities and ambiguities of their individual situation' (Parker 1995:2).

Nursing as art and/or science has been addressed somewhat differently at different times and in different contexts. A continuing thread nonetheless exists, which demonstrates the significance that nursing has given as a discipline and a profession to both science and art, and the nature of their relationship in nursing. Modern secular professional nursing since its beginnings in the nineteenth century has been and continues to be a complex set of practices that contains many anomalies and contradictions. The art and science of nursing manifests itself within a broader and changing social, cultural and political agenda. Nursing's social mandate acknowledges the art and science of nursing. The challenge for nurses in the contemporary healthcare context is to exercise that mandate judiciously and creatively.

REFLECTIVE QUESTIONS

1 What do you think are the main reasons nursing has come to be viewed as an art?

2 Why has nursing made consistent attempts to align itself with science?

3 How do you think the art and science of nursing can interrelate in the current contexts of healthcare?

RECOMMENDED READINGS

Carper B 1978 Fundamental patterns of knowing in nursing. Advances in Nursing Science 1:13–23

Chinn PL, Maeve MK, Bostick C 1997 Aesthetic inquiry and the art of nursing. Scholarly Inquiry for Nursing Practice 11(2):83–100

Johnson JL 1996 The perceptual aspect of nursing art: sources of accord and discord. Scholarly Inquiry for Nursing Practice: An International Journal 10(4):307–327

Peplau HE 1988 The art and science of nursing: similarities, differences, and relations. Nursing Science Quarterly 1(1):8–15

REFERENCES

Aranda S 2008 Designing nursing interventions. Collegian 15:19–25

Australian Nursing and Midwifery Council (ANMC) 2006 National competency standards for the registered nurse, 4th edn. ANMC, Canberra

Berriot-Salvadore E 1993 The discourse of medicine and science. In: Davis NZ, Farge A (eds) A history of women in the West: Vol. 3. Renaissance and enlightenment paradoxes. Belknap Press, Cambridge, Massachusetts

Buchanan T 1999 Nightingalism: haunting nursing history. Collegian 6(1):28–33

Capra F 1982 The turning point: science, society and the rising culture. Simon & Schuster, New York

Carper B 1978 Fundamental patterns of knowing in nursing. Advances in Nursing Science 1:13–23

Chinn PL, Maeve MK, Bostick C 1997 Aesthetic inquiry and the art of nursing. Scholarly Inquiry for Nursing Practice 11(2):83–100

Chinn PL, Watson J (eds) 1994 Art and aesthetics in nursing. National League for Nursing, New York

Cohen JS 1991 Two portraits of caring: a comparison of the artists, Leininger and Watson. Journal of Advanced Nursing 16:899–909

Darbyshire P 1994a Understanding caring through arts and humanities: a medical/nursing humanities approach to promoting alternate experiences of thinking and learning. Journal of Advanced Nursing 19(5):856–863

Darbyshire P 1994b Understanding the life of illness: learning through the art of Frida Kahlo. Advances in Nursing Science 17(1):51–59

Dickens C 1910 Martin Chuzzlewit. Macmillan, New York

Donahue P 1996 Nursing: the finest art. Mosby, St Louis

Fawcett J 1984 The metaparadigm of nursing: present status and future refinements. Image: Journal of Nursing Scholarship XVI(3):84–89

Fineout-Overholt E, Johnston L 2007 Evaluation: an essential step to the EBP process. Worldviews on Evidence-Based Nursing First Quarter:54–59

Flaskerud JH, Halloran EJ 1980 Areas of agreement in nursing theory development. Advances in Nursing Science 3(1):1–7

Gortner SR 1983 The history and philosophy of nursing science and research. Advances in Nursing Science January:1–8

Hinshaw A 2000 Nursing knowledge for the 21st century: opportunities and challenges. Journal of Nursing Scholarship 32:117–123

Holden RJ 1991 In defence of Cartesian dualism and the hermeneutic horizon. Journal of Advanced Nursing 16(11):1375–1381

Jennings BM 1986 Nursing science: more promise than threat. Journal of Advanced Nursing 11(5):505–511

Johnson DE 1961 The behavioural system model for nursing. In: Riehl JP, Roy C (eds) Conceptual models for nursing practice, 2nd edn. Appleton Century Crofts, New York

Johnson JL 1993 Toward a clearer understanding of the art of nursing. Unpublished doctoral dissertation. University of Alberta, Edmonton

Johnson JL 1994 A dialectical examination of nursing art. Advances in Nursing Science 1(1):1–14

Johnson JL 1996 The perceptual aspect of nursing art: sources of accord and discord. Scholarly Inquiry for Nursing Practice: An International Journal 10(4):307–327

Kritek PB 1985 Nursing diagnosis in perspective: response to a critique. Image: Journal of Nursing Scholarship 17(1):3–8

Lafferty PM 1997 Balancing the curriculum: promoting aesthetic knowledge in nursing. Nurse Education Today 17:281–286

Levine M 1971 Holistic nursing. Nursing Clinics of North America 6(2):253–263

Munhall PL 1982 Nursing philosophy and nursing research: in apposition or opposition? Nursing Research 31:176–177, 181

Nelson S 1995 Humanism in nursing: the emergence of light. Nursing Inquiry 2(1):36–43

Pape TM 2003 Evidence based nursing practice: to infinity and beyond. Journal of Continuing Education in Nursing 34(4):154–161

Parker J 1990 Professional nursing education in the university context. Meredith Memorial Lecture, La Trobe University, Melbourne

Parker J 1995 Searching for the body in nursing. In: Gray G, Pratt R (eds) Scholarship in the discipline of nursing. Churchill Livingstone, Melbourne

Parker J 2001 The implications of international health policy trends on nursing education: an Australian perspective. Policy, Politics, and Nursing Practice 2(2):142–148

Parker J 2002 Evidence based nursing: a defence (editorial). Nursing Inquiry 9(3):139–140

Parker J, Gibbs M 1998 Truth, virtue and beauty: midwifery and philosophy. Nursing Inquiry 5(3):146–153

Parker J, Johnston L, Faulkner R 2000 Evidence-based nursing: integrating research into practice. In: Greenwood J (ed) Nursing theory in Australia: development and application, 2nd edn. Prentice Hall, Sydney, pp 396–412

Parker J, Rickard G 1999 Nursing town and nursing gown: time, space and the reinvention of nursing through collaboration. Clinical Excellence for Nurse Practitioners 3(1):36–42

Peplau HE 1988 The art and science of nursing: similarities, differences, and relations. Nursing Science Quarterly 1(1):8–15

Rogers M 1970 Theoretical basis of nursing. FA Davis, Philadelphia

Roy C 1980 The Roy adaptation model. In: Riehl J, Roy C (eds) Conceptual models for nursing practice. Appleton Century Crofts, New York

Smith FB 1982 Florence Nightingale, reputation and power. Croom Helm, London

Snow CP 1964 The two cultures: and a second look. New American Library, New York

Trembath R, Hellier D 1987 All care and responsibility: a history of nursing in Victoria 1850–1934. Florence Nightingale Committee, Australia, Melbourne

Watson J 1985 Nursing: human science and human care. Appleton Century Crofts, Norwalk, Connecticut

Heroines, hookers and harridans: exploring popular images and representations of nurses and nursing

Philip Darbyshire

LEARNING OBJECTIVES

After reading this chapter, students will be able to:

- explain the importance of nursing's image for contemporary nursing
- describe the various prevalent stereotypes of the nurse and nursing, and try to explain the persistence of these
- debate the issue of whether nurses really wish to abandon the 'overworked angel' image
- explain the difficulties involved in proposing a 'realistic' portrayal of nurses and nursing, and
- propose a strategy or small-scale project that could help promote alternative media representations of nurses and nursing.

KEY WORDS

Images, iconography, media, stereotypes, portrayal, mythical, realism

INTRODUCTION

Since the mid-1970s, there has been a burgeoning interest in the study of popular images of nurses and nursing; it seems that every conceivable aspect of the image of nurses has been scrutinised. Writers have focused on images of nurses and nursing on television (Anonymous 2003, Buresh & Gordon 1995, Holmes 1997, Kalisch et al 1983, Lenzer 2003), in cinema (Darbyshire 1995, Fiedler 1988, Jones 1988, Kalisch & Kalisch 1983c, Kalisch et al 1982), in novels and short stories (Hunter 1988, Jones 1988, Summers 1997), in news coverage (Berry 2004, Delacour 1991, Doolan 2000, Dunn 1985, Ferns & Chojnacka 2005, Kalisch & Kalisch 1984, Mason 2002, Takase et al 2002), in advertisements (Lusk 2000, Regan 2005), in greeting cards (Smith 2003), on the internet (Kalisch et al 2007) and elsewhere. Why such fascination with the image of nurses? With the possible exception of doctors, why is there no comparable body of inquiry literature regarding the image of teachers, social workers, physiotherapists, accountants, occupational therapists or other professional groups?

In this chapter, I will explore some of the early history and iconography of nurses and nursing in order to clarify the origins of many of the issues and 'images of nursing' which are so hotly contested and debated today. The 'so what?' question is important here. Why, when there are so many other pressing issues and concerns facing nursing and healthcare, should we worry about nursing's image? At one fundamental level, this matters because how we see and understand ourselves as nurses impacts on how we think and work as nurses (Takase et al 2002, 2006). Furthermore, understanding how and why nursing's image has been shaped and formed helps us understand vital lessons about how the world works. Delacour argues that:

> Certainly it is important that we analyse the process through which dysfunctional images and discourses are maintained. Moreover, it is useful to regard reading media as a politically situated and critical activity for the nursing profession (Delacour 1991:413).

Developing a critical and questioning view of our historical and contemporary representations is thus important for every nurse's personal and professional development. What we should strive for is to move beyond a 'knee-jerk' response that this or that image is good or bad, and to develop the critical thinking and analytic qualities that help us understand the production, meaning(s) and possible effects of popular images of the nurse and nursing.

Perhaps of even greater concern is that in so many media 'medical shows' and stories, nurses and an informed, valuable nursing voice is airbrushed out. As The Kaiser Family Foundation report, 'As seen on TV: health policy issues in TV's medical dramas', from the United States showed:

> ... the shows portrayed doctors as dominating discussions around health policy issues. Nurses, social workers, and other members of the health care team hardly existed in policy scenes (www.kff.org/entmedia/John_Q_Report.pdf) (pp 27–8).

NURSING'S EARLY ICONOGRAPHY

Representations and images of nursing are as old as nursing and healing themselves. By tracing the origins of modern nursing back to antiquity and to the earliest accounts of babies, pregnant women, family and other members of early communities being cared for, usually by women, we can see that, 'The nurse as saintly domestic is no modern invention' (Kampen 1988). The earliest Greco–Roman depictions were almost entirely of 'baby nurses' and the image of the 'modern' nurse as tender of the sick or wounded was not to appear until the fourteenth century (Kampen 1988).

With the emergence of religious orders and associated charitable services came a new iconography of nursing which showed women extending their care practices from the immediate household and family arena to the care of strangers. This was not always welcomed, however, and the Middle Ages in Europe especially saw the slaughter of many 'wise women' who were burnt as witches (Darbyshire 1985). Commenting on fifteenth century depictions of 'nurses' working with the sick, Kampen makes the significant observation that:

> Several features common to scenes of nursing sisters help to define the nature of their role: they nurse patients who are most often men lying in bed, they work in a distinctive location that does not look like a house, they wear distinctive costumes, their activities are domestic and religious rather than specifically medical, and most important, they are never subordinated to patients and doctors (Kampen 1988:23).

It is salutary to think that, with the exception of the last phrase, this description would have fitted any typical Victorian infirmary almost 500 years later. So powerful is this depiction of nurses as tenders of the prostrate sick, reinforced no doubt by the iconographic imagery of Florence Nightingale wending her ethereal way through the wards of Scutari Hospital during the Crimean War, that nursing has often been seen in the public mind as being exclusively focused on this particular form of acute care nursing. McCoppin and Gardner (1994) noted how this one-dimensional view of nursing and nurses can occlude the view of all other forms and areas of nursing, which can somehow be deemed to be 'less than' or 'other than' 'real nursing', which of course was deemed to be practised exclusively at the bedsides of sick people:

> The stereotypical view of nurses as working only in acute care, high technology areas often portrayed in the media makes it very difficult to provide the alternative view of nurses working within the community which is more difficult to make 'attention grabbing' (McCoppin & Gardner 1994:156).

It is not only the various forms of community nursing which may be seen as less than 'real nursing', but also the myriad other 'nursings', such as working in mental health, health promotion, school nursing, working with people with learning/intellectual disabilities and many others. This masking of what, even in 1985, was more than half of the whole nursing workforce (Dunn 1985) is significant as it can help narrow and restrict students' and other nurses' perceptions of what nursing fundamentally 'is'. For example, in Kiger's study of student nurses in Scotland, she found that: 'The picture of adult medical-surgical nursing as typical of real nursing persisted throughout [the students' concept of] working with people' (Kiger 1993).

The 'real nurse as general nurse' is, however, only one of many distortions and misrepresentations that have plagued nursing since its inception. Why nursing should be such a fertile ground for image construction and manipulation is a hugely complex issue and one that has been discussed and argued over many years. One way of beginning to understand the heady brew of images, social constructions, myths and contradictions and 'realities' which form the image(s) of nurses and nursing is to look more carefully at the persistence and power of the major stereotypes of nurses which still exist in either blatant or more subtle forms even today.

NURSING'S STEREOTYPES

Perhaps it could be considered something of a backhanded compliment that there are so many stereotypes associated with nursing. At least we are not seen as bland and instantly forgettable! Major stereotypes can, however, be so unrelentingly negative in their connotations and so wholly untenable in their relationship to any notion of a 'reality' of nursing. (This notion of a single nursing reality is itself contentious and I shall return to this later.) The problem with any stereotype is that it can become so pervasive that its effects become more than merely an annoyance. As Delacour observes:

> … even stereotypes regarded as dubious may, after a measure of exposure, become internalized and naturalized, they are thereby metamorphosed into categories of the normal, the real, and the healthy and desirable (Delacour 1991:413).

If the sole problem with nursing stereotypes was just that some get-well cards, tabloid newspaper stories or 'X-rated' films portrayed nurses as oversexualised bimbos, then perhaps we could laugh it off, but when the effects of stereotyping are more serious, then there is more at stake than nursing's collective need to 'lighten up'.

The images and perceptions of nursing, both within the profession and in society in general are important for several reasons. We live in an era where image and the marketing of image has never been more important, and while we can certainly maintain that the 'core business' of nursing is caring for the health and wellbeing of people, we would be foolish to ignore the importance of nursing's image. If we are to attract creative, committed, intelligent and passionate people into nursing, then nursing needs to be seen as every bit as worthwhile and challenging a career as any other in the fields of healthcare or social service. The persistence of hackneyed old stereotypes does nothing to enhance the attractiveness of nursing as a career.

Muff (1982:211) has suggested six 'major nursing stereotypes': angel of mercy, handmaiden to the physician, woman in white, sex symbol/idiot, battleaxe, and torturer. Dunn (1985:2) credits the average tabloid newspaper with even less imagination, being interested in only three types of nurse: angel, battleaxe and nymphomaniac.

Angels with pretty faces

If nursing iconography has an enduring stereotypic image, it must surely be the nurse as 'angel'. While much of the earliest artwork and imagery of nurses showed nurses ministering to the sick in various quasi-religious ways and settings, nurses in Australia, even in the late 1800s, were 'redefining the image of nurses as motivated primarily by self-sacrifice' (Bashford 1997). However, it was Florence Nightingale's story that captured the public imagination and stimulated a swathe of hagiographic accounts (which critic Leslie Fiedler called 'shameless schlock' (Fiedler 1988:103)), and movies such as *The White Angel* and *The Lady with the Lamp* (Jones 1988, Kalisch & Kalisch 1983b). So powerful were these images of the angelic presence which lit up the wards of Scutari with her lamp, that Florence Nightingale has become easily identified as the soul or spirit of nursing and as the embodiment of selfless, devoted, compassionate care that borders on the saintly. Despite some of the more critical and balanced scholarship concerning the life and work of Florence Nightingale (e.g. Hektor 1994), the stereotype of the nurse as selfless angel is still prevalent, especially in the public imagination.

There are several difficulties here. At first glance it may seem no bad thing to think that society views nurses as 'angels'. Who wouldn't like to be thought of in such a 'positive' light? Which nurse would not like to think that she was capable of such profound caring, which could earn such adoration? Is this not just being held in high regard by society? Don't we feel good when opinion polls put nurses near the top of the list for perceived honesty, trustworthiness and hard work? Salvage (1983) perceptively pointed out that nurses often collude in sustaining the 'selfless angel' stereotype while professing to scorn it. As she noted, 'The trouble is we are secretly flattered by the myths, especially those emphasising dedication and high-minded self-sacrifice' (Salvage 1983:14).

However, buying into the 'angels' stereotype may be a Faustian bargain, for there is a price to pay for this. 'Angels' may be saintly, but such perfection is impossible for mere mortal nurses to achieve or maintain; nurses are, after all, only human. Nor do angels seem to require any education or experience; their sanctity is more of a divine gift. For real nurses, however, becoming a skilled and competent nurse is hard work. We may be born with particular dispositions and talents (although some would dispute even this), but we cannot be 'born nurses'. That will take more than an accident of birth. Such shafts of grace as we achieve are often hard won through our sustained engagement in the lives of those people who place their trust in us.

Doctors' handmaidens

If the 'angel' myth is a remnant of nursing's religious order origins, then the unquestioning obedience of the doctor's handmaiden owes much to nursing's military origins. This stereotype touts the image of the nurse as a kind of 'lady in waiting', or the doctor's 'right-hand woman'. For decades this has been a hugely influential media view of nursing. Essentially, the nurse is there to provide faithful and obedient service to the doctor and, like the 'angel' myth, this view has often been sustained by nurses themselves, who were flattered by the idea that 'their' doctors or 'their' consultant says that he or she could not manage without them. In her analysis of nurses' image in post-war Britain, Hallam (1998) noted also that: 'Within the broadcasting environment, nursing's professional discourse of "service" was interpreted as service to medicine, nurses themselves did little to challenge the picture' (Hallam 1998:37).

In this sense, the 'handmaiden' stereotype may be less mythical than nursing would like to acknowledge. While nationally and internationally, particular nurses and nursing projects/initiatives have led healthcare advances (often in collaboration with medical colleagues), there are still many nurses who work with doctors who seem to not recognise nurses' ability and responsibility to make an equal contribution to care, and who assume that the nurse's role is to make coffee, not decisions. Despite claims of teamwork and 'multidisciplinary' cooperation, some nurses continue to work in 'teams' where teamwork is lots of people doing what one person says, and that one person is usually a doctor.

The battleaxe or monstrous figure

For images to be powerful and long lasting they must be capable of being both sustained and subverted. The battleaxe figure is in many ways a magnificent subversion of other stereotypes of the nurse. It is what Hunter (1988) calls, in a slightly different context, the translocated ideal. Where the 'angel' is often portrayed as pretty, feminine, Caucasian, slim, caring, white-clad for purity, fun, deferential and loved by patients, the battleaxe or matron figure was almost the exact opposite—tyrannical, fearsome, asexual, cruel, monstrously large, dark-clad, and set on crushing all fun and individuality. On a BBC radio program that I compiled several years ago, I listened to a recording of a 1960s radio quiz show where one of the male panellists joked that the tragedy of nurses is that they were one day destined to become matrons. Matrons, like other nurses who refuse to fit the accepted stereotype of the pretty, kind, compliant nurse, are banished to the moral margins of societal acceptance where they become objects of fear or ridicule.

Think here of 'bad' nurses like Charles Dickens' Sairey Gamp (Summers 1997), Ken Kesey's 'Big Nurse/Nurse Ratched' from *One Flew Over the Cuckoo's Nest* (Darbyshire 1995), Annie Wilkes from Stephen King's *Misery* and the more comic figures of Hattie Jacques from the *Carry On* film series (Ferns & Chojnacka 2005) or Matron Dorothy from Australia's 1990 television series, *Let the Blood Run Free* (Delacour 1991). The 'battleaxe' stereotype cries out for a feminist analysis that reveals the fate of any nurse who does not comply with the mythical norms of the ideal nurse and who challenges male power (usually patients and doctors). Worse than this, perhaps, is that the battleaxe figure is a powerful woman who is unattracted to them (Darbyshire 1995), thus proving that she cannot be a 'real' nurse, as one of the most prevalent and damaging stereotypes is the nurse as an easily available sex bomb.

Naughty nurses and nymphomaniacs

When I was lecturing in Scotland, I would discuss the question of nurses' image with the first year students who had just begun their course. I asked them what a common reaction would be at a party if they happened to mention that they were nurses. After the laughter and ribaldry had settled, it was clear that a common, if not thankfully universal, reaction from some men was a 'knowing grin' and some suggestion that a night of unbridled sexual abandon might lie ahead. For this reason, many of the students said that they would make up an occupation rather than 'admit' to being a nurse. Why is the 'naughty nurse' stereotype so prevalent? Why are there no 'naughty lawyer' sexual stereotypes? Why are there no pornographic films made about the adventures of a group of occupational therapy students? Why don't sex shops sell physiotherapist uniforms? What is it about nurses that make them such a target?

This is a deep and complex issue, but consider the following points in relation to Hunter's (1988) notion of a 'translocated ideal'. Nursing is utterly implicated in social power relations, between nurses and doctors, nurses and other nurses, nurses and patients, nurses and relatives, and more. When patients enter hospital, the traditional power relations are reversed and they find themselves vulnerable and dependent, rather than strong and in control. At a societal level (for not every male patient will see his situation in this way), one way of redressing this balance is to metaphorically (or perhaps even practically) sexualise the encounters between nurses and patients.

We also know that nurses' practices in relation to patients' bodies are part of this process. Nurses are exceptionally privileged in that we are intimate body workers. Nurses have access to people's most private body areas and bodily functions (Lawler 1991). One of the most important and demanding practices that a nurse develops is the ability to work with patients' intimate body parts without sexualising the encounter. To transgress this boundary would be both embarrassing and dangerous. In an almost-too-painful-to-watch scene in Dennis Potter's television play, *The Singing Detective*, a nurse has to anoint with cream the genital areas of the hero, 'Philip Marlowe', as he has extremely debilitating psoriasis and cannot do this for himself. As the nurse applies his cream he becomes sexually aroused and despite trying desperately to divert his thoughts, he develops an erection. The nurse, however, wants to get the procedure done and continues creaming, causing him to ejaculate and suffer an agony of humiliation.

Fagin and Diers (1983:117) are clear on the damaging implications of conflating sexualisation and intimate body work: 'Thanks to the worst of this kind of thinking, nursing is a metaphor for sex. Having seen and touched the bodies of strangers, nurses are perceived as willing and able sexual partners.' The 'naughty nurse' stereotype also encourages the subversion of another ideal—that of the saintly purity of the nurse as 'angel'. Beneath the pristine white uniform, tightly bunched and restrained hair, and sheepish obedience to authority, lies the pornographer's win–win scenario. Either the nurse is *really* a 'sex-bomb' being barely held in check by the rules and regulations of the institution and awaiting the slightest excuse to release all of this pent-up passion, or she *really* is completely subservient to (male) authority, in which case she will willingly agree to every sexual demand. If you think that these scenarios are far-fetched, consider a feature that ran several years ago in the United Kingdom tabloid newspaper, *The Sun*, which aroused furious opposition, and not only from nurses and their organisations. The feature had the headline, 'Calling all you naughty nurses', and read:

> Yes, we know you're out there. Lots and lots of people tell stories about those saucy times when temperatures soared in the wards. Who hasn't heard about the time the young nurse turned a bed bath into a saucy romp? And delighted male patients are always revealing how they got some very special medicine from the attractive sister when the screens were drawn. So come on folks. Let's hear from the naughty night nurses—and their happy patients—about the fun times in Britain's hospitals. We're opening our own special phone line between 10 a.m. and 6 p.m. today. Ring the number below and tell us your stories.

Such was the wave of protest from nursing organisations and others that the feature was withdrawn within days. Sadly, such 'saucy nurse' stories remain a staple of tabloid journalism (Ferns & Chojnacka 2005).

NURSING'S IMAGE: BLAME THE MEDIA?

For any nurse who wants to place the blame for the worst excesses and misrepresentations of nursing's image, then the media in general offer a clear, if rather too easy, target. Too easy perhaps because we assume that the media is almost automatically the most pervasive form of image transmission. Yet a study of 1155 people in the United States found that less than 10% of the respondents felt that they obtained their information from the media. Most said that their opinions came from first-hand impressions gained during visits to a hospital (Begany 1994, Delacour 1991).

Delacour (1991:418) makes the important point that often it is not only the ways in which nursing is portrayed but also, more than that, it is that nursing is 'symbolically annihilated by the mass media' and virtually ignored. To test this claim, it would be interesting to keep a local and a national newspaper for a month or two with a view to checking how many health stories included authoritative comments from nurses compared with doctors. Many nurses would say that they could confidently predict the results of such a survey well in advance.

Considerable research has been undertaken into the role of the media in constructing and shaping nursing's image. In the United States in particular, the team of Philip and Beatrice Kalisch in the 1980s produced numerous books and papers on many different aspects of this question (Kalisch & Kalisch 1983a, 1983c, 1984, 1987, Kalisch et al 1982).

This criticism of the media in general continues unabated. Holmes (1997:137), for example, advises that we should (perhaps) give up watching medical 'soaps' on television as they are 'anodyne and legitimating rather than transformative and critical'.

While 'soaps' may well be 'anodyne', there are probably few viewers of Grey's Anatomy or All Saints who bemoan that the show is no longer as 'transformative and critical' as it used to be. Blaming genres for not being what we would wish them to be is surely tilting at windmills. To simply stop watching 'soaps' because we disagree with aspects of their portrayal of nurses and nursing is scarcely a mode of engagement. Nor is it particularly astute to imagine that the media exist to 'accurately' (or should it be positively/flatteringly?) depict nurses and their work. Much as we may dislike the notion, the mass media exists primarily as a profit-making business. It is not nursing's tame public relations machine.

There is also an argument to be made that criticisms of the portrayals of nurses often seem to misunderstand the different genres of representation. For example, criticising a film like Carry On Nurse, or a television series like SCRUBS, for giving a false image of nurses and nursing makes little sense. These are not documentaries and their purpose was never to represent the 'reality' of nursing. They are comedies, and they work by upsetting or translocating our understandings and expectations of medicine or nursing. Condemning a Carry On film for not being a true-to-life account of nursing is like criticising Thursday for not being a beautiful mountain range.

Stanley's detailed and carefully nuanced analysis of nurses in feature films avoids the simplistic characterisation of portrayals of nurses as being 'good/bad'–'angel/ devil' (Stanley 2008). While a 'blame the media' approach has a seductive simplicity, it is unlikely to achieve any significant results. However, working with the media in order to help create more 'realistic' portrayals of nursing's work has been reported to help (Buresh & Gordon 1995). In the early days of the filming of the medical soap ER, there was virtually no consultation with nurses or ER departments. Emergency room nurses in the United States, however, did more than complain or stop watching—they became proactive and contacted the producers regularly with comments and criticisms, but also with offers of help, story line ideas, and the names of subspecialty ER nurses who were willing to help the show 'get it right'.

NURSING'S IMAGE: DEPICTING 'REALITY'?

In a news report, the warning of Joanne Rule, former head of the RCN (UK) public relations office was repeated: 'if nursing were to succeed finally in shaking off the "angel" image it so professes to hate, it might be replaced by an image that it hated even more' (Rule 1995). One of the significant difficulties in challenging potentially damaging images of nursing is that it is very difficult to give an agreed account of what a 'good portrayal' should look like. As Bashford noted in her study of how early Australian nurses challenged their systems:

> … resistance was never straightforward. Often, rather than new discourses offering empowering new subject positions, they produced confusion, contradiction and insecurity. Women were asked to think about their work in religious terms in one moment and in one context, in scientific terms in another, and as a type of professionalism in another (Bashford 1997:74).

This historical dilemma will seem blindingly contemporary to today's nurses who are struggling with very similar issues around nurses' 'expanded role' and what this means for nursing's identity/identities. The other difficulty in looking for a 'realistic' image of nurses is that it would be a precious and narcissistic stance for nursing to adopt which stated that the only acceptable portrayals of nurses and nursing were those that were 'positive'. (And for 'acceptable', ask: Acceptable to whom? To me personally? To nurses at my hospital? To nursing in general?) It would be reassuring to think that nursing was a little more secure in its role and purpose than to require constant flattery from an unrelenting diet of uncritical media comments and compliments. This quest for the 'positive' portrayal of nursing has been questioned by Hallam who argued that:

> This search for a positive image of nursing identity poses two crucial problems. On the one hand, it tends to presume a professional consensus in terms of what this image is or could be ... the positive image approach can also be critiqued from the viewpoint of media reception, it conceptualises readers and viewers as uncritical receivers of messages who unquestioningly digest the authority of the image (Hallam 1998:33).

Similarly, Cheek has observed that 'the task is not to look for real and authentic representations of nursing, but rather to look for the speaking and representation that is done about nursing' (Cheek 1995:239). This is not to say, however, that no 'positive' images and accounts of nurses and nursing can be found. For example, in his account of his serious injury and recovery, surgeon and rehabilitation specialist Tony Moore describes the artistic and technical expertise of the intensive care nurses who gave him a blanket bath:

> They worked like a ballet corps in slow motion, softly moving me forwards, to the side, sponging, touching, towelling with clean tenderness, and when one gently washed my genitals I felt nothing but the compassion of her care (Moore 1991:11).

Richard Selzer was another surgeon who found himself a patient in intensive care following legionnaires' disease. He is hugely embarrassed by his dependency and incontinence, but again, his nurses are memorably skilled in what he calls 'the forgiveness of the flesh' (Selzer 1993). Unlike the unfortunate 'Philip Marlowe' in *The Singing Detective*, Selzer's nurses spare him the embarrassment and pain that could so easily become part of his intimate body care. One nurse who makes such a profound difference to Selzer's care and recovery is Patrick, whom Selzer describes as being 'the sort of nurse who can draw the pus out of a carbuncle with his gaze alone, and turn it into a jewel' (Selzer 1993:56). Selzer is emphatic that the power of skilled nurse caring is not merely 'nice to get', but that it is actually transformative. He describes his being carried back to bed by Patrick following a tub bath as the moment when his 'molecules rearranged themselves'. He says: 'It is the true moment of cure' (Selzer 1993:93).

Read these authors' accounts of their care and then consider that bathing patients is deemed by some to be basic nursing care—where for 'basic' read 'unimportant and thus able to be undertaken by virtually anyone'. There are many other 'positive' accounts in literature and popular culture of nurses and nursing which are valued, appreciated and have a markedly beneficial effect on the recipient. However, care is needed not to fall into the trap of 'collecting' these accounts as a kind of trophy for nursing. If we are to cultivate and develop our questioning and critical powers, then the positive accounts also need to be questioned and discussed.

NURSING'S IMAGE: FROM AFFRONT TO ACTION

During the past few decades, there has been a plethora of research and discussion regarding nursing's image and the portrayals of nursing. We are now much more aware of the forces that shape and maintain many of popular culture's images of nurses and nursing. Perhaps the next few decades will see nurses moving from this position of greater awareness to one of more positive action. By this I mean that it is no longer enough to be outraged at the 'negative images' and stereotypes that we will continue to encounter. Indignation or 'refusing to watch' are not strategies for change. Nor will it be enough to merely call for negative images of nurses to be withdrawn or 'banned'.

The most pressing task ahead is for nurses and nursing to use the media in a much more 'streetwise' way than we have in the past (Buresh & Gordon 2006). If we do not like the images that are being presented, then we have a responsibility to provide alternatives. If we think that media reports and stories about nursing are inaccurate or inadequate, then we need to interest the media in alternatives. If we feel that the media completely ignores a particularly important program, service or aspect of nursing, then why not alert them to this and highlight the importance of what it is that they are missing. No media like to feel that they are missing something interesting or important, especially in their local area.

Delacour (1991) lists excellent questions that we should ask about the images and representations of nurses and nursing:

> Who has speaking rights? Who says what? Which position? On behalf of whom? Who is silenced? What are the assumptions? What is privileged in the text? What is ignored, glossed over or marginalised? What is the target audience and how is the reading/viewing position constructed to promote a 'preferred' reading? Which genre and its codes and effects? What type of publication/program and resultant status of discourse? How are power and knowledge articulated? How are gender, sexuality, roles and relationship, race, class, deviance and normality constructed? Which rhetorical devices? Which linguistic features (Delacour 1991:419)?

These are questions that do not naively assume the existence of a right or wrong image, but that begin the task of unpacking and exploring this complex yet highly revealing area wherein we can learn so much about ourselves, our society and those for whom we care. To these questions we should add some others that will help us be more active in redressing nursing's image. Questions such as: What images would we want to see in the media? How can we show the positive power of nursing to local and national media? Why would/should the media be interested in this program/innovation/nursing development? How can we 'sell' this idea or story to them in such a way that they can't ignore it? Whose expertise and support could we call upon to help us do this? (Belcher 2003, Buresh & Gordon 2006, Clark 1989, Monahan 1996, National Nursing and Nursing Education Taskforce 2006, Strasen 1992, Waters 2003).

CONCLUSION

We now know a great deal about representations of nurses and nursing in the various media and popular culture. As nurses, our task now is not simply to 'adapt' to, or merely observe and comment on future changes, but also to get out there and make the changes happen.

REFLECTIVE QUESTIONS

1 Discuss with a group of your peers the reactions that you have encountered, both favourable and unfavourable, when you have told people that you are a nurse/student nurse and how you feel about such reactions.

2 Use Delacour's list of questions to assess and question some selected images of nurses/nursing (e.g. a film, documentary, novel, medical 'soap').

3 Plan how you would go about creating your own media story about nurses or nursing. What would you choose as the issue? Would it be a nurse-led clinical initiative, an ethical dilemma, a particularly successful patient outcome, an exciting new approach in nursing education, or a particular nurse who is doing something really special in an area? How would you go about interesting the media in the story and how would you present it?

4 Visit 'Nursing Advocacy.org' for the most comprehensive online campaigns and resources related to nursing's public image (www.nursingadvocacy.org).

5 Visit www.philipdarbyshire.com.au and listen to 'The professionals', a feature program on nursing's image as portrayed in the BBC Radio archives. Discuss if and how you think nursing would be portrayed differently in the current decade.

RECOMMENDED READINGS

Bloomfield J 1999 The changing image of Australian nursing. Online. Available: www.clininfo.health.nsw.gov.au/hospolic/stvincents/stvin99/Jacqui.htm

Buresh B, Gordon S 2006 From silence to voice: what nurses know and must communicate to the public. Cornell University Press, New York

Darbyshire P 'The professionals'; nursing as portrayed in the archives of BBC Radio. Online. Available: www.philipdarbyshire.com.au

Davis C, Schaefer J 1995 Between the heartbeats: poetry and prose by nurses. University of Iowa Press, Iowa City

Donahue MP, Donahue PM 1996 Nursing: the finest art. Mosby-Year Book, St Louis

Friedman L 2004 Cultural sutures: medicine and media. Duke University Press, Durham

Gordon S 2005 Nursing against the odds: how health care cost-cutting, media stereotypes, and medical hubris undermine nursing and patient care. Cornell University Press, New York

Jones A 1988 Images of nurses: perspectives from history, art, and literature. University of Pennsylvania Press, Pennsylvania

REFERENCES

Anonymous 2003 American nurses speak out over portrayal in ER. Nursing Standard 18(14–16):5

Bashford A 1997 Starch on the collar and sweat on the brow: Self sacrifice and the status of work for nurses. Journal of Australian Studies 52:67–80

Begany T 1994 Your image is brighter than ever. RN 57(10):28–34

Belcher D 2003 Nurses making a difference. Bridging the gap between nurses and the media: the grassroots. Center for Nursing Advocacy. American Journal of Nursing 103(5):130

Berry l 2004 Is image important? Nursing Standard 18(23):14–16

Buresh B, Gordon S 1995 Taking on the TV shows. American Journal of Nursing 95(11):18–20

Buresh B Gordon S 2006 From silence to voice: what nurses know and must communicate to the public. Cornell University Press, New York

Cheek J 1995 Nurses nursing and representations: an exploration of the effect of viewing positions on the textual portrayal of nursing. Nursing Inquiry 2(4):235–240

Clark G 1989 To be or not to be: it's time to market nursing's image. In: Gray G, Pratt R (eds) Issues in Australian nursing 2. Churchill Livingstone, Melbourne, pp 175–92

Darbyshire P 1985 Bedpans or broomsticks? Nursing Times 81(Nov 6–12):44–45

Darbyshire P 1995 Reclaiming 'Big Nurse': a feminist critique of Ken Kesey's portrayal of Nurse Ratched in One Flew Over the Cuckoo's Nest. Nursing Inquiry 2(4):198–202

Delacour S 1991 The construction of nursing: ideology discourse and representation. In: Gray G, Pratt R (eds) Towards a discipline of nursing. Churchill Livingstone, Melbourne, pp 413–33

Doolan E 2000 Nursing: image politics and the media. British Journal of Perioperative Nursing 10(9):474

Dunn A 1985 Images of nursing in the nursing and popular press. Bulletin of the Royal College of Nursing (UK) History of Nursing Group 6:2–8

Fagin C, Diers D 1983 Nursing as a metaphor. The New England Journal of Medicine 309(2):116–117

Ferns T, Chojnacka I 2005 Angels and swingers matrons and sinners: nursing stereotypes. British Journal of Nursing 14(19):1028–1032

Fiedler L 1988 Images of the nurse in fiction and popular cultures. In: Jones A (ed.) Images of nurses: perspectives from history art and literature. University of Pennsylvania Press, Pennsylvania, pp 100–12

Hallam J 1998 From angels to handmaidens: changing constructions of nursing's public image in post-war Britain. Nursing Inquiry 5(1):32–42

Hektor L 1994 Florence Nightingale and the women's movement: friend or foe? Nursing Inquiry 1:38–45

Holmes C 1997 Why we should wash our hands of medical soaps. Nursing Inquiry 4(2):135–137

Hunter K 1988 Nurses: the satiric image and the translocated ideal. In: Jones A (ed.) Images of nurses: perspectives from history, art, and literature. University of Pennsylvania Press, Pennsylvania, pp 113–27

Jones A 1988 Images of nurses: perspectives from history, art, and literature. University of Pennsylvania Press, Pennsylvania

Kalisch B, Kalisch P 1983a An analysis of the impact of authorship on the image of the nurse presented in novels. Research in Nursing and Health 6(1):17–24

Kalisch B, Kalisch P 1983b Anatomy of the image of the nurse: dissonant and ideal models. American Nurses Association Publications G-161 3-23. Online. Available: www.nursingadvocacy.org/images/kalisch/anatomy_of_the_image_of_the_nurse_ocr.pdf 20 Sept 2008

Kalisch B, Kalisch P 1983c Heroine out of focus: media images of Florence Nightingale. Part 1: popular biographies and stage productions. Nursing and Health Care 4(4):181–187

Kalisch B, Kalisch P 1984 An analysis of news coverage of maternal-child nurses. Maternal-Child Nursing Journal 13:77–90

Kalisch B, Kalisch P, McHugh M 1982 The nurse as a sex object in motion pictures. Research in Nursing and Health 5(3):147–154

Kalisch BJ, Begeny S, Neumann S 2007 The image of the nurse on the internet. Nursing Outlook 55(4):182–188

Kalisch P, Kalisch B 1987 The changing image of the nurse. Addison Wesley, Menlo Park, California

Kalisch P, Kalisch B, Scobey M 1983 Images of nurses on television. Springer, New York

Kampen N 1988 Florence Nightingale: a prehistory of nursing in painting and sculpture. In: Jones A (ed.) Images of nurses: perspectives from history, art, and literature. University of Pennsylvania Press, Pennsylvania, pp 6–39

Kiger A 1993 Accord and discord in students' images of nursing. Journal of Nursing Education 32(7):309–317

Lawler J 1991 Behind the screens: nursing somology and the problem of the body. Churchill Livingstone, Melbourne

Lenzer J 2003 ER blamed for nursing shortage. British Medical Journal 327:1294

Lusk B 2000 Pretty and powerless: nurses in advertisements 1930–1950. Research in Nursing and Health 23(3):229–236

McCoppin B, Gardner H 1994 Tradition and reality: nursing and politics in Australia. Churchill Livingstone, Melbourne

Mason DJ 2002 Invisible nurses: media neglect is one cause of the nursing shortage. American Journal of Nursing 102(8):7

Monahan BB 1996 The nurses' media handbook: a reference for nurses planning to meet the media. Massachusetts Nurse 66(5):2, 6, 12

Moore T 1991 Cry of the damaged man. Picador, Sydney

Muff J 1982 Handmaiden, battle-axe whore: an exploration of the fantasies, myths and stereotypes about nurses. In: Muff J (ed.) Socialization, sexism and stereotyping: women's issues in nursing. Wareland Press, Illinois, pp 113–52

National Nursing and Nursing Education Taskforce 2006 Media and communication principles for nursing and midwifery. Online. Available: www.nnnet.gov.au/downloads/rec9_commprinciples.pdf 10 Sept 2008

Regan M 2005 Virgin's nurses and the public image of nursing. Nursing Philosophy 6(3):110–121

Rule J 1995 Nurses may live to regret the 'angel' image era has ended (news item). Nursing Management 2(6):5

Salvage J 1983 Are you in the PINC? Distorted images. Nursing Times 79(1):13–15

Selzer R 1993 Raising the dead: a doctor's encounter with his own mortality. Penguin, Harmondsworth

Smith L 2003 Image counts: greeting cards mail it in when it comes to accurately portraying nurses. Online. Available: http://include.nurse.com/apps/pbcs.dll/article?AID=2003310010351 25 Sept 2008

Stanley D 2008 Celluloid angels: a research study of nurses in feature films. Journal of Advanced Nursing 64(1):84–95

Strasen L 1992 The image of professional nursing: strategies for action. Lippincott, Philadelphia

Summers A 1997 Sairey Gamp: generating fact from fiction. Nursing Inquiry 4(1): 14–18

Takase M, Kershaw E, Burt L 2002 Does public image of nurses matter? Journal of Professional Nursing 18(4):196–205

Takase M, Maude P, Manias E 2006 Impact of the perceived public image of nursing on nurses' work behaviour. Journal of Advanced Nursing 53(3):333–343

Waters A 2003 Image makeover brings in recruits for US nursing. Nursing Standard 17(43):9

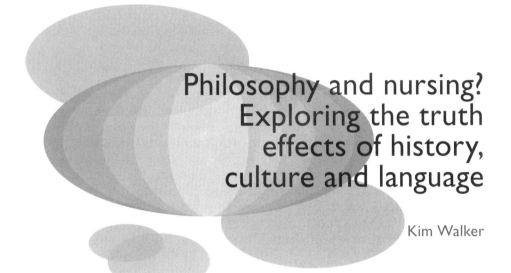

Philosophy and nursing? Exploring the truth effects of history, culture and language

Kim Walker

LEARNING OBJECTIVES

By reflecting on this chapter, readers will be able to:

- articulate the complexity of the relationships between philosophy and nursing
- identify the ways that history, culture and language have been influential in shaping nursing as a practice and scholarly discipline
- describe the major philosophical frameworks and how they inform thought and action generally, and
- appreciate how nurses might begin to engage philosophy as a way of reflecting on nursing's relation to the truth.

KEY WORDS

Philosophy, essentialism, naturalism, humanism, holism, anti-intellectualism, feminism, gender, postmodernism

[T]he things which seem most evident to us are always formed in the confluence of encounters and chances, during the course of a precarious and fragile history … they reside on a base of human practice and human history; and … since these things have been made, they can be unmade, as long as we know how it was that they were made (Foucault, cited in Kritzman 1988:37).

[W]hat is philosophy today—philosophical activity, I mean—if it is not the critical work that thought brings to bear on itself? In what does it consist, if not in the endeavour to know how and to what extent it might be possible to think differently, instead of legitimating what is already known (Foucault, 1991:13)?

PHILOSOPHY AND NURSING?

A strange combination indeed! What interest would nurses have in philosophy, which is, after all, something usually seen as the province of bespectacled professors locked away in their ivory towers? Undoubtedly though, philosophy in many guises has informed nursing from its very beginnings, but sometimes without our consent or complete understanding of the consequences. Therefore, it is for me a fascinating challenge to explore the most significant philosophical positions that have shaped—and continue to inform—our profession in order to better understand why contemporary nurses might think and act the way they do. This is the cut and thrust of this chapter: a journey *into* philosophy *out* of nursing, but simultaneously a journey *into* nursing *out* of philosophy.

My history as a nurse is tightly bound up with a life as someone who has always asked difficult questions of the world and who, consequently, has spent more years than he cares to remember struggling with seemingly countless contradictions and inconsistencies lived out between articulating philosophies of nursing and engaging in it as a practice (Walker 1993). In living through and finding ways to better understand these things, I have journeyed through diverse and often complex philosophical territories—journeys, it could be argued, that have provided me with the credentials to contribute to this text.

Therefore, in this chapter, I want to explore with you the ways many different philosophies—each with their own histories and effects—have variously enabled and disabled what passes for the 'truth' of nursing. And this is why philosophy is perhaps best thought of as 'a way of reflecting not so much on what is true and false but *on our relationship to the truth*' (Foucault, cited in Lotringer 1989:201, emphasis added). Throughout, I attempt to show how certain truths about what it is to be a nurse and 'do' nursing have been decided *for* us, but not necessarily *by* us. These truths have generally made it difficult for nursing to position itself as a serious discipline (in terms of its 'body of knowledge') and authoritative profession (in terms of nurses' capacity to make decisions on their own behalf and be recognised for their contribution to the wellbeing of humankind). But it is our *relationship* to these truths and the effects they create in the minds and actions of ourselves and others that we need most to interrogate. Let me begin this work by putting forward a couple of truths to which I subscribe.

Nursing first and foremost is a practice; it only comes to true (or material) expression in action. Moreover, nursing, as an intractably social and relational activity, is bound up in and manifests itself by way of ceaseless acts of communication and interaction with others. Language, history and culture are at the core of this activity and they are the most significant phenomena through which we construct and interpret our worlds. Philosophy is primarily a linguistic and cultural phenomenon in the sense that it is about words and ideas shared by certain people in specific circumstances. There is no other place to start thinking philosophically about nursing than nursing's origins in history, culture and language. This discussion will lead us nicely towards a more sophisticated analysis of how philosophy might be embedded in nurses' everyday talking and moving-about-in-the-world as active agents in that world's creation. With luck, it will encourage you to read more on this fascinating topic, and, if that is the case, then I have achieved more than I could hope for!

WHAT'S IN A NAME? LANGUAGE AND THE POWER TO DEFINE

We make sense of the world by differentiating objects and ideas from each other by means of the way in which something means something only because it is not something else. Moreover, the relation between an object or idea and its name is complex and multiple; that a 'nurse' is the creature we have come to know as 'nurse' is unquestionably a function of history (in this case, the history of the origins of words), culture (the interplay of people in societies of shared practices and understandings) and the politics of knowledge (how some ideas and truths come to dominate at the expense of others). Language is the slippery medium burdened with the responsibility for allowing humans to communicate through shared vocabularies—generated by our various formal and informal educations—about our lived experiences and the interpretations we ascribe to them in order to render our lives both accessible and meaningful.

If we reflect on the complexity of the linguistic structures we employ to engage with one another, it becomes easier to appreciate what a miracle effective communication really is. Most *words* have more than one form and one meaning; most *sentences* can be made sense of in a number of ways depending on syntax, grammar and context; all *stories* contain within them multiple possibilities for interpretation; and all stories are themselves framed within even more sophisticated *narrative structures* we call myth, metaphor, discourse and ideology, to mention the more common of these.

The sheer complexity of language and its expression renders the communicative act between human beings far more dense and opaque than we usually care to acknowledge, and we let language 'have its way with us' much more often than we ought to allow. In other words, we seldom stop to ask questions at a deep level about what is said and why because we normally operate only on the surface of language and its various structures and mechanisms. Not so on these pages, however! Against this brief introduction to the sophistication of language, let's move on with our journey into philosophy by taking a closer than usual look at the word 'nurse'.

If we consult the *Oxford English Dictionary* and carefully examine the various entries we discover that 'nurse' is both a noun and a verb. A noun that at the same time enacts its very meaning as a verb limits the potential for confusion, namely: a nurse nurses. Superficially, this congruence between noun and verb seems logical and constructive. At a deeper level, however, it is unhelpful in so far as it leaves no room for alternate understandings of what a nurse might be and/or do. So we are left with two terms that define themselves only in relation to themselves—a kind of linguistic bind or tautology, which, as you will come to discover, is all but bereft of philosophical and practical worth.

As a noun, 'nurse' first appeared in late Medieval England at which time (1450) its primary meaning was: 'A woman employed to suckle, and to take charge of, an infant'. It also meant 'One who takes care of, looks after, or advises another'. A little later (1526), this definition was extended slightly to incorporate: 'A person, usually a woman, who attends or waits upon the sick; now *esp.* one trained for this purpose'. Already it becomes obvious that the nurse is in no way a neutral term; it is highly charged socially, politically and emotionally.

If we examine the word as a verb, again we see the notion of a woman suckling an infant (1535), fostering, tending, cherishing (a thing) (1542), and waiting upon or attending to (a person who is ill) (1736). Finally, in 1861, the verb at last makes explicit the meaning it has today: 'to perform the duties of a sick-nurse'. This last meaning and its appearance in the English language 12 months after the establishment of the first Nightingale schools of nursing in 1860 (see Cuff & Gordon Pugh (1924:3) for more) highlights the profoundly incestuous relationship between language and reality: this is what I mean by the power to define and why history and culture are important to the politics of 'naming'. In the preface to her *Notes on Nursing*, Nightingale makes the following very telling statement:

> Every woman … has, at one time or another of her life, charge of the personal health of somebody, whether child or invalid—in other words, every woman is a nurse (Nightingale 1969:3).

As exemplified in Nightingale's definition, to be a nurse is to be a woman first. This idea reinforces both the necessity and centrality of nursing as a human caring activity that has always fallen to women. But it also seriously disables the potential for nursing to be anything but *merely* women's work (in a world that even today values men's work in every way more than women's). This is a double bind—the grip of which will likely never relent in its capacity to constrain the possibilities for nurses to exercise power in any way commensurate with, for example, medicine's capacity to do so.

THE ESSENTIAL NURSE

Embedded within the discussion above are the manifestations of a particular philosophical position, namely *essentialism*. This philosophy allows someone to claim the 'truth' that 'a man is a man down to his very thumbs, and a woman is a woman down to her little toes' (Thomson & Thomson 1911:4); or that women are 'longer lived' than men because 'their constitution has staying powers, probably wrapped up with femaleness' (Thomson & Thomson 1911:7). In other words, there is something *inherently* or essentially female about women and equally something *inherently* or essentially male about men; this is what is called an 'essence' and it is self-evident, irreducible to any other form and is permanent and incontestable. Clearly, essentialism is a very politically conservative posture and this has been significant for nursing because it has relegated nurses to an inferior position in the order of things in what is a still overtly patriarchal society in the developing and developed worlds.

Essentialism has a close cousin in another philosophical viewpoint: *biological determinism* (anatomy and physiology exclusively determine whether we are male or female; boys/men have a penis; girls/women have vaginas; function follows form). Essentialism draws on this determinism very strongly to posit an essence—or a universal, immutable and sex-specific set of qualities and behaviours—of maleness and femaleness, as I suggested above.

But essentialism is also closely related to another significant philosophical stance, both embraced by and reflected in early conceptions of nursing: *naturalism*. Consider the following remarks from the previously cited Thomson and Thomson text, *The Position of Woman: Actual and Ideal*:

> It seems consistent that men should fight, if there is fighting to be done; and that women should nurse, if there is nursing necessary. Man hunted and explored, women made the home and brought up the children ... [a] woman is *naturally* a teacher of the young, a domesticator, a gardener, and so on (Thomson & Thomson 1911:15, emphasis in the original).

Furthermore, these authors justify their remarks:

> When we say that this or that occupational differentiation is natural to women we do not simply mean it is sanctioned by convention. We mean that it is congruent with *femaleness*, that it occurs in many races and countries, and that it has stood for a long time the test of eliminative selection (Thomson & Thomson 1911:15–16, emphasis added).

Naturalism also posits a timeless and universal femaleness and maleness inherited since the origin of the species and it is simply 'God-given' in the great order of beings (reflect, for example, on the concept of 'human nature' and how much of human behaviour we rationalise by this concept without giving it another thought). Indeed, naturalism still exerts enormous influence in the ways the world of work is carved into hierarchies of who is 'naturally' better equipped to do certain types of work and who not; consider that it was only in the last couple of decades that women were able to become airline pilots because of the fear that their hormonal fluctuations might render them temporarily unable to be in command of their emotions and therefore endanger the lives of their passengers. The very idea of a woman in charge of an airplane was for a very long time anathema to the airline industry (not to mention the travelling public) and probably still is to many.

If we examine nursing education texts throughout the last century, we can see the significance of essentialism, naturalism and biological determinism in the ways nursing has been inextricably linked to the female of the species and how this has shaped the form and content of nursing education and, ultimately, what a nurse is and does (e.g. Brackman Keane 1969, Burbridge 1935, Cuff & Gordon Pugh 1924, Hansen 1958, Nixon & Wakeley 1948, Watson 1908). This reality explains why even in the early twenty-first century only about 10% of the world's nurses are men. And by now you should be better able to appreciate how—as Nietzsche (cited in Hayman 1997:38) puts it: 'Every philosophy conceals another philosophy'.

By way of advancing the analysis of how philosophies insert themselves into nursing, I draw on the work of a very significant thinker whose philosophical writing has deeply influenced my own, namely Michel Foucault (1926–84). Much of Foucault's early intellectual project was to explore how 'knowledge' (and philosophy as a form of knowledge) came to be constructed in specific forms for equally particular circumstances (e.g. the law, science, psychiatry) (Foucault 1970, 1972). In his work he analysed the various forces and structures at play in the development of the modern or civilised Western world, and advanced the still quite radical notion that truth and its effects is intimately connected to knowledge production, which in turn is bound up in the exercise of power (Foucault 1978, 1980, 1984).

These three things—knowledge, truth and power—all interact with and through language in such a way so as to produce certain disciplines (such as science and the law). These disciplines, in turn, generate an authority for themselves by enabling those subscribing to the discipline to speak of and define the disciplines' territory, address specific audiences and, in so doing, compete for supremacy of position among the various disciplines. In the process, the disciplines' disciples would have us believe that certain truths are more significant than others; indeed, how some are absolute.

This is how science as a discipline (or specific body of knowledge and practices), for example, has come to dominate our contemporary times as the most revered form of knowledge. Indeed, it is held to be the truth of all things for many communities of professionals. Nursing too has been seduced by the authority of science and has been very concerned to define itself as a science in order to augment its authority and prestige. There is also a chapter in this text dedicated to exploring this notion of nursing as a science (Ch 3), and I will not enter this debate directly (although as you read into this chapter you will discover how certain philosophies closely linked with science have influenced and expedited nursing's development as a science).

(HU)MANKIND AND ITS PHILOSOPHIES OF SELF-DEFINITION AND WORLDLY DEFINITION

Undoubtedly, given the historical epoch in which modern nursing was conceived, much of nursing's theory and philosophical development has been strongly humanist in orientation. *Humanism* is perhaps the most influential philosophy of the last 400 years because of the ways it has shaped government, religion, politics and much else besides. Humanism, in a word, posits that human beings are the sovereigns of their kingdom, which is to say, the world as we know it. Human beings are able to claim sovereignty because they, unlike any other member of the animal kingdom, are possessed of an intelligence, which provides the higher order functions such as language and the capacity for rational thought. Unequivocally, humanism posits that the human beings *are* the rational authors of their own lives because they possess a stable, coherent and self-same identity, which enables their capacity to act purposefully on the world around them to their own benefit (see Johnson 1994, Lather 1991, McLaren 1988, Rogers 1980, Weedon 1997).

Humanism is especially attractive to a profession such as nursing, which clearly has human beings and their interests, needs and wants as the main focus of, and reason for, its very existence. However, humanism is also a gendered philosophy, which again creates problems for nursing's unproblematic appropriation of it as a defining force in curriculum and practice. Reflect for a moment on the concept of 'mankind': why is it that the term for the collective of men and women, of humanity, is gendered male? Why wasn't humanity collectively called 'womankind', for example. Consider how strange to the ear it sounds, and also how unusual it is that 'mankind' sounds so seemingly natural. (Wouldn't 'humankind' be so much more appropriate?) As Irigaray reminds us:

> Man seems to have wanted, directly or indirectly, to give the universe his own gender as he wanted to give his own name to his children, his wife, his possessions. This has significant bearing on the sexes' relationships to the world, to things, to objects.

In fact, anything believed to have value belongs to men and is marked by their gender. Apart from possessions in the strict sense that man attributes to himself, he gives his own gender to God [le Dieu], to the sun [le soleil], and also, in the guise of the neuter, to the laws of the cosmos and of the social or individual order. He doesn't even question the genealogy of his attribution (Irigaray 1993:31–32).

Nursing then, as a female gendered profession, has always to contend with the ever-present reality of patriarchy: a world created by men, for men and to whom women are sometimes and only vaguely equal but, mostly, are not. Note too that even in the liberal feminist position, which puts woman as man's equal, the norm to which the female gender has to aspire is still the male version! Humanism is therefore best understood as a philosophy in the service of patriarchy, and to illustrate just how influential humanism has been in nursing let me cite from a couple of the numerous American scholars who led the development of nursing theories from the 1950s through to the late 1980s (a period when humanist thought was especially influential in a number of other disciplines, including psychology, education and organisational theory). As you will see, these nurse scholars share an abiding commitment to situating the unique, individual human being at the heart of their theories around which invariably wind the core concepts of environment, health and nursing.

For Imogene King (1981, 1987) and her interpersonal/systems interaction model of nursing, humans are 'open systems interacting with environment' (King 1981:10) and are viewed as 'rational, sentient, reacting, social, controlling, purposeful, time-oriented, and action-oriented' beings (King 1987:107). Calista Roy takes a similar line in her work when she asserts that the individual 'shares in creative power; behaves purposefully, not in a sequence of cause and effect; possesses intrinsic holism; and strives to maintain integrity and realise the need for relationships' (Barone & Roy 1996:66). Moreover, the individual in society is best understood in the context of the 'purposefulness of human existence; unity of purpose of humankind; activity and creativity for the common good; and value and meaning of life' (Roy & Andrews 1999:83).

Clearly, the autonomous, self-defining human being is accorded primacy in these statements, which exemplify the logic of humanism and its emphasis on the significance of human relationships, sentience and rationality, and the forward-thrust of human life. And as you have just read, another important philosophical position is given voice in these theorists' work: *holism* or the idea that the whole is greater than the sum of its parts. The idea of the 'whole' or complete human being is another important facet of the philosophy of humanism, and the philosophy and language of holism currently dominates the rhetoric of healthcare policy and practice. Holism is particularly appealing for a human-centred service because it allows practitioners to imagine they are taking into account every aspect of their clients' needs and wants. Holism defines the human as a 'bio–psycho–social–spiritual being'. You will already have come across this language I'm sure.

Holism is the philosophical opposite of *reductionism*: the idea that every whole can be broken up into its constituent parts. Medicine, for example, is essentially a reductionist science in that the human mind–body complex is reduced to ever-smaller components, as medical knowledge seeks to understand the total or whole organism by breaking it into its various organ systems and structures, examining their tissues and cells, and eventually looking at the cells and their components at the microscopic level. Modern medicine has made reductionism into a highly sophisticated science from which the various medical specialties and subspecialties arise—for example, neurology (the study of the nervous system) or neuroendocrinology (the study of the hormones of the nervous system).

Medicine—as a science—is essentially founded on the philosophy of *empiricism*, or the notion that the only true knowledge is derived from the strict application of experimental method. Empiricism encourages reductionism in the way it insists on increasingly rigorous examination of cause-and-effect relationships at ever-finer levels of discrimination. Hence, we have the appearance of disciplines such as microbiology (the study of pathological organisms) and microphysics (the study of atomic particles). These disciplines strongly influence the development of nursing as a science and without them it would undoubtedly look more like an art or craft than the highly technologically driven and biomedically oriented profession it is today.

Nursing has become ever-more reductionist throughout the twentieth century, as it too has been obliged to follow medicine down this philosophical and practical path; the trouble is that reductionism inherently devalues the total organism. Reductionism sits very awkwardly with nursing's need to be seen to be caring for a whole human being. So we live with a considerable tension in nursing—preaching one philosophy (holism), while mostly practising its absolute antithesis (reductionism). This paradox has come about largely through the influence of another significant philosophical position: *Cartesianism*.

Rene Descartes was an Enlightenment philosopher (1596–1650) deeply committed to the project of harnessing scientific thought and method in order to better understand and intervene in the world. He coined the now famous phrase: *I think, therefore I am*. This maxim became the founding principle of what it is to be a modern human being and further endorsed humanism as the defining philosophy for society's men and women.

Cartesianism was forged on the anvil of another important philosophical doctrine dominant early in the 'Age of Enlightenment': *rationalism*, the notion that the only way to truth is through the deliberations of the rational human mind. Rationalism is the opposite of empiricism (which privileges the apprehension of data through the senses (of seeing, hearing, and so on) rather than relying on the operations of the mind alone; the debate between empiricists and rationalists about which is the surer way to the 'truth' is never-ending). Descartes' key insight was that the only thing he could not doubt as a rational thinking creature was the fact that his thinking *proved* his existence as a sentient (feeling) human being. He could be sure of his capacity to reason, but he could not be sure of what his senses (via his body) told him; consequently, he regarded the body 'as a source of interference in, and a danger to, the operation of reason' (Grosz 1994:5). This led him to assert that the 'mind and body are distinct entities. In his view, the mind exists in time only, whereas the body, unlike the mind, is physical and has extension in space' (Benner & Wrubel 1989:33).

This idea that the thinking mind is completely separate from a non-thinking body (Cartesianism or its other frequently cited name, dualism) is responsible for the way modern medicine and healthcare still tend to treat problems of the mind with one science (psychology/psychiatry) and problems of the body with another (medicine/surgery). In contemporary healthcare we even go so far as to treat people with problems of the mind in one institution (the psychiatric hospital/clinic) and problems of the body in another (the general/acute hospital).

Descartes' then-radical ideas also spawned a related philosophy: *mechanism*. Descartes thought the world and human beings could be analysed and their problems and illnesses diagnosed by understanding the world and body as a machine (the clock to be precise). Just as the clock has a variety of interconnected parts, each of which needs to be delicately attuned to the others in order for the clock to function smoothly, so too, the world and human beings could be understood. When something fails or doesn't work properly, it is merely a matter of locating the malfunction and putting it right. Modern surgery certainly makes sense of the human body in this way. So too, it can be argued, does nursing, given that philosophical frameworks for clinical practice are themselves predicated on strongly medical models of health and illness, which are, in turn, reductionist, mechanistic and, ultimately, Cartesian.

For a compelling example of how Cartesianism, reductionism and mechanism influence the everyday practice of nursing, I suggest you read Fassett and Gallagher's (1998) fascinating tale *Just a Head: Stories in a Body*. This text brings to vivid expression the issues discussed above, and is a salutary reminder of the perils these philosophies inflict on real-life human actors and those charged with their care.

By now I expect you are a little perplexed by all these 'isms' and the incredible interconnectedness of them all. Without doubt, this is why the study of philosophy is not only strenuous, but also profoundly rewarding (intellectually speaking). As humankind has sought ever-more sophisticated frameworks for making sense of themselves and their worlds, scholars have begun to appreciate how no one truth about those worlds is capable of defining them without the support of many others.

Of course, certain truths (as I hope you are beginning to realise) capture people's imaginations and win their hearts more than others. This depends entirely on how, where and when one is positioned in the world. Living in Enlightenment Europe (from the early sixteenth to the late eighteenth centuries) would have been a very exhilarating experience because this is when much of the science and technology we presently enjoy, as well as the philosophical material I have been discussing, came into being. It has only been in the last century that serious critiques and challenges to many of the 'philosophies' espoused over these pages—to the 'received truths' they have generated—began to appear. These received truths became influential simply with the passing of time, the force of continued use and in the absence of better alternatives; indeed, together they form a powerful set of theoretical traditions that have been very resistant to critique. In what follows, however, I will undertake exactly such a critique as we edge our way towards the close of this chapter.

THE TYRANNY OF 'ISMS': POSTMODERN PHILOSOPHY AS LIBERATOR

I want now to make clear the philosophical ideas that have informed my writing and, in doing so, will return us to the place from which we began. For as must by now be fairly obvious to you, there is a sort of circuitous and mutually reinforcing logic operating between all these different but related philosophical positions. You will recall I mentioned early in the chapter how nursing hasn't always been aware of how philosophy inserts itself into our everyday thinking and behaving, and this is partly the reason why. The philosophies I have been unpacking here are experienced only subliminally by most of us in the sense that we have assimilated them into our ways of thinking to the point where we really cannot think at all without their influence.

Postmodern philosophy, however, provides us with a rather neat reality check in respect of this problem. I have found it enormously useful as I have grappled with how I (and others) have come to be the nurses we are, and why. In bringing to a close this admittedly superficial and rather attenuated discussion on nursing and the politics of truth, I would like to suggest a way forward for nursing's relationship to philosophy, which has been rather fraught with a certain ambivalence, if not hostility. The gender issue that has surfaced repeatedly in this reading of nursing and its relationship to philosophy is at the root of my concerns. So let me explain. Elizabeth Grosz, an Australian feminist scholar, reminds us:

> As a discipline, philosophy has surreptitiously excluded femininity, and ultimately women, from its practices through its usually implicit coding of femininity with the unreason associated with the body (Grosz 1994:4).

Tracing the influence of particular philosophies on nursing as we have here, it might have struck you that there is a peculiar logic at play within and/or between them. Either the philosophy is inflexible because its truth claims rest on the basis of its (seeming) self-evidence (essentialism, naturalism, biological determinism) or a philosophy is wedded to a particular thinker's ideas (Cartesianism, dualism and mechanism). Conversely, the philosophy may be the product of a chronologically sequential line of thinkers over an extended period that mutually reinforces the veracity of its propositions over this time and thereby cements its worth in the collective psyche of humanity (empiricism, rationalism, science). Or, differently again, one philosophical viewpoint might sit uncomfortably in relation with, and often be all but cancelled out by, its opposites (holism versus reductionism; empiricism versus rationalism).

Postmodern philosophy is a creature born of these tensions to which I have just given voice. Postmodernism (yes, another 'ism') attempts to understand how these tensions arise and what effects they invoke. Postmodernism is not one philosophy, but a hybrid of many, and its value lies in its insistence that Truth (as absolute and unimpeachable) is a necessary figment of the philosophical imagination that is now rather bankrupt in the sense that clearly—and as this text illustrates—*multiple* truths abound—not all of which are useful, some of which are plainly dangerous, but also many of which can be decidedly illuminating of the human condition and help advance its development.

Postmodernism has received plenty of flak ever since it first appeared on the cultural landscape in the early 1960s. Its antagonists argue that it is philosophically and politically corrupt because it disallows any single claim to the truth in favour of all truths being relative to each other and therefore disputable and fragile. This *relativism* is said to be exceedingly unhelpful because it does not help people adjudicate between competing claims to the truth and therefore disenfranchises them in many ways. I agree postmodernism in its extreme relativistic forms is problematic for these reasons, but this is not the version to which I subscribe. Some truths are more helpful than others and we need to be able to figure out how to differentiate between them and make decisions on the basis of our analyses. It has been the work of this chapter to show how certain philosophical positions have produced a set of truths about what nursing is and what it is to be a nurse. Others, too, have been busy this last decade or so exploring nursing from postmodern positions, and shedding light on complex and fascinating issues and concerns hitherto unthought (e.g. Anderson 2004, Brennan 1998, Latimer 1998, Parker 2004, Parker & Gibbs 1998, Pryce 2004, Whittaker 1998).

Postmodern philosophy, then, is best thought of as a radical questioning of all that has passed in the name of philosophy. Such questioning temporarily decentres the authority of previous philosophies and, in doing so, opens the way for new and hopefully more constructive ways of reflecting on our relationship to the (many) truths that shape our everyday worlds (Caputo 1997, Elam 1994). Why does Grosz voice her concern above in relation to philosophy's exclusion of femininity and women from its development and ongoing construction? Once again, the answer lies in the problem of gender.

Postmodern philosophers have uncovered a powerful effect of knowledge production they call 'binary logic' or 'dichotomous thinking'. As Grosz tells us:

> ... feminists and philosophers seem to share a common view of the human subject as a being made up of two dichotomously opposed characteristics: mind and body, thought and extension, reason and passion, psychology and biology (Grosz 1994:3).

You will now be familiar with how this logic manifests in some of the philosophies we have been discussing on these pages. As Grosz continues to explain, this

> ... bifurcation of being is not simply a neutral division of an otherwise all-encompassing descriptive field. Dichotomous thinking necessarily hierarchies and ranks the two polarised terms so that one becomes the privileged term and the other its suppressed, subordinated, negative counterpart ... [b]ody is thus what is not mind, what is distinct from and other than the privileged term (Grosz 1994:3).

It is equally significant that this mind/body opposition is linked to a whole series of related oppositions which, by association, can function in place of the mind/body pairing. For example, as Grosz puts it:

> [T]he mind/body relation is frequently correlated with the distinctions between: Reason and passion, sense and sensibility, inside and outside, self and other, depth and surface, reality and appearance, mechanism and vitalism ... temporality and spatiality, psychology and physiology, form and matter, and so on (Grosz 1994:3).

What is absolutely crucial to this hierarchy of opposing terms is that the first term (e.g. mind) is assigned the male gender—and, as Irigaray reminded us earlier (1993), man, in his sheer arrogance, has assigned his name to everything of value. Consequently, the second, subordinated term in the logic of binaries is relegated the female gender. This is how the great gender divide actually works: not only is it merely a reflection of the inequality of the species in terms of who gets to do what in the world (as my earlier discussion emphasised), it actually produces this inequality because it is deeply reinforced at the level of language. Indeed, language subtly authorises so much of what we do without our ever realising it, and this is why I have insisted on the uncontestable centrality of language as not just reflecting the world so we can give it meaning, but, rather, that it brings the world into view in highly particular ways.

Thus the female of the species is associated with the human body, whereas the male claims the human mind; similarly, reason is linked with the mind and with men, passion with women and the body. Intellectual work is therefore most properly men's work, whereas caring (which is intimately associated with the body) is consigned to women. And these distinctions are non-negotiable and irreversible. This is why

Grosz (1994) can claim that philosophy has largely neglected to include women in its development because it simply never entered men's minds to do so. Women, men have argued, are much less well-suited to engage in intellectual work, but are naturally, essentially and biologically best suited to nurture, suckle, care for and assist others in the care of their bodies. And so we are returned to our definitions of nursing and to Nightingale's injunction that to be a nurse is first to be a woman!

TOWARDS A FEMINIST POSTMODERN PHILOSOPHY FOR NURSES

Ironically, nursing and *feminism* have never been happy companions. This is partly because, as 'naturally' women's work, feminists have been rather disinclined towards the study of nursing, seeing little point in making so obviously female gendered an occupation the object of their philosophical gaze (which of course merely reflects and endorses the largely misogynist leanings of masculinist philosophy and its history). Nurses, too, have generally been reluctant to embrace feminism because it exposes the inequities and tensions conjured up in the very idea that nursing is naturally women's work. To be sure, many, if not most, nurses have wanted to believe the truth that nursing is all but exclusively women's work because it has matched their (largely uncritical) version of what it means to be a woman in the first place. That said, feminism and postmodern philosophy can and must be considered as an ally for nurses and nursing. This is because feminism squarely places women on the philosophical and political agenda and lets nothing escape its scrutiny as it pursues ever-more cogent truths about what it means to be a woman.

Postmodernism, in step with feminism, seeks to unsettle the hard-baked certainties of previous philosophical positions by pointing out the often shaky and untenable foundations on which they rest. Therefore, combining feminism and postmodernism seems a sensible way to proceed if nursing and philosophy are to have a more meaningful relationship and if nurses are to better understand and critique the repressive and less enabling philosophies that have previously kept us in our places (namely, doctors' 'handmaidens' and patients' 'angels of mercy'). However, this journey to another philosophical home for nursing is not likely to be easy.

Perhaps the most significant obstacle we have in this endeavour is the deep and perennial anti-intellectualism nursing's history and culture has produced (Walker 1997). This anti-intellectualism is born of the same binary thinking explored above. If a nurse's very raison d'être is wound around her (essentially/naturally/biologically determined) feminine capacity to care for and nurture others, and that caring/nurturing work is closely related to people's bodies while it also requires the fairly heavy investment and cooperation of nurses' own bodies (nursing being generally hard physical labour), then you can appreciate how purely intellectual work (i.e. philosophy) is not likely to receive much attention let alone a high priority in nursing. Undoubtedly, it is difficult to know quite how to inspire nurses to even 'think philosophically' let alone engage in the task of producing philosophical writings, and perhaps this is not what is at issue anyway.

As Silverman (1994:233) tells us, 'philosophy begins in wonder for it has to have something to wonder about'. A place to begin such a project of 'wondering' in nursing is to ask how and why nursing has been restricted by definitions—not all of them written by nurses—about who or what a nurse is (and can be) and what she or he does (or could do). The work of this chapter has been to start this process of asking questions about our identity and the powerful and largely intangible influences that have come to shape our sense of what it means to be a nurse. As you might now be more aware, in many ways nurses have not been the rational authors of their lives the philosophers, such as Descartes, would have us believe, because the script for life as a nurse was 'always already' written for us by others (who certainly were not always nurses).

As nurses and nursing engage with the vicissitudes of life in the twenty-first century and with the legacy of our history now more explicit and available to all, perhaps we can begin to imagine a relationship with philosophy that enables us to re-vision and re-fashion ourselves in ways that truly reflect the contribution our knowledge, skills and actions have on those in our care. While I have brushed over the whole issue of 'caring' as a philosophy for nursing (and there is another chapter in this text devoted to this idea (Ch 6)), there can be no doubt in my mind at least that a feminist and postmodern philosophy of caring holds considerable promise for nursing in terms of providing guidance and intellectual nourishment to the profession. As I said in the closing words to my chapter in the first and second editions of *Contexts of Nursing*, and which are certainly no less relevant now:

> The most appropriate philosophical discourse for nursing is one that is demonstrably feminist in that it places gender firmly on the agenda; [it must also be] overtly critical in that it asks difficult questions about all those concerns with which nursing has been struggling for so long. But it must do this within a context that helps us devise strategies for change at the level of *practice*. Indeed, the relationship between nursing and philosophy must begin with the practice of nursing and end there. Why else, if nursing is 'in the "truth" of things', a practice discipline, would we bother (Walker 2000:64)?

REFLECTIVE QUESTIONS

1 How and why are the times in which nurses find themselves influenced by the history of philosophy?

2 Why is our thinking and acting not always apparent to us and sometimes even in conflict?

3 How can we challenge the received wisdoms through which we live, in order to live differently, if not better, than perhaps we do?

RECOMMENDED READINGS

Caputo JD (ed.) 1997 Deconstruction in a nutshell: a conversation with Jacques Derrida. Fordham University Press, New York

Elam D 1994 Feminism and deconstruction: Ms. en abyme. Routledge, London

Foucault M 1980 Power/knowledge: selected interviews and other writing 1972–1977. Gordon C (ed.) Pantheon, New York

Foucault M 1984 The Foucault reader. Rabinow P (ed.) Pantheon, New York

Johnson P 1994 Feminism as radical humanism. Allen & Unwin, Sydney

REFERENCES

Anderson M 2004 Lesson from a postcolonial-feminist perspective: suffering and the path to healing. Nursing Inquiry 11(4):238–246

Barone SH, Roy C 1996 The Roy adaptation model in research: rehabilitation nursing. In: Walker PH, Neuman B (eds) Blueprint for use of nursing models: education, research, practice, and administration. National League for Nursing, New York, pp 64–75

Benner P, Wrubel J 1989 The primacy of caring: stress and coping in health and illness. Addison Wesley, Menlo Park, California

Brackman Keane C 1969 Essentials of nursing: a medical-surgical text for practical nurses. WB Saunders, Philadelphia

Brennan S 1998 Nursing and motherhood constructions: implications for practice. Nursing Inquiry 5(1):11–17

Burbridge GN 1935 Lecture for nurses. Infectious Diseases Hospital, Melbourne

Caputo JD (ed.) 1997 Deconstruction in a nutshell: a conversation with Jacques Derrida. Fordham University Press, New York

Cuff HE, Gordon Pugh WT 1924 Practical nursing including hygiene and dietetics. William Blackwood, Edinburgh

Elam D 1994 Feminism and deconstruction: Ms. en abyme. Routledge, London

Fassett D, Gallagher MR 1998 Just a head: stories in a body. Allen & Unwin, Sydney

Foucault M 1970 The order of things: an archaeology of the human sciences. Tavistock Publications, London

Foucault M 1972 The archaeology of knowledge. Tavistock Publications, London

Foucault M 1978 The history of sexuality, volume one. Pantheon, New York

Foucault M 1980 Power/knowledge: selected interviews and other writing 1972–1977. Gordon C (ed.) Pantheon, New York

Foucault M 1984 The Foucault reader. Rabinow P (ed.) Pantheon, New York

Foucault M 1991 Notes on Marx: conversations with Duccio Trombadori. Goldstein RJ, Cascaito J (trans.). Semiotext(e), New York

Grosz E 1994 Volatile bodies: toward a corporeal feminism. Allen & Unwin, Sydney

Hansen HF 1958 Study guide: a review of practice nursing. WB Saunders, Philadelphia

Hayman R 1997 Nietzsche: Nietzsche's voices, Phoenix, London

Irigaray L 1993 Je, tu, nous: toward a culture of difference. Routledge, New York

Johnson P 1994 Feminism as radical humanism. Allen & Unwin, Sydney

King I 1981 A theory for nursing: systems, concepts, process. Wiley, New York

King I 1987 King's theory of goal attainment. In: Parse RR (ed.) Nursing sciences: major paradigms, theories and critiques. WB Saunders, Philadelphia, pp 107–13

Kritzman LD 1988 Politics philosophy culture: interviews and other writings 1977–1984. Routledge, New York

Lather P 1991 Getting smart: feminist research and pedagogy with/in the postmodern. Routledge, London

Latimer J 1998 Organising context: nurses' assessments of older people in an acute medical unit. Nursing Inquiry 5(1):43–57

Lotringer S 1989 Foucault live (interviews, 1966–84). Semiotext(e), New York

McLaren P 1988 Schooling the postmodern body: critical pedagogy and the politics of enfleshment. Journal of Education 170(3):53–83

Nightingale F 1969 Notes on nursing: in what it is, and what it is not. Dover Publications, New York

Nixon JA, Wakeley C 1948 Text-book for nurses: anatomy, physiology, surgery and medicine. Oxford University Press, London

Parker J 2004 Nursing on the medical ward. Nursing Inquiry 11(4):210–217

Parker J, Gibbs M 1998 Truth, virtue and beauty: midwifery and philosophy. Nursing Inquiry 5(3):146–153

Pryce A 2004 'Only odd people wore suede shoes': careers and sexual identities of men attending a sexual health clinic. Nursing Inquiry 11(4):258–270

Rogers C 1980 A way of being. Houghton Miflin, Boston

Roy C, Andrews HA 1999 The Roy adaptation model, 2nd edn. Appleton & Lange, Stamford

Silverman HJ 1994 Textualities: between hermeneutics and deconstruction. Routledge, New York

Thomson JA, Thomson M 1911 The position of woman: bibliogically considered. In: Cuff HE, Gordon Pugh WT (eds) The position of woman: actual and ideal. William Blackwood, Edinburgh, pp 1–28

Walker K 1993 On what it might mean to be a nurse: a discursive ethnography. Unpublished doctoral dissertation. La Trobe University, Melbourne

Walker K 1997 Dangerous liaisons: thinking, doing, nursing. The Collegian 4(2):4–14

Walker K 2000 Why philosophy? Nursing and the problem of truth. In: Daly J, Speedy S, Jackson D (eds) Contexts of nursing: an introduction. MacLennan & Petty, Sydney

Watson JK 1908 A handbook for nurses. Scientific Press, London

Weedon C 1997 Feminist practice and poststructuralist theory. Basil Blackwell, Oxford

Whittaker R 1998 Re-framing the representation of women in advertisements for hormone replacement therapy. Nursing Inquiry 5(2):77–86

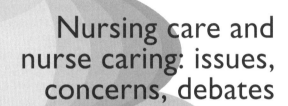

CHAPTER 6

Nursing care and nurse caring: issues, concerns, debates

Debra Jackson and Sally Borbasi

LEARNING OBJECTIVES

This chapter will:

- introduce caring as a professional concept that is entwined with understandings about nurses and nursing
- explore caring as a theoretical concept
- discuss perceptions of nurse caring from the perspective of patients/clients
- provide an overview of issues related to care and cure
- critique caring as the basis of the discipline of nursing, and
- contemplate threats to nurse caring.

KEY WORDS

Caring, clinical nursing, cure, work, patients/clients

NURSING AND CARING

The concept of caring is intertwined with nursing—some literature even states that caring and nursing are synonymous (Hayes & Tyler-Ball 2007, Wilkin & Slevin 2004)—and has been identified as central to the theory and practice of nurses. For many years, nurse theorists have developed theories of nursing in which caring is positioned as a major foundational element (Leininger 1984, 1986, Watson 1985, Watson et al 2005). Efforts to theorise caring, and understand it as a concept that is able to be compatible with, and integral to, the practice of nursing, have occupied a lot of energy in nursing for a number of years, and continue to attract the attention of nurse scholars from all over the world (e.g. Finfgeld-Connett 2008, Sumner 2008). The close relationship of nursing and caring is able to be seen in the many definitions and perspectives of nursing that position caring as inherent and central to the nursing role (e.g. Benner 1984, Leininger 1984, Sumner 2008, Swanson 1993, Watson 1988, Watson et al 2005).

Initially, the concept of caring may appear to be simple and uncomplicated, and indeed, general dictionary definitions of caring define it in simple terms. It is a generic word and one that is widely used in the general lexicon—meaning that it is not 'owned' specifically by nursing and nor does it apply only to nurses and nursing. However, when used in relation to nursing, the concept of care cannot be oversimplified. Terms such as *nursing care* and *nurse caring* carry certain meanings and understandings. In these contexts, care is a complex, multidimensional concept that is positioned as the characteristic that distinguishes nursing, and sets it apart from other health-related activities (Jackson & Borbasi 2000). Although a caring perspective is not unique to nursing, it is widely accepted that nursing has an essential role to care for the health of individuals, families and communities, and many believe the care given by nurses has the potential to restore health (Benner et al 1999, Watson & Foster 2003).

In this chapter we introduce caring as a professional concept, and acquaint you with some of the major arguments and viewpoints associated with caring in general and nurse caring in particular. In writing this chapter we have drawn on a substantial body of international literature that reflects some of the major perspectives of nurse caring that have been published over the past 20–30 years. It is necessary to cover literature over this long period in order to develop an appreciation of the longitudinal and international nature of the debates and discussions around caring. Furthermore, you will see that many of the issues remain unresolved, and that this is one debate that will continue into (and likely even beyond) your own nursing careers.

CARING AS A THEORETICAL CONCEPT

The complexity around such a seemingly uncomplicated and simple concept such as caring can be seen when one considers the plethora of literature devoted to it. Even a cursory database search on caring will generate copious literature on the subject. Try it! Upon examining this literature you will also see that this is a discussion that has spanned generations of scholars and that each generation builds on the work of previous scholars. You will also see it reveals a multitude of definitions, and various positions on the ways that caring can be conceptualised. Several theories of nursing have been developed from the standpoint of defining and describing caring practices. Leininger (1986) believes caring is the essence of nursing, but dismisses the idea of nurses' care motivated by a sense of duty. Rather, she considers caring as learned because it is an integral part of cultural life. However, factors within various cultures (e.g. gender) may either curtail or facilitate the use of care knowledge by nurses.

Watson (1988), another well-known luminary on the subject, writes of a science (and practice) of caring, and conceptualises caring as the ethical and moral ideal of nursing. In 1990, Rawnsley noted that caring:

> … has been proposed to be a philosophy and science, an ethic, an interactive set of client expectations and nursing behaviours, expert nursing practice, the hidden work of nursing and a synonym for nursing itself (Rawnsley 1990:42).

If we look at feminist and nurse Falk Rafael's (1996:3–17) work, she suggested caring could be considered either 'ordered caring', 'assimilated caring' or 'empowered caring' (p 4). Ordered caring she proposed as problematic for nurses because it is about merely following orders; 'it allows only a severely limited scope of caring, one that is devoid of knowledge, power or ethics' (Falk Rafael 1996:11). To illustrate this point, she draws on the example of the kindness and gentleness shown by nurses towards psychiatric patients as they were led towards the Nazi gas chambers. Assimilated caring was described as a form of caring in which the feminine construct of caring is grounded in (male) scientific discourses. This appropriation of a male construct is proposed as giving legitimacy to the essentially female activity of caring. Falk Rafael positioned empowered caring as the most desirable and effective form of caring. This form of caring, she asserted, was grounded within a feminist perspective, and involves the use of power, knowledge and ethics. Falk Rafael (1996) proposes the acronym of CARE (credentials, association, research, expertise) to encapsulate the elements of this empowered caring.

REFLECTION

Do you think the work that Falk Rafael published in 1996 about caring is still relevant today?

Another theorist you may have found through your literature searching proposed holistic caring as a form of nurse caring (Williams 1997). Williams regards this as a global concept with four dimensions that she names physical caring, interpretive caring, spiritual caring and sensitive caring. No doubt known to you, holism is a concept crucial to the effective practice of nursing, and is a term used to describe the nurse's belief that a 'patient is a person with social, physical, mental, and spiritual components' (Williams 1997:61–62). Holism is positioned as central to notions of professional caring, and is so intrinsic to this, it is often taken for granted—viewed as a 'given', and therefore often not described or examined in discussions on professional caring. The use of a holistic perspective is said to facilitate an ethos that recognises the uniqueness and value inherent in individuals, and allows for the provision of individualised nursing care. More recently, a theory of 'nursing as caring' has been offered by Boykin and Schoenhofer (2001) who consider human beings as a species to be innately caring, and that reaching one's full potential in terms of caring is a lifelong process.

Through the literature, there is general agreement about the difficulties associated with defining and positioning caring (Bassett 2002, Paley 2001, Sumner 2008). What is more, it has even been suggested that the task of rescuing the concept of caring from its elusivity is impossible, a situation Paley (2001) attributes to problematic suppositions about the nature of knowledge. Nevertheless, even accounting for the difficulties associated with defining caring, the importance of exploring how nurses have theorised and attempted to understand the elusive nature of a concept so central to their practice cannot be underestimated.

Let's look at more of the literature. Many nurses consider caring as being primarily a relationship between nurse and others in which experiences are shared. Consider Pearson (1991:199), for example; he describes the broad, global human concept of caring as 'investing oneself in the experience of another sufficiently enough to become a participant in that person's experience'. Sullivan and Deane (1994) assert that nurse caring prizes human relationships, and is informed by principles of sharing, sincerity, concern and moderation. Wolf et al (1994:107) propose that nurse caring has several tangible dimensions, including 'respectful deference to others, assurance of human presence, positive connectedness, professional knowledge and skill, and attentiveness to the other's experience'.

In addition, caring is understood to have intellectual as well as emotional aspects (Kapborg & Bertero 2003), and in 1992 Pepin suggested two dimensions of caring: love and labour. Love is said to consist of affective (i.e. pertaining to feelings) concepts such as altruism, compassion, emotion, presence, connectedness, nurturance and comfort, and it is this aspect of caring that has dominated the nursing literature (Pepin 1992). Labour refers to the element of care related to toil and service, and encompasses roles, functions, knowledge and tasks. Though Pepin (1992) suggested that this latter dimension of caring has received much less attention in the nursing literature, a number of these issues are discussed in some depth in nursing discourses on topics such as competency and clinical expertise (e.g. Hardy et al 2002). When considering the concepts of emotion and labour it would be remiss not to mention the concept of 'emotional labour'. This term emanated from sociology and pertains to workers who are required to display emotions that are in keeping with organisational requirements, rather than how the person—the individual nurse—truly feels (Mann & Cowburn 2005, Staden 1998). Research has shown this to be an under-appreciated and stressful aspect of nurses' caring work (Henderson 2001, Mann & Cowburn 2005).

REFLECTION

Do you think these theories are relevant in today's world? If yes, why? If no, why not?

EXPERIENCING NURSE CARING: WHAT DO PATIENTS SAY?

Upholding the theory that caring is a concept central to the practice of nurses is not only important for the profession, but is also highly significant for the recipients of that care. It makes sense that if nurses are to claim they are caring professionals, they are obliged to find out what nurse caring means to patients, and how nurses can demonstrate care for patients. Somewhat ironically it has been the more recent rise of quality improvement processes that has spearheaded the interest in patients' views about the care they receive in healthcare settings, and this movement has not been led by nurses, but economists. Another determinant of mounting interest in patients' satisfaction with care is the fact that patients are no longer ill informed, passive recipients of health services, but increasingly informed and active consumers who expect a certain standard of care and are not afraid to litigate should their expectations not be met.

REFLECTION

- Have you ever been a recipient of a health service?
- What approach/es do you take if the 'care' you receive falls short of your expectations?
- What are your expectations of 'care'?
- Are you able to articulate them?
- If you *have* experienced being a patient, would you say that your perceptions of what constitutes caring were different from those you hold when you practise as a nurse or nursing student?

If we continue our literature searching, it can be seen that patients' views of professional caring may be very different from those proposed by nurses. Nurses often (but not always) embrace psychosocial models of caring, while studies of patients often (but not always) suggest that patients value caring that is more technical or task-orientated in nature. For example, one study exploring the caring behaviours of hospital nurses from patients' perspectives found physical caring behaviours such as 'monitoring' were ranked much higher than aspects of caring such as 'trusting relationships', which could be considered to be affective or psychosocial in nature (Greenhalgh et al 1998; similarly Webb 1996). Indeed in 1996, Webb cautioned nurses against placing too much emphasis on the psychological elements of care, at the expense of physical or technical aspects of care. In light of burgeoning technological intervention, this advice appears sound. Yet, the difference in perceptions of caring between nurses and patients warrants consideration.

In Western industrialised societies, technological skills and expertise are viewed as high status, and the domain of 'professionals'. In times of vulnerability, such as when people are ill, people like to feel assured they are in the care of competent health professionals, and perhaps view technological proficiency as evidence of such competence and expertise. The interpersonal aspects of caring so highly idealised by nurses may be viewed by patients as 'non-professional' caring—the type of caring available to them within their own social worlds, and not something they necessarily seek within a context of professional caring.

Other factors may also play a part in how patients experience or view nurse caring. For example, a Norwegian study demonstrated a gender-related difference in satisfaction with the quality of nursing care between young female patients when compared to young male patients (Foss 2002). In this study, the young female patients perceived nurses to be less committed and caring, to have less time and to be less skilled than did the male patients.

Similarly, a Jordanian study (Ahmad & Alasad 2004) that surveyed patients for their opinions of nursing care discovered that male patients tended to have a more positive experience of nursing care than their female counterparts. The most important predictors for satisfaction with care in Ahmad and Alasad's study, however, related to the nurse's ability to meet the patient's information needs, the amount of information provided and the time nurses spent with patients. Demonstrating respect and courtesy towards family and friends was considered another major predictor. Patients appreciated those nurses who 'told them what to expect in the next shift, took interest in them as persons, provided them with privacy and perceived them as friends'. The authors concluded that the best aspects of nursing care are a 'happy atmosphere, patients' privacy and individualised care' (Ahmad & Alasad 2004:239).

REFLECTION

• What are your views on the findings by Ahmad and Alasad (2004)?

• Would you tend to agree/disagree with them?

In Sweden a study was conducted into patient satisfaction with nursing care at night (Oleni et al 2004). A number of nurses and patients were surveyed for their opinions. The study found a significant difference between nurses' and patients' assessments of patient care requirements in terms of nursing intervention. The nurses' assessments of nursing care were more positive than patients' perceptions. Patients scored lower for the concepts of information and participation, observation and monitoring, and night rest. Again this study demonstrated the importance patients attach to nurses providing them with appropriate and adequate information in order to better place the patient to influence and take responsibility for the care they receive. Patients were less positive about nursing observation and monitoring, and almost a quarter of them were dissatisfied with their ability to rest at night.

If we look at the findings from a review of predominantly quantitative observational studies related to patient satisfaction with the care provided by nurses, patient satisfaction was revealed as contingent on a number of factors (Johansson et al 2002). These included technological competence, as well as being responsive, kind, attentive, calm and encouraging. Insufficient information was shown to be 'perhaps the most common cause of dissatisfaction' (Johansson et al 2002).

Even as we write this chapter the world of healthcare is changing and the way patient care is organised and delivered is undergoing constant reformation. Because it is a commodity limited in resources yet high in demand, the healthcare arena and all who service it are under duress to do more with less. Nurses everywhere are experiencing heavy workloads, long hours and increasingly complex professional demands. This is not a context conducive to the provision of personalised care and considered information giving.

Yet in the world of healthcare today it would appear the pendulum is returning to nursing interventions based on feeling as being more important for patient satisfaction than medical–technical interventions (Johansson et al 2002). As a recent study of patient experience revealed, it is the ability of nurses being able to show that the patient is an important person and that nurses really *care about* them that epitomises the best nurse caring behaviours (Mok & Pui Chi Chiu 2004:482).

Caring behaviour considered paramount to patient and family includes the creation of a natural and constructive relationship between nurse and patient—indeed, the capacity to 'feel kinship' with the patient is attributed to the best nurses and the value of physical contact, especially if it has a comforting effect, should never be underestimated (Johansson et al 2002). Hayes and Tyler-Ball (2007) undertook a study of trauma patients' perceptions of nurse caring, and found that the patients found it difficult to separate their care experiences into care received in different areas of the hospital. Rather, patients formed a picture or view of the hospitalisation experience, and this meant that overall perceptions of very good care would be compromised by a single negative episode of care.

Alongside moves to patient-centred care has been a concomitant effort to involve the family in care. Family-centred nursing has become an important foci for nurses' research and has a well-formulated philosophy and standards. In Australia, its proponents are working hard to implement some of its central tenets, although there is resistance in some quarters. The Insititute for Family Centred Care in North America has a well developed website promoting its cause (see www.familycenteredcare.org/faq.html).

To conclude this section we would like to use the words of one of Australia's eminent leaders in nursing, Professor Judy Lumby, who at the beginning of this century stated: 'ultimately it is the patient who must judge whether we care' (Lumby 2001:144). In a technologised world that values profit over people, it is hard to imagine that a nurse who exhibits caring behaviour could fail to make a difference.

CARE AND CURE

As you are no doubt aware, in a relatively short space of time, rapid developments in medical science, nursing knowledge and related health technologies have acted to dramatically improve patient outcomes and prolong life. We are now told that the human genome project and similar advances in science will lead to predicted increases in human life expectancy by as much as 25 years, and living into our hundreds will become commonplace (BBC World Service 2000).

In most parts of the world, these same technologies have radically and permanently changed the face of healthcare, and this has been the catalyst for a discussion in nursing and health that has become known as the 'care/cure' debate (e.g. Baumann et al 1998, Graham 2008, Webb 1996). This is a debate that has raged for quite a number of years. Johnston and Cooper (1997) suggest that the healthcare system in the United States was designed to cure illness and disease, rather than care for people and their health. This is the case for many Western healthcare systems, and provides a challenge for those whose main imperative is to care.

Clearly, caring alone will not meet all the health needs patients have but, as Webb (1996) pointed out, curing strategies may be insufficient unless accompanied by a caring dimension. In recent times a number of nursing scholars have published work on the concept of nursing as a therapeutic activity in its own right and the need for effective therapeutic relationships if the patient is to be 'cured' (Ersser 1997, Freshwater 2002, Johns 2001, Ramjan 2004). Williams (1997) too has suggested caring is, in itself, essential to cure. She proposes that caring nurse behaviours have been demonstrated to have positive effects in terms of patients' wellness and, conversely, non-caring behaviours by nurses have been shown to negatively affect patient wellbeing and recovery.

Writing from a medical perspective, Graham (2008:310) highlights the importance and value of family-centred primary care models within service contexts, which he names as 'cult of cure' systems. However, the concepts of care and cure historically have been constructed as binary and oppositional. Moreover, the difference between the roles of nurse and physician is often centred on ideas of the nurse as caring and the physician as curing. Sullivan and Deane (1994; similarly, Caffrey & Caffrey 1994) suggest caring (as nursing) is viewed as a traditionally feminine activity, and has not been conferred the power and status of male-defined activities, of which the physician/curer may more easily lay claim.

Indeed, if we look back over time, we can see it was Florence Nightingale herself who appeared to reject the idea that nurses can have an essential curing role. In her book *Notes On Nursing* (Nightingale 1859–1946:74), she states 'nature alone cures', but goes on to say 'what nursing has to do is to put the patient in the best position for nature to act upon him [sic]' (p 75). More recently, in defining professional caring, several scholars have contended these two concepts are not truly antagonistic (e.g. King & Norsen 1994, Leftwich 1993). Nurses identify elements of both caring and curing, and certain science-based skills and knowledge are highly valued as essential to caring (Carper 1978, Wolf et al 1994). Furthermore, patients themselves expect nurses to have a high level of professional proficiency and technical skill, which are associated with 'cure', and construct these as key aspects of professional caring (Borbasi 1996, Ray 1987, Wolf et al 1994).

King and Norsen (1994) contend that notions of 'care/cure' as solely the domain of either nurse (care) or physician (cure) are not helpful or acceptable, as nurses and physicians have both curing and caring dimensions to their practice areas (see also Leftwich 1993). In a similar vein, Webb (1996) urges nurses to overcome the cure/care dichotomy between medicine and nursing, and argues it is no longer important to distinguish the care given by specific professional groups but to focus instead on establishing clear goals of care. Rather than regarding notions of care and cure as being polarised or at opposite extremes then, it is more accurate to say the notions of care/cure are compatible and complementary. Both are acknowledged and accepted as key aspects of nursing's agenda, and both are reflected in the theories of professional caring constructed by nurses (Wolf et al 1994). Moreover, in today's health service we are seeing an increasing emphasis on multidisciplinary approaches to caring.

Having acknowledged that nursing is a composite of care and cure, it is perhaps ironical to note that the circumstances within which nurses find themselves working today probably mitigate against both. While some patients may be fortunate enough to be cured, technological and pharmacological advances have meant many are merely 'contained' in a state of chronic illness (Rizza et al 2008). Often these patients are aged with multiple co-morbidities, which makes caring for them extremely complex and, by the same token, nurses, because they are so occupied with administering medical treatments, may overlook the nurse caring behaviours so important to patient satisfaction and wellbeing. Have we perhaps reached a stage where neither cure nor care is winning out?

CARING AS THE BASIS OF THE DISCIPLINE OF NURSING

In addition to being complex and multidimensional, caring is also controversial, for among members of the profession, the debates about the centrality of caring to nursing continue (Cloyes 2002, Paley 2001, Sumner 2008). There are conflicting trains of thought and these challenge the relevance and appropriateness of caring as a foundational aspect of nursing. Stockdale and Warelow (2000) raise concerns about the inconsistencies around care and caring, and the ill-defined nature of caring. They point out the difficulties associated with adopting care as the essence of nursing, when there is not a universal accepted definition from which nursing can continue to develop.

All would agree that nurses do have a curative (as well as a caring) orientation, and in 1987 Kitson argued that if nurses choose to align themselves with care rather than cure, with the nurturing processes rather than with technology and treatment, then they will need to identify how to organise and put into operation those skills they possess. Successful execution of the caring role is, she believes, 'intimately bound up with having the necessary space to practice, sufficient room to manoeuvre and to be able to explore new areas of knowledge and expertise' (Kitson 1987:324).

In a major and very influential piece of work, Dunlop (1986) questioned whether a science of caring is even possible and resolves that, if it is, it will have to take a hermeneutical form (based on hermeneutics)—a 'form that in many ways does violence to our traditional ideas of science', but one that 'challenges the male hegemony of science' (Dunlop 1986:669). In a philosophical critique, Walker (1995) has also highlighted the problem of nurses' attempts to represent nursing as both a discourse of science and a discourse of caring.

The emergence of differing perspective(s) about the nature of nursing has not been without debate, and there are nurses who believe that an emphasis on alliance to concepts such as caring and holism, with their attendant rejection of the natural sciences, will do more harm than good to nursing's attempts to become a credible academic discipline. Indeed, in some quarters there is strident scepticism. Writing in 2002, Paley positions the ideology of caring as 'a slave morality', and goes on to state that:

> It represents an attack on the 'medical-scientific model', motivated by resentment, and designed to establish nursing's superiority. Its effects have been debilitating, and it has prevented nursing from becoming a 'noble' (that is, properly scientific) discipline (Paley 2002:25).

However, meeting the demands of the caring imperative concerned with cure requires that nurses have considerable specialist knowledge of a range of scientific disciplines such as pharmacology, anatomy, physiology, biochemistry, immunology, microbiology and physics. A sound scientific knowledge base is undeniably essential for nursing, given the need for continued development of the discipline and the need to meet the demands of increasingly technological societies; none would argue that competency in the scientific disciplines is not an essential aspect of nursing knowledge and integral to the caring imperative claimed by nursing.

THREATS TO CARING

From much of what we have said so far, it can be seen that the concept of caring is inherently incompatible with the underlying objectives of many of the organisational structures in which nurses find themselves today. In many parts of the (Western) world, healthcare is not intrinsically altruistic; nor is it based on any real system of equity (Lumby 2001). Rather, healthcare tends to be resourced on a fee-for-service basis, and access to healthcare services is therefore linked very strongly with an individual's ability to pay for such services. Healthcare is increasingly looked at with entrepreneurial, rather than philanthropic, eyes. To investors, provision of healthcare services may represent an opportunity for profit, and even 'whilst appropriating the language and images of nursing for business purposes, many entrepreneurs treat professional nursing care as a commodity to be whittled away until it becomes impotent' (Jackson & Raftos 1997:38). Although, to be sure, nurses comprise the largest occupational/professional group within the healthcare system; the system itself is based on a set of values that directly challenges and compromises the very essence of nursing.

In the past it was thought that large, impersonal institutions, by their very nature, may devalue caring by providing little incentive or opportunity for nurses to demonstrate behaviours associated with caring, or failing to provide an environment where caring could be expressed (Morse et al 1990). Align that with today's healthcare system, shaped as it is, by overarching economic influences such as cost containment and profit margins, and we have even less of a platform for caring work (Jarrin 2006). Economic imperatives have been the catalyst for reexamining the whole concept of 'patient care', and attempts have been made to reconceptualise traditional care delivery in order to come up with ways of doing more with less resources (Caplan & Brown 1997, Johnston & Cooper 1997, Ray 1989). These new approaches in provision of care are sometimes presented as strategies to improve patient care but, as Williams (1997) suggests, frequently they are more concerned with institutional cost saving than on quality patient care (similarly, Duffield & Lumby 1994, Lumby 2001).

This positioning of the wealth of an individual as a major indicator for allocation of (increasingly scarce) health resources is, by its very nature, incompatible with nursing's caring imperative, which places a high value on the individual (Chinn 1989, Morse et al 1990, Williams 1997). Care is most likely viewed by nurses as a resource to be allocated on the basis of need rather than ability to pay. These tensions are inherent in the working life of many nurses, and compromise the ability of nurses to provide care in the way idealised by the profession.

This key philosophical difference between nursing's caring imperative, and the underlying ethos of many (Western) healthcare systems, throws nurses and health administrators into a permanent state of possible conflict, and has the potential to become a source of professional tension for nurses (Jackson & Raftos 1997, Jarrin 2006, Johnston & Cooper 1997, Kralik et al 1997). As a result, many nurses leave nursing disillusioned with a 'system' that inhibits nurse caring behaviour. As we have experienced on an international scale, this contributes to critical shortages of nursing staff, which places the system, including patients and remaining staff, under even greater duress (Hinshaw 2008).

Two decades ago Ray (1989) attempted to reconcile the seemingly irreconcilable by proposing a theory of caring compatible with the bureaucratic cultures existing within large organisations. She suggested it is essential the discipline of nursing comes to terms with the corporatisation of healthcare, and that a failure to do this would be disastrous for nursing.

The transformation of American and other Western healthcare systems to corporate enterprises emphasising competitive management and economic gain seriously challenges nursing's humanistic philosophies and theories and nursing's administrative and clinical practices. The recent refocusing of nursing as a human science and the art and science of human caring places nursing in a vulnerable position. When pitted against the new goal of corporate advancement in healthcare delivery, nursing faces a loss of self-identity and an increased risk of alienation and confusion in this competitive arena (Ray 1989:31).

Using a grounded theory approach, Ray generated a 'theory of the dynamic structure of caring in a complex organization' (Ray 1989:31), and proposes this as a means by which nurses can practise within bureaucratic health structures without compromising nursing's caring imperative. This theory proposes several 'structural caring categories', which Ray names as political, economic, legal, technological/physiological, educational, social, spiritual/religious and ethical (Ray 1989). However, Caffrey and Caffrey (1994) suggest that caring will never be accommodated as a core value while profit remains a primary motive of healthcare systems. That these comments are still so salient, and that many of these issues continue to confound us, shows the longitudinal nature of the debate.

Insidiously, over the last few years, further threats to nurse caring have emerged, largely in the form of unregulated healthcare workers and the implementation of education and training programs for new breeds of healthcare practitioners. While nurses may have expanded and extended their roles at upper echelons in the health system, they need to be constantly on guard at the rear end: never more so than in a time of cost constraint and massive shortfalls in registered nurse numbers (Hinshaw 2008). It may well be that nursing, as we know it today, will shortly be overrun by workers who will do the job, but do it without any regard to caring as nurses have conceptualised it.

CONCLUDING THOUGHTS

Caring is proclaimed and understood as the basis of modern nursing, and as you are discovering, nurses have produced vast amounts of literature on aspects of care and caring, and how they may be applied in a nursing context. However, while the concept of professional caring is difficult to articulate, it is recognised as being a complex concept involving the development of a range of knowledge, skills and expertise. Professional caring has similarities with non-professional, or informal, caring and applies knowledge derived from various discipline areas to promote the health and wellbeing of people.

The major perspectives of caring recognise the importance of various types of knowledge and, with few exceptions, all allude to the expressive, artistic and scientific perspectives said to construct nursing. Other common themes that characterise the constructions of caring adopted by nurses are holism, compassion, empathy and communication. Evidence suggests that patients, too, view caring as a perceptible concept, and highly value it as an essential and healing aspect of their professional encounters with nurses. However, in contrast to the ways nurses view caring, reflection on what is known about patients' attitudes to nurse caring suggests that, above all, patients want a nurse who demonstrates caring through clinical and technical competence, as well as through interpersonal skills and, increasingly, a person who keeps them informed along each step of their illness trajectory, including informing family and friends.

Accepting caring as the basis of nursing practice and scholarship is not without problems. Issues of autonomy and power are ill at ease with the concept of caring.

Servitude and altruism are intrinsically linked to caring, and these do not sit well with nursing's move to professionalism. To provide adequate care takes time and time costs money. Many nurses work within organisational structures whose primary motivation lies with the cost containment or the accumulation of wealth, rather than a mandate to heal—these economic factors may compromise or even be antithetical to nursing's imperative to care.

The caring imperative, therefore, represents a potential source of stress and occupational conflict for nurses. While it is argued that the need for nursing to place caring as a central concept has never been greater, there are concerns that the caring components of nursing are deemed unsophisticated and hence inferior to the therapeutic interventions of medicine and other allied health service providers. There is the potential for caring to become overlooked—to dissipate.

Despite the many creative theories of nurse caring, the tasks of establishing coherent and clear connections between caring and notions such as professionalism, scholarship and autonomy remain incomplete. Nurses are left with many issues to consider and debate. Even as the healthcare system as we know it today is shaped, reshaped and shaped again, in the years to come the conundrum of caring as the basis of nursing practice and scholarship will no doubt continue to captivate and confound nurses.

REFLECTIVE QUESTIONS

1 Think for a moment about why you chose nursing as a career. Did the desire to care for people have any role in your decision making?

2 Take some time to reflect on your experiences of caring for and being cared for. Based on your experiences to date, how would you define caring?

3 Think about some of the ways you show care to the significant people in your life. Do you think that any of these ways of showing care will be the same or similar to how you will show care to your patients/clients as a nurse?

4 Some people view nursing and caring as being synonymous. Do you think this is good for nursing? Why? Why not?

RECOMMENDED READINGS

Dunlop M 1986 Is a science of caring possible? Journal of Advanced Nursing 11(3):661–670

Hayes J, Tyler-Ball S 2007 Perceptions of nurses' caring behaviours by trauma patients. Nursing Administration Quarterly 14(4):187–190

Hinshaw AS 2008 Navigating the perfect storm: balancing a culture of safety with workforce challenges. Nursing Research 57(1) Supplement 1:S4–S10

Lumby J 2001 Who cares? The changing health care system. Allen & Unwin, Sydney

Sumner J 2008 Is caring in nursing an impossible ideal for today's practicing nurse? Nursing Administration Quarterly 32(2):92–101

REFERENCES

Ahmad M, Alasad J 2004 Predictors of patients' experiences of nursing care in medical-surgical wards. International Journal of Nursing Practice 10(5):235–241

Bassett C 2002 Nurses' perceptions of care and caring. International Journal of Nursing Practice 8(1):8–15

Baumann A, Deber R, Silverman B, Mallette C 1998 Who cares? Who cures? The ongoing debate in the provision of health care. Journal of Advanced Nursing 28(5):1040

BBC World Service 2000 Who wants to live forever? Online. Available: www.bbc.co.uk/worldservice/people/highlights/000822_116.shtml 22 Aug 2000

Benner P 1984 From novice to expert: excellence and power in clinical nursing. Addison Wesley, Menlo Park, California

Benner P, Hooper-Kyriakidis P, Stannard D 1999 Clinical wisdom and interventions in critical care: a thinking-in-action approach. WB Saunders, Philadelphia

Borbasi SA 1996 Living the experience of being nursed: a phenomenological text. International Journal of Nursing Practice 2(4):222–228

Boykin A, Schoenhofer SO 2001 Nursing as caring: a model for transforming practice. Jones & Bartlett, Publishers, National League for Nursing Press, Sudsbury, Massachusetts

Caffrey R, Caffrey P 1994 Nursing: caring or codependent? Nursing Forum 29(1):12–17

Caplan G, Brown A 1997 Post-acute care: can hospitals do better with less? Australian Health Review 20(2):43–52

Carper B 1978 Fundamental patterns of knowing in nursing. Advances in Nursing Science 1(1):13–23

Chinn P 1989 Awake, awake. Advances in Nursing Science 11(2):1

Cloyes K 2002 Agonizing care: care ethics, agonistic feminism and a political theory of care. Nursing Inquiry 9(3):203–214

Duffield C, Lumby J 1994 Caring nurses: the dilemma of balancing costs and quality. Australian Health Review 17(2):72–83

Dunlop M 1986 Is a science of caring possible? Journal of Advanced Nursing 11(3):661–670

Ersser S 1997 Nursing as a therapeutic activity: an ethnography. Avebury, Aldershot

Falk Rafael A 1996 Power and caring: a dialectic in nursing. Advances in Nursing Science 19(1):3–17

Finfgeld-Connett D 2008 Qualitative convergence of three nursing concepts: art of nursing, presence and caring. Journal of Advanced Nursing 63(5):527–534

Foss C 2002 Gender bias in nursing care? Gender-related differences in patient satisfaction with the quality of nursing care. Scandinavian Journal of Caring Sciences 16(1):19–26

Freshwater D (ed.) 2002 Therapeutic nursing: improving patient care through self-awareness and reflection. Sage, London

Graham R 2008 Medicine and children with special health care needs: conflict with the cult of cure. Journal of Developmental and Behavioural Pediatrics 29(4): 309–310

Greenhalgh J, Vanhanen L, Kyngas H 1998 Nurse caring behaviours. Journal of Advanced Nursing 27(5):927–932

Hardy S, Garbett R, Titchen A, Manley K 2002 Exploring nursing expertise: nurses talk nursing. Nursing Inquiry 9(3):196–202

Hayes J, Tyler-Ball S 2007 Perceptions of nurses' caring behaviours by trauma patients. Journal of Trauma Nursing 14(4):187–190

Henderson A 2001 Emotional labour and nursing: an under-appreciated aspect of caring work. Nursing Inquiry 8(2):130–138

Hinshaw AS 2008 Navigating the perfect storm: balancing a culture of safety with workforce challenges. Nursing Research 57(1) Supplement 1:S4–S10

Jackson D, Borbasi S 2000 The caring conundrum: potential and perils for nursing. In: Daly J, Speedy S, Jackson D (eds) Contexts of nursing: an introduction. MacLennan & Petty, Sydney

Jackson D, Raftos M 1997 In uncharted waters: confronting the culture of silence in a residential care institution. International Journal of Nursing Practice 3(1):34–39

Jarrin OF 2006 Results from the nurse manifest 2003 study: nurses' perspectives on nursing. Advances in Nursing Science. Philosophy and Ethics 29(2):E74–E85

Johansson P, Oleni M, Fridlund B 2002 Patient satisfaction with nursing care in the context of health care: a literature review. Scandinavian Journal of Caring Sciences 16(4):337–344

Johns C 2001 Reflective practice: revealing the [he]art of caring. International Journal of Nursing Practice 7(4):237–245

Johnston C, Cooper P 1997 Patient-focused care: what is it?. Holistic Nursing Practice 11(3):1–7

Kapborg I, Bertero C 2003 The phenomenon of caring from the student nurse's perspective: a qualitative content analysis. International Nursing Review 50(3):183–192

King K, Norsen L 1994 The care/cure, nurse/physician dichotomy doesn't do it anymore. Image: Journal of Nursing Scholarship 26(2):89

Kitson AL 1987 Raising standards of clinical practice—the fundamental issue of effective nursing practice. Journal of Advanced Nursing 12(3):321–329

Kralik D, Koch T, Wootton K 1997 Engagement and detachment: understanding patients' experiences with nursing. Journal of Advanced Nursing 26(2):399–407

Leftwich R 1993 Care and cure as healing processes in nursing. Nursing Forum 28(3):13–17

Leininger M 1984 Care: the essence of nursing and health. Slack, New Jersey

Leininger M 1986 Care facilitation and resistance factors in the culture of nursing. Topics in Clinical Nursing 8(2):1–12

Lumby J 2001 Who cares? The changing health care system. Allen & Unwin, Sydney

Mann S, Cowburn J 2005 Emotional labour and stress within mental health nursing. Journal of Psychiatric and Mental Health Nursing 12:154–162

Mok E, Pui Chi Chiu 2004 Nurse–patient relationships in palliative care. Journal of Advanced Nursing 48(5):475–483

Morse J, Solberg S, Neander W, Bottorf J, Johnson J 1990 Concepts of caring and caring as a concept. Advances in Nursing Science 13(1):1–14

Nightingale F 1859–1946 Notes on nursing. Harrison Book Company, London

Oleni M, Johansson P, Fridlund B 2004 Nursing care at night: an evaluation using the Night Nursing Care Instrument. Journal of Advanced Nursing 47(1):25–32

Paley J 2001 An archaeology of caring knowledge. Journal of Advanced Nursing 26(2):188–198

Paley J 2002 Caring as a slave morality: Nietzschean themes in nursing ethics. Journal of Advanced Nursing 40(1):25–35

Pearson A 1991 Taking up the challenge: the future for therapeutic nursing. In: McMahon R, Pearson A (eds) Nursing as therapy. Chapman & Hall, London

Pepin J 1992 Family caring and caring in nursing. Image: Journal of Nursing Scholarship 24(2):127–131

Ramjan LM 2004 Nurses and the 'therapeutic relationship': caring for adolescents with anorexia nervosa. Journal of Advanced Nursing 45(5):495–503

Rawnsley M 1990 Of human bonding: the context of nursing as caring. Advances in Nursing Science 13(1):41–48

Ray M 1987 Technological caring: a new model in critical care. Dimensions in Critical Care Nursing 6(3):173–179

Ray M 1989 The theory of bureaucratic caring for nursing practice in the organizational structure. Nursing Science Quarterly 13(2):31–42

Rizza R, Eddy D, Kahn R 2008 Care, cure and commitment: what can we look forward to? Diabetes Care 31(5):1051–1060

Staden H 1998 Alertness to the needs of others: a study of the emotional labour of caring. Journal of Advanced Nursing 27(1):147–156

Stockdale M, Warelow P 2000 Is the complexity of care a paradox? Journal of Advanced Nursing 31(5):1258–1264

Sullivan J, Deane D 1994 Caring: reappropriating our tradition. Nursing Forum 29(2):5–9

Sumner J 2008 Is caring in nursing an impossible ideal for today's practicing nurse? Nursing Administration Quarterly 32(2):92–101

Swanson K 1993 Nursing as informed caring for the well-being of others. Image: Journal of Nursing Scholarship 25(4):352–357

Walker K 1995 Courting competency: nursing and the politics of performance in practice. Nursing Inquiry 2(2):90–99

Watson J 1985 Nursing: the philosophy and science of caring. Colorado Associated University Press, Boulder, Colorado

Watson J 1988 Nursing: human science and human care. A theory of nursing. National League for Nursing, New York

Watson J, Foster R 2003 The Attending Nurse Caring Model: integrating theory, evidence and advanced caring—healing therapeutics for transforming professional practice. Journal of Clinical Nursing 12(3):360–365

Watson J, Jackson D, Borbasi S 2005 Contemplating caring: issues, concerns, debates. In: Daly J, Speedy S, Jackson D, Lambert V, Lambert C (eds) Professional nursing: concepts, issues and challenges. Springer Publishing, New York

Webb C 1996 Caring, curing, coping: towards an integrated model. Journal of Advanced Nursing 23:960–968

Wilkin K, Slevin E 2004 The meaning of caring to nurses: an investigation into the nature of caring work in an intensive care unit. Journal of Clinical Nursing 13(1):50–59

Williams S 1997 Caring in patient-focused care: the relationship of patients' perceptions of holistic nurse care to their levels of anxiety. Holistic Nursing Practice 11(3):61–68

Wolf Z, Giardino E, Osborne P, Ambrose M 1994 Dimensions of nurse caring. Image: Journal of Nursing Scholarship 26(2):107–111

CHAPTER 7

The growth of ideas and theory in nursing

Sarah Winch, Amanda Henderson and Debra Creedy

LEARNING OBJECTIVES

At the completion of this chapter, the reader will be able to:

- define the term theory
- describe the terms modernity and postmodernity
- identify the dominant historical and societal trends within the nursing profession
- explain how these trends influence the practice of nursing and accompanying knowledge development, and
- differentiate the contribution of theory to research and research to theory.

KEY WORDS

Theory, modernity, postmodernity, knowledge, practice

INTRODUCING THEORY

This chapter aims to help you critically understand the relevance of theory to inform the ongoing development of nursing knowledge and contribute to the improvement of nursing practice. Clinical practice informed by theory gives nurses the necessary foundation to enlighten and restructure healthcare and improve quality of care at all practice levels. We begin with a brief overview of the philosophies, models and theories that underpin contemporary nursing theories. The next section emphasises nursing practice with a focus on knowledge utilisation, with theory and research as tools of practice.

Broadly, we can state that theory refers to any attempt to explain or represent a phenomenon, and ranges from the highly abstract and large scale, to the specific. Theories act as a lens by which to view the world. If you change the thickness of the lens and its shape, then what is being viewed is seen differently, in more or less detail, or expanded or reduced in size. Theories also act like a kaleidoscope, where turning the end of the instrument creates different patterns forming from the same small elements that are present. Theory and the application of theory to human understanding and social phenomena results in key elements (we shall call them variables and ideas) that underpin our understanding of the person and society being emphasised in different ways. Likewise, key philosophical ideas such as the nature of truth, evil and justice may be viewed differently.

When we focus on the process and practice of nursing, the central phenomena that require explanation are the nurse, the nursed and the care setting, including practices, processes and organisation. Nursing theories help us make sense of processes and practices. They explain why and when nursing takes place, provide an understanding of how the practice of nursing proceeds and also assist with practice change through critique. In this way nursing theories help us understand the practice of nursing, how we interact with the nursed and how we structure our nursing actions to provide nursing care.

NURSING AS SOCIAL PROCESS: THE ROLE OF SOCIAL THEORY IN UNDERSTANDING NURSING

Nursing can be viewed as a social and cultural product of society. That is, nursing is an interactive process that always takes place within a social context. Our common understanding of nursing involves a nurse and the nursed (the patient, consumer or client) interacting within a socially and politically constructed system (healthcare facility or provider) that directs actions and responses.

Knowledge of the role of social theory is valuable when we seek to answer the 'how' and 'why' questions about nursing and the social context from which it arises. The field of social theory is comprehensive, as it spans all of the social sciences and the humanities. In the following section we provide an overview of two major ways that social theory contributes to nursing. These are: an analysis of modernity and its contribution to the type of world we live in; and a critique of the social milieu that constructs and defines nursing.

Modernity and postmodernity: how social theory informs the way we think

Modernism, and postmodernism, are terms that hold a number of meanings in different contexts. For example, they may refer to specific styles of literature, art and architecture in the nineteenth and twentieth centuries. Or, as we explore here, they

EXAMPLES OF WELL-KNOWN NURSING THEORISTS (TOMEY & ALLIGOOD 1998)

- Faye Glenn Abdellah: 21 nursing problems
- Patricia Benner: stress and coping in illness
- Anne Boykin and Sarvina O Schoenhofer: the theory of nursing as caring
- Joyce J Fitzpatrick: rhythm model
- Dorothy Johnson: behavioural system model
- Imogene King: general system's framework/theory of goal attainment
- Katharine Kolcaba: theory of comfort
- Madeleine Leininger: theory of cultural care, diversity and universality/ transcultural nursing model
- Myra Levine: conservation model
- Ramona T Mercer: maternal role attainment
- Betty Neuman: nursing systems model
- Margaret Newman: theory of health as expanding consciousness
- Florence Nightingale: environmental adaptation theory
- Dorothea Orem: self-care framework
- Ida Jean Orlando: theory of the nursing process discipline
- Rosemarie Parse: theory of human becoming
- Josephine Paterson and Loretta Zderad: humanistic nursing theory
- Hildegard Peplau: theory of interpersonal relations
- Martha E Rogers: science of unitary human beings
- Nancy Roper, Winifred W Logan and Alison J Tierney: the elements of nursing: a model of nursing based on a model of living
- Callista Roy: adaptation model
- Jean Watson: theory of human caring
- Ernestine Wiedenbach: the helping art of clinical nursing

can elicit two different ways of thinking, both of which are fundamental to how we understand nursing.

First, we review modernity and postmodernity as a particular set of philosophical beliefs. These provide a useful philosophical framework that we can use to analyse practice-specific theories by tracing the traditions from which they emerge. Our second understanding relates to how nursing as a social process happens within the different time frames that represent the modern and postmodern eras. This provides a broad social and historical context that explains the nature of nursing and the transformations to nursing practice that are initiated through social change. In a later section, we examine modernism and postmodernism as broad cultural configurations that influence how society is organised.

Modernity and the Enlightenment

For many theorists, modernity encompasses a large historical period that emerged in Europe dating from the Renaissance to the present. Philosophical ideas on the nature of knowledge and modern method (Rene Descartes), science as power (Frances Bacon), the state and the science of human nature (Thomas Hobbes) and modern politics and power (Niccolo Machiavelli) construct the early basis of modernity. Later, in the eighteenth century, many of these ideas had their full intellectual flowering in a time known as 'the Enlightenment'. The goal of the Enlightenment project was to replace the ignorance, tradition and superstition present in the church-dominated societies of the Middle Ages, with knowledge that was based on science and reason. This far-reaching period of intellectual development is still prominent in much of contemporary thinking in nursing and other disciplines.

Ideas on the nature of human life that stem from the Enlightenment period reflect a particular belief about the self and the human condition. The modernist concept of 'the self' is a unified, rational, autonomous and essential entity. This means that 'the self' can be observed and studied. It is free, capable of thought and of independent action. This is a description of human beings as active agents doing things for reasons and shaping the world to their own ends. These core ideas about the nature of the self are central to many nursing theorists who see patients and nurses as autonomous beings who are able to be influenced in their behaviours to promote health and wellbeing or to address deficits caused by illness.

The Enlightenment period crystallised a belief in universal goals and human progress towards an ideal through the application of value-neutral knowledge. Knowledge derived from the empirical or natural sciences can be applied to society to increase human progress and happiness, while knowledge from the human sciences can be used to transform society into a scientific, rational culture. These ideas, which Yeatman (1991) terms 'rational utopianism', underpin modernist emancipatory politics (i.e. the search for truth and progress through value-free, objective knowledge).

For researchers working within this framework (and this includes most nurses), it is important to select the correct research method, as this endorses 'truth' and provides theory that is an objective reflection of a securely grounded world (Hollinger 1994). Society and history are seen as a whole, able to be grasped through totalising methodologies and explained by grand and comprehensive explanations (meta-narratives). In nursing these would take the form of theories of caring or grand theories of nursing.

Research methods based on modernist assumptions promote the ideas of objectivity, and most importantly value neutrality. In this way a society based on science and universal values can be assumed to be truly rational and emancipatory. As such, theory is an objective representation of social reality. Ideas from the Enlightenment period have led to positivism, scientism and an emphasis on technological reason. For example, although ideas about ageing have been present in the wider literature since ancient times, the Enlightenment constructed the idea of 'old age' through medicine, science and philosophy as an essential part of life. Modernity spawned practices of calculation, division and ranking of the population. It was then possible to separate older age as a distinct developmental stage (Katz 1995). As such, all human institutions and practices, including hospitals and nurses, can be analysed by science and improved. This central belief is very much a part of healthcare and service provision today.

Modernity is also about order and rationality (logical thinking underpinned by science). This order and stability are maintained in modern societies through the means of 'grand or master narratives'. These are stories about the practices and beliefs present in a society. A 'grand narrative' in Australian culture may be that the family is a 'haven' and a 'central building block' of society. Generally, if we support families to function well, they will raise the next generation properly, and care for their sick and elderly. Contemporary healthcare and social policy reflects this type of grand narrative. For example, aged care policy, such as home and community care, is based on supporting families (often aged spouses) to care for their partners. Likewise, early discharge policy and short stays in acute care hospitals rely on a well-organised, functioning family to provide supportive care.

Postmodernity

The central theme of modernity is a belief in the idea of progress in human life through the application of value-free knowledge gained in an objective way (science). However, as the German philosopher Jurgen Habermas and others have established, the twentieth century experience of the Holocaust and nuclear devastation shattered confidence and faith in scientific progress (Harvey 1989). Postmodernism (which in our discussion here includes the related although not identical category of poststructuralism) presents an altogether more pessimistic view of the world in general. It seeks to critique or deconstruct grand narratives to reveal the contradictions and instabilities that are inherent in any social organisation or practice. For example, in Australia, community nurses know that the grand narrative involving the family as a source of comfort and support is not always true. Postmodernism, while rejecting grand narratives, prefers 'mini-narratives', or stories that explain small practices and local events, rather than large-scale universal or global concepts. These 'mini-narratives' are always locally based on particular situations and do not claim to be universal or generalisable to other contexts, and have great application in promoting understanding of aspects of nursing practice.

Drawn from a complex mix of ideas from theorists such as Hegel, Nietzsche and Weber, the postmodern position is associated with concepts such as irrationality, play, deconstruction, antithesis and indeterminacy (Gillan 1988). In a sense, these are the opposite of the science-based rationality that underpins modernism. Critics of the Enlightenment, such as the well-known philosopher Nietzsche, argue that truth, knowledge and rationality are not immutable and science itself may rest on faith (Hollinger 1994). Postmodernism, taken to its extreme, refutes all claims to truth and reduces theory to narrative or storytelling. Postmodernism abandons the dualism of facts and values, objectivity and subjectivity, descriptions and interpretations, and gives all methodologies a political emphasis, while contextualising all claims, methods and values. Moreover, postmodernism does not accord 'reason' a central and transcendental status.

From the Enlightenment onwards, the idea of the 'subject' has had a central place in thought about the special nature of humanity. For key Enlightenment thinkers, the autonomous subject was the central tenet of civil society. By stark contrast, many postmodern thinkers dispute the concept of the sovereign individual or subject, viewing these ideas about the subject as a form of grand narrative that requires deconstruction itself. For postmodernists, individuals are subjects, constituted through a variety of practices and knowledges or discourses in society in which they are positioned at any one point in time. The modernist, humanist concept of a unified, rational, autonomous and essential self is seen as illusory and results from regular positioning within a common, frequently used discourse (Grosz 1993).

Postmodernity has influenced several thinkers and observers of nursing practice, including Winch (2005), who argues that this type of analysis can provide a highly analytical view of nursing practice. This view links the minutiae of nursing work with formation of identity (of the subject), and the monitoring and fashioning of patient conduct within broader historical, social and political processes and institutions.

Characterising modern healthcare institutions

The second way by which we may understand modernism and postmodernism is to view them broadly as historical cultural configurations that influence how society is organised. In two to three centuries, modern industrial capitalism altered earlier farming or rural societies and set the scene for the society we know in Australia today. In line with the massive social change from the modern to the postmodern, nursing as a social process or cultural product has also been transformed.

Jameson (1984) outlines three primary phases of capitalism in Western industrialised nations that have produced particular cultural practices associated with modernism and postmodernism. These provide a framework for how we may understand healthcare and nursing. The first predates both modernism and postmodernism and is termed *market capitalism*. This occurred in the eighteenth through to the late nineteenth centuries in Western Europe, England and the United States. This phase is associated with particular technological developments such as the steam-driven engine. It is in this phase that nursing began to emerge as a central form of healthcare responsible for cleanliness and hygiene, with the growth of the clinic and the asylum. The work of the nursing theorist Florence Nightingale is prominent in this period.

The second phase, termed *monopoly capitalism*, occurred from the late nineteenth century until the mid-twentieth century, and is associated with modernism, industrialism, the growth of cities, the nuclear family, democracy and social legislation. It is in this phase that we see the growth of particular institutions such as the modern hospital, the development of the health professions and the rise of medicine as the dominant and most powerful form of healthcare.

The third phase, the one that we currently occupy, is a form of multinational or *consumer capitalism*, a postindustrial or postmodern society. Developing after World War II, the third phase encompasses all of the second phase but emphasises new technologies, marketing, selling and consuming commodities, and the growth of the internet. It is in this era that multinational pharmaceutical companies have grown very powerful, seeking to influence medical care and the consumption of particular drugs, ordered through medical practitioners and marketed in some countries, such as the United States, directly to the consumer. Modern managerialism has also crept into healthcare and influenced nursing work, with a focus on healthcare targets and clinical pathways. Health services are now managed as businesses, with patients as consumers.

Our consideration of the modern and postmodern has ranged over a wide number of issues, of which there is no clear agreement among social theorists, philosophers or nursing thinkers. Some argue that we live in truly postmodern times, and we must abandon the quest for truth and justice through the application of science. Others still believe that society is evolving to become a more logical and rational place, despite the odd setback. Nursing over this period of time has ebbed and flowed with the dominant social and cultural practices of the time. What is clear is that the work that nurses do is essential in a civil society. What is less certain in a postmodern, postindustrial time is how that work may be fragmented or reorganised and what nursing may look like in the future.

IMPLICATIONS FOR THE DEVELOPMENT OF A BODY OF KNOWLEDGE

Social theory has influenced how nurses inquire into their profession. This inquiry has explored ways to study human beings, what counts as 'evidence', reflection on practice and analysing the profession itself. Prevailing ideas and theories have been instrumental in how nurses approach and conduct their practice and accordingly the development of professional knowledge. This section provides a brief overview of some of the more dominant ideas and theories that have influenced the discipline of nursing. These influences are significant determinants of how nursing is presently understood and practised.

The contribution of scientific inquiry

From the Enlightenment period onwards, science and reason were perceived to be methods to obtain value-free knowledge in a neutral manner. Prior to the Enlightenment, nursing work had been undertaken by untrained religious people and local women with experience of caring for family members or having babies (Ehrenreich & English 1973). A structured, logical analysis of human behaviour began with John Locke (1690) in *An Essay Concerning Human Understanding*. Locke espoused the belief that all ideas originate in experience. The inherent premise was that a newborn infant must acquire his or her ideas of this world by observing what goes on around him or her. The limits of understanding are therefore set by the limits of sense and reason. This argument was readily adopted as the dominant philosophy on all aspects of intellectual life during the eighteenth century (Miller 1985). This argument was termed *empiricism*. It referred to the idea that what was known was only possible through sensory experience. Knowledge could therefore be validated (Mitchell 1987).

Florence Nightingale (1820–1910) gave shape and form to what was to become the discipline of nursing by using the scientific methods proposed from the Enlightenment period. Tutored in mathematics as a child, Nightingale systematically collected data and analysed this statistically (Cohen 1984). Nightingale's explanation of the phenomena of concern to nursing marks the beginning of systematic inquiry and the development of a knowledge base (Newman 1983). She applied 'scientific inquiry' to illness generally to derive specific nursing interventions. Nightingale is best known for her carefully collected information in relation to the environment, namely the concepts of ventilation, warmth, light, diet, cleanliness and noise (Tomey & Alligood 1998). Through careful observation, keen documentation and subsequent analysis of these factors, she sought insights into causal relationships on which nursing could make a difference.

Nightingale also needed to persuade influential politicians who championed her cause. She used the dominant method of the day to progress this, namely observation, to collect objective data and logic/reasoning instead of religion and superstition (Ehrenreich & English 1973). Since Nightingale, nurses have approached their practice in a structured and systematic manner. As a discipline, nursing has sought theory in an attempt to describe, explain, predict and control. Nurses have borrowed theory from a range of other disciplines to assist in understanding the core phenomena inherent in nursing. In many situations nurses have modified and adopted theory from these disciplines in an attempt to develop a nursing-specific theory.

The dominance of empiricism in the practice of nursing

Physiological theories based in scientific methods of inquiry were well advanced by the second half of the nineteenth century and provided information about how the body worked (Miller 1985). The biomedical model, the basis of contemporary acute medical practice, arose from this form of investigation. This model views people as biological beings, made of cells, tissues and organs that achieve homeostasis, an internal mechanism that keeps physical and chemical parameters of the body relatively constant. Consistent with the notions of reason and causality that accompanied modernity, how the body functioned could be likened to a machine (Benner & Wrubel 1989, Pearson et al 2005).

The biomedical model has continued to dominate healthcare during the twentieth century (Aronowitz 1998), and has become the dominant paradigm in many areas of practice, not only for the medical profession but also for nurses (Pearson et al 2005). For example, during the initial establishment of intensive care areas, nurses frequently learnt with doctors about how the physiological body responded in situations of illness (Fairman 1992). Nurses, who had become responsible for the physical body, were learning more about the physiological responses that accompanied health problems. Potentially, this knowledge was instrumental in assisting health restoration, nurses could act quickly using this information and interventions based on biomedicine could be appropriately administered.

Increasing knowledge of human physiology has resulted in a plethora of methods and tools to diagnose and prescribe treatment. These methods have largely been dictated by the medical profession, creating a hierarchy based on science in which nursing knowledge has been coerced (Henderson 1994). This situation has arisen primarily because healthcare is directed by medicine and provision of care by nurses is largely organised to support interventions directed by the medical profession.

The extensive use of the biomedical model has similarly led to an emphasis on technical-related aspects of the nursing role. This can be partially explained by the observation that during clinical interactions the body is essentially objectified. In the physical interaction the patient experiences his or her body as a scientific object beneath the dispassionate gaze consistent with scientific investigation (Leder 1984). This has inadvertently led to a devaluing of assisting the individual through the experience of their illness (Pearson et al 2005). When disease is conceptualised as the aberrant dysfunction at the tissue, cellular or organ level, the biomedical model is an efficient theoretical framework to explore this function (Benner & Wrubel 1989).

This perspective has been contested by many contemporary nursing theorists working from a postmodern perspective. These theorists (e.g. Rosemarie Parse, Martha Rogers, Jean Watson and Patricia Benner) are interested in the non-technical, or more caring, relational aspects of the nursing role, which examine the minutiae of the daily practice of nursing work and the patient's experience of illness from their own perspective. They argue that this is more akin to the reality of nursing as it is actually practised. Nurses can make an important contribution in such dimensions of patient care. They have a capacity to recognise and explore an individual's spirituality, feelings, situated meaning and ethical concerns that accompany the individual's journey through the illness trajectory, which are lost in a purely biomedical or scientific approach. The work of these postmodern scholars has resulted in a growing appreciation of the experience of illness and also recognition of tacit nursing knowledge (Benner & Wrubel 1989).

THE META-PARADIGM OF NURSING: IDENTIFYING A DISTINCT BODY OF KNOWLEDGE

In line with the emergence of organised society and the modern-day hospital (Bullough & Bullough 1972), during the phase we have identified as *monopoly capitalism*, nursing knowledge grew through a complex mix of practice, science, social and behavioural theories and tradition. This resulted in a body of healthcare knowledge that is respected independently of medicine, although not necessarily seen as equal or as valuable. During the push to obtain professional status, nurses recognised the need to identify core proponents that would assist in the continuous debate and refinement of a unique body of knowledge. To assist with this, a meta-paradigm was sought by which to organise and direct the knowledge that would become nursing's unique focus.

A meta-paradigm of any discipline is a statement or group of statements identifying the relevant phenomena to the discipline (Fawcett 1984). It originates from the term paradigm, used to describe accepted practices and techniques through which a discipline accumulates and refines its knowledge base. According to Kuhn (1970), a paradigm assists in the articulation and refinement of the phenomena being explored. Exploration of the scholarly arguments, as they pertain to nursing, identifies four central recurring themes that can arguably be described as constituting a meta-paradigm for nursing. The components of the paradigm are identified as: nursing (as an action); client (human being); environment (of the client and nurse–client); and health. The nurse interacts with the client and the environment for the purpose of facilitating the health of the client (Fawcett 1984, Newman 1983).

These four components facilitate the description and explication of theories in nursing. For example, the model proposed by Roper et al (1990), which addresses clients' activities of daily living, is a development on earlier notions of understanding health. This model recognises the integral part of psychosocial wellbeing on health, and appropriately ensures consideration of environmental factors, including communication and capacity to develop relationships. These components of the meta-paradigm are essential because what is meant by nursing is largely influenced by the meanings and the importance attributed to it (Newman 1983). Insights into potential meaning may be derived through an understanding of the shifts and developments in how two of these components are understood, the client and the environment.

Understanding the client

Words referring to the person receiving the nursing care have changed in line with some of the broad cultural configurations that we mentioned previously. Historically, nursing language uses the term 'patient' to refer to the nursed. In modern times (i.e. the postindustrial age), we have exchanged this term for 'client' and, in some cases, 'consumer'. This interesting change of language is meant to confer an attitude of active participation of the person receiving care.

These changes in nomenclature about the person being nursed are, in part, related to how the individual being nursed is actually viewed—that is, how they are understood as a human being and a person. How the individual is approached and how nursing care is attended to has largely been influenced by how the human body has been conceptualised, which has in turn influenced what practices are perceived to constitute nursing.

According to the biomedical model, health was the maintenance of the body's biological functioning. However, with increasing knowledge about the human body, the conceptualisation of the individual, and accordingly health, has broadened. Methods of scientific inquiry have not only been used to describe the internal operation of the biological body, but also human behaviour. Consistent with empirical research, initially human behaviour was likened to a stimulus–response model—for example, if a person was hungry, they sought food. Subsequent to these initial observations and experiments, it was recognised that there was a cognitive component to human behaviour. Individuals could think, plan and make decisions on remembered information.

Acceptance of the cognitive component of the individual has been very influential in broadening the scope of nursing work. The impact of psychological wellbeing on overall health status meant that nurses could have a sphere of influence apart from the technical interventions accompanying tests, procedures and other intrusions into the body.

Aspects of the human condition relating to stress and anxiety are core concepts repeatedly studied in nursing. These concepts frequently accompany deviations of health when experienced by clients, and they are an area in which nurses are readily able to make a difference (Devine & Cook 1986). Many nursing theories have been developed in response to the potential of psychological issues that affect individuals with deviations in their health condition. Theorists using this approach include Peplau and Travelbee (Tomey & Alligood 1998).

PEPLAU AND THE THEORY OF INTERPERSONAL RELATIONS IN NURSING

In the theory of interpersonal relations in nursing, Peplau (1987) emphasises the importance of the nurse–client relationship. The relationship develops through interlocking and overlapping phases. These are: the orientation phase; the working phase (subdivided into identification and exploitation); and the resolution phase. It 'is educative and therapeutic when nurses and patient can come to know and respect each other as persons who are alike, and yet different, as persons who share in the solution of problems' (Peplau 1987).

However, during the early part of the twentieth century, the limitations of experimental research in explaining the human condition were exposed by Sigmund Freud. The work of Freud is powerful in challenging the notion of accepted empiricism. Freud, through recognition of the subconscious of individuals, exposed another form of knowledge that was not acquired through empirical studies (Miller 1985). Freud's work demonstrated the importance of the unconscious and instinctual forces in human conduct (Miller 1985). The recognition of this knowledge is influential in postmodernity—there is now acknowledgment that we can learn more about ourselves and how we function within the world apart from rigorous empiric methods. Meanings are understood as specific to the individual or a small group of individuals as 'mini-narratives'.

Understanding the environment

From the inception of this chapter, we have argued that the social and cultural environment produces nursing and structures nursing action. Nursing does not occur in a vacuum. Despite this fundamental premise, the various conceptualisations of the environment remain the most ill defined of all the central concepts of the espoused meta-paradigm (Brodie 1984). Kleffel (1991) similarly reviews the perspective of the environment, and concludes that the concept of the environment is important as a domain of nursing knowledge, as it is the nature of the environment as it is conceived in global terms that impacts on nursing.

We have seen how the nature of nursing and transformation of nursing practice can be initiated through shifts in social thoughts and ideas that emerge from the global environment, such as the growth of science as an explanation (from the Enlightenment) or the different ways that nursing work has been produced across the broad epochs of monopoly and postindustrial capitalism. Let us now take a specific example that affects nursing practice and that has become prominent in the postindustrial era—that is, growth of the business model of healthcare.

Among the competing discourses involved in the complex production of healthcare in Western industrial nations, the strength of the business-model-driven healthcare system is paramount. The roots of modern managerialism with its stress upon healthcare targets, admissions, discharges and care pathways can be traced to the industrial revolution. This factory-style production of nursing work is a form of Taylorism (Lundy 1996). Taylorism involves taking a professional skill set and breaking it up into component parts, which can then be further classified according to a particular skill level. Workers with less training can participate in what is hitherto a complete professional activity. This provides definite economic benefits, as less of the more highly trained professionals are required. For the nurses working on the factory line, producing regimented segments of nursing care according to prescribed pathways, the scope of what we would term professional nursing practice, is stymied. In a climate that Hofstadter (1963) has termed *unreflective instrumentalism*, there has been a loss of the complexity of nursing and the ability for the high level of analysis and reflection necessary for a practice-based profession to provide the highest level of care.

In this type of business-driven healthcare environment, Ackroyd and Bolton (1999) argue that while nurses do retain autonomy from managers, the context of nursing is controlled via the supply of patients. By increasing the number of patients, managers control the time that nurses have to treat. This means that nurses have to work harder if they want to give what they feel is an appropriate level of care. In this way, key parameters of nursing activity are gradually lost to the profession that may wish to control the quality of its work. Thus we can see that awareness of the environment in which nurses work is revealing—as the environment prescribes the conditions not only in which development of knowledge occurs, but also how that knowledge can be applied.

Concomitantly, it is argued that the nursing profession is starting to mature and that professional nurses have started to examine their behaviours, how these have emerged and manage their situation to better suit the profession. Nurses are beginning to acknowledge the complexity of the knowledge operating within the profession (Street 1992) and are learning how to best draw on this knowledge. Street (1992) advocates for critical inquiry—that is, the capacity for self-reflection and collaborative analysis to effect rational change. For nurses to enact this, she advocates nurses draw on the work of Habermas (1971), who argues that individuals should act from raised awareness, rather than coercion or habit, as previously recognised in nursing behaviour.

IMPLICATIONS FOR CONTEMPORARY NURSING PRACTICE: THEORETICAL PLURALISM

Nursing has been informed and influenced by many different ideas and trends within modern society. These are evident in the education, practice and research of nursing. The involvement of nurses in understanding their professional practice is imperative so that the foundations upon which they base their practice are not hidden beliefs, but are made overt so that their effects can be considered and further developed to better meet the health needs of the broader community.

The difficulty with the development of theory in nursing is the notion that 'one size fits all'—that is, one theory should account for all the 'truths' in nursing (Emden & Young 1987). Theoretical pluralism as described by Dickoff and James (1984), however, permits the nurse to select and apply the theoretical model appropriate to the particular practice setting and client situation. This approach also allows and acknowledges that the selection and application of a variety of nursing theories and models depends on the depth and breadth of knowledge of the individual nurse. For example, the conceptual and theoretical framework adopted by nurses in a community health clinic may be different from the framework adopted by nurses working in an acute care hospital.

How theory informs the development of the discipline of nursing is somewhat ambiguous—it is essentially an interactive process with research. Arguably, theory and research occur along a continuum, in that research can test the validity of theoretical concepts (Chinn & Jacobs 1987). Alternatively, there is a growing emphasis on research formulating theory (Emden & Young 1987). Data derived from practice are conceptualised; theories are then formulated and inform the intellectual structure organising practice (Benner 1984). Ideally, theory development and research are interactive processes.

Many nursing theories have been largely informed through dominant societal trends, rather than emerging from limitations experienced within the practice of nursing. It is therefore not surprising that nurses have not embraced theory in their practice. Similarly, it is recognised that much of nursing research does not attempt to substantiate nursing theory (Donaldson & Crowley 1978). The challenge for nursing is for practitioners to have a comprehensive understanding of ideas, how they have contributed to their practice and how nurses can derive the best outcomes from a systematic organisation of these ideas into theories that inform their own spheres—namely, research, knowledge and practice.

CONCLUDING THOUGHTS

The ways you think about people and about nursing have a direct impact on how you approach people, what questions you ask, how that information is processed, and what nursing activities are included in the care offered. The utilisation and application of nursing theory (in the form of philosophies, models and theories) help you think critically for professional practice. Theory and research together lead to systematic inquiry, which informs practice and thus directs nursing care.

REFLECTIVE QUESTIONS

1 To what extent is theory development crucial to nursing and nursing practice?

2 How does the Western industrial healthcare environment affect nursing work in the twenty-first century?

3 How does the conceptual shift of postmodernity affect the development of nursing knowledge in practice?

4 What local situations and conditions operate in your sphere of practice that influence the nursing care you provide?

RECOMMENDED READINGS

Alligood M, Marriner-Tomey A (ed.) 2002 Nursing theory: utilization and application, 2nd edn. Mosby, St Louis

Hollinger R 1994 Postmodernism and the social sciences: a thematic approach. Sage, London, pp 169–77

Pearson A, Vaughan B, FitzGerald M 2005 Nursing models for practice, 3rd edn. Butterworth Heinemann, London

REFERENCES

Ackroyd S, Bolton S 1999 It is not Taylorism: mechanisms of work intensification in the provision of gynaecological services in a NHS hospital. Work Employment and Society 13(2):369–387

Aronowitz RA 1998 Making sense of illness. Cambridge University Press, Cambridge

Benner P 1984 From novice to expert: excellence and power in clinical nursing. Addison-Wesley, Menlo Park, California

Benner P, Wrubel J 1989 The primacy of caring. Addison Wesley, Menlo Park, California

Brodie JA 1984 Response to Dr J Fawcett's paper. Image: Journal of Nursing Scholarship 16(3):87–98

Bullough B, Bullough V 1972 A brief history of medical practice. In: Friedson E, Lorber J (eds) Medieval men and their work. Aldine-Atherton, Chicago, pp 86–102

Chinn P, Jacobs MK 1987 A model for theory development in nursing. Advances in Nursing Science 1(1):1–11

Cohen IB 1984 Florence Nightingale. Scientific American March:128–136

Devine EC, Cook TD 1986 Clinical and cost saving effects of psychosocial educational interventions with surgical patients: a meta-analysis. Research in Nursing and Health 9:89–105

Dickoff J, James P 1984 Toward a cultivated but decisive theoretical pluralism. In: McGee M (ed.) Theoretical pluralism in nursing science. University of Ottawa Press, Ottawa

Donaldson SK, Crowley DM 1978 The discipline of nursing. Nursing Outlook February:113–120

Ehrenreich B, English D 1973 Witches, midwives, and nurses. Writers and Readers Co-operative, London

Emden C, Young W 1987 Theory development in nursing: Australian nurses advance global debate. Australian Journal of Advanced Nursing 4(3):22–40

Fairman J 1992 Watchful vigilance: nursing care, technology and the development of intensive care units. Nursing Research 41:56–60

Fawcett J 1984 The meta-paradigm of nursing: present status and future refinements. Image: Journal of Nursing Scholarship 16(3):84–86

Gillan G 1988 Foucault's philosophy. In: Bernauer J, Rasmussen D (eds) The final Foucault. MIT Press, London

Grosz E 1993 Bodies and knowledges: feminism and the crisis of reason. In: Alcroff L, Potter E (eds) Feminist epistemologies. Routledge, New York, pp 187–216

Habermas J 1971 Knowledge and human interest (transl. by JJ Shapiro). Beacon Press, Boston

Harvey D 1989 The condition of postmodernity. Basil Blackwell, Oxford

Henderson A 1994 Power and knowledge in nursing practice: the contribution to Foucault. Journal of Advanced Nursing 20(5):935–939

Hofstadter R 1963 Anti-intellectualism in American life. Alfred A Knopf, New York, pp 233–71

Hollinger R 1994 Postmodernism and the social sciences: a thematic approach. Sage, London

Jameson F 1984 Postmodernism: or the cultural logic of late capitalism. New Left Review 146:53–92

Katz S 1995 Disciplinary texts: rhetoric and the science of old age in the late nineteenth century and early twentieth century. Australian Cultural History 14:109–126

Kleffel D 1991 Rethinking the environment as a domain of nursing knowledge. Advances in Nursing Science 15:307–315

Kuhn TS 1970 The structure of scientific revolutions. University of Chicago Press, Chicago

Leder D 1984 Medicine and paradigms of embodiment. Journal of Medicine and Philosophy 9:29–43

Lundy C 1996 Nursing beyond Fordism. Employee Responsibilities and Rights Journal 9(2):163–171

Miller GA 1985 Psychology: the science of mental life. Penguin, London

Mitchell GD 1987 A new dictionary of sociology. Routledge & Kegan Paul, London

Newman MA 1983 The continuing revolution: a history of nursing science. In: Chaska NL (ed.) The nursing profession: a time to speak. McGraw Hill, New York, pp 385–93

Pearson A, Vaughan B, Fitzgerald M 2005 Nursing models for practice, 3rd edn. Butterworth Heinemann, Oxford

Peplau HE 1987 The art and science of nursing: similarities, differences and relations. Nursing Science Quarterly 1:8–15

Roper N, Logan W, Tierney A 1990 The elements of nursing, 3rd edn. Churchill Livingstone, Edinburgh

Street A 1992 Inside nursing. State University Press, New York

Tomey A, Alligood MR 1998 Nursing theorists and their work, 4th edn. Mosby,
   St Louis
Winch S 2005 Ethics, government and sexual health: insights from Foucault. Nursing
   Ethics 12(2):177–186
Yeatman A 1991 Postmodern critical theorising: introduction. Social Analysis 30:3–9

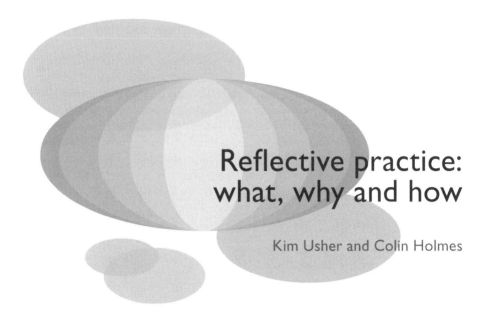

CHAPTER 8

Reflective practice: what, why and how

Kim Usher and Colin Holmes

LEARNING OBJECTIVES

After reading this chapter, students should have gained:

- an understanding of the importance and benefits of reflection to a practice-based discipline such as nursing
- insight into the nature of reflection and the ideas of its leading theorists
- an appreciation of the link between self-awareness and professional self-monitoring
- an understanding of the strategies that assist with reflection—for example, reflective writing, journalling, critical incident analysis, clinical supervision, and forms of creative expression, and
- insight into the legal and ethical issues surrounding the keeping of professional journals.

KEY WORDS

Reflection, reflective practice, journalling, critical incident analysis, self-awareness

INTRODUCTION

The context in which nursing occurs has changed markedly in the last two decades. As a result of advances in nursing and medical knowledge, and reduced government spending (which has led to a reduction in hospital beds, shorter hospital stays, and more rapid patient turnovers), workers in healthcare institutions are spending much more of their time dealing with acutely ill patients who require specialised care (Usher et al 2001). This can cause feelings of concern or confusion, but we must also recognise that it offers us an opportunity to reconceptualise our profession by making it more responsive and reflective of the needs of society (Lauder et al 2004). The role of the nurse is also influenced by cultural, social, economic, historical and political constraints that all affect the ways in which nurses approach and react to certain situations (Taylor 2000). It is a given that society expects nurses to practise safely and to undertake what is necessary to remain current. Reflection helps us to self-correct where the notion of continuous improvement becomes habitual to our practice (Usher et al 2008).

As a consequence of the changing healthcare arena, today's nursing graduates must not only be clinically competent practitioners, but also need to be adept at *critical thinking* in order to understand the complexities of the world and the rapidly changing practice arena, even though this can itself be challenging (Johns 2004, Usher et al 1999). Critical thinking, or the practice of questioning, is necessary so that practitioners integrate relevant information from various sources, examine assumptions, and identify relationships and patterns (Parker & Clare 2000). *Reflective practice* and critical thinking are often used interchangeably, but, while not identical, there is a reflexive relationship. After all, as Lumby (2000:338) explains: 'to adopt a critical approach to the world, it is necessary to reflect on the world and one's experiences in it'.

We begin this chapter by introducing you to the *why* of reflection, and explaining why *reflection* is a useful strategy for undergraduate nursing students, as well as registered nurses. We will also provide an overview of the related legislation that requires the use of reflective thinking in practice by registered nurses and makes it a requirement for all students exiting undergraduate university degrees. The next section of the chapter addresses the *why* and *what* of reflective practice, including an overview of the definitions of reflection.

WHY BE REFLECTIVE?

Every workplace presents a complex environment to the new recruit. It is often difficult to understand and appears to abound with multiple decisions, each coupled to a host of different ways in which the desired outcomes could be achieved. Nursing is no different. When you first enter a nursing context, perhaps during your first clinical placement, you will be confronted by discrepancies, such as those between 'ideal' and 'real' practice, and you will experience or witness difficult interpersonal relationships. It is important that these situations do not distract you from your nursing goals or from seeking to provide the best possible care. Reflection can help you during these times, as it will assist you to recognise and set aside the emotional content and enable you to learn from otherwise negative experiences. Reflection can take on an even more important role when you find yourself faced with difficult working conditions and environments (Usher et al 2008). It will help you identify alternative ways you could react in the future, hopefully resulting in more positive outcomes.

Johns (1998) explains how reflection offers a way to bring to the surface the contradictions between what you intend to achieve in a situation and how you actually practise. In other words, being faced with contradiction opens the possibility for change and offers the practitioner the opportunity to achieve desired practice. One of the outcomes of reflection is thus a process of continuous monitoring and improvement of practice. Reflection is a legitimate activity or process, as it can generate knowledge in the way that nursing theory, for example, can.

Regulatory authorities in Australia have embraced the need for practitioners who are reflective, and require that all nurses engage in some form of reflective activity. This is indicated by their adoption of the Australian Nursing and Midwifery Council (ANMC) competency standards for registered nurses (2005). These are a set of competencies representing the minimum core standards for registration as a nurse in Australia. The competencies are organised into four domains: professional practice; critical thinking and analysis; provision and coordination of care; and collaborative and therapeutic practice. The domain of relevance to reflection includes self-appraisal, professional development, research for practice, reflecting on practice, feelings and beliefs, and the consequences of these for individuals. These competencies have been extended to apply to enrolled nurses and also specialty groups, such as critical care nurses and nurse practitioners. The National Competency Standards for the Midwife (Australian Nursing and Midwifery Council 2006) also has reflective and ethical practice as one of its four domains, and the codes of professional conduct for nurses and for midwives in Australia likewise require that they practise reflectively and ethically (Australian Nursing and Midwifery Council 2008a, 2008b).

The Nursing Council of New Zealand has also incorporated reflection as a key competency for registered nurses. Reflection in the New Zealand registered nurse competencies is included under 'Competency 1.5: Practices nursing in a manner that the client identifies as being culturally safe' (Nursing Council of New Zealand 2007). The Nursing Council of New Zealand also has competencies for enrolled nurses, midwives and nurse practitioners. Further information about these competencies is available from the following websites:

- Australian Nursing and Midwifery Council competencies and codes of professional conduct for registered nurses: www.anmc.org.au
- Competencies for the registered nurses' scope of practice in New Zealand: www.nursingcouncil.org.nz

Encouragement for reflection is also echoed in the education sector, in the 'Review of higher education financing and policy (final report): learning for life', or the 'West Report' as it is commonly known (Department of Employment, Education, Training and Youth Affairs 1998), where reflection is listed as an expected attribute of graduates from all undergraduate university degrees in Australia. In other words, it is a requirement of your undergraduate education that you exit the program of study with the ability to reflect. As a result, all undergraduate degree coordinators are now charged with the responsibility of ensuring their graduates have been provided with the opportunity to develop the skill of reflection.

WHAT IS REFLECTION OR REFLECTIVE PRACTICE?

Reflection comes from the verb *reflectere*, which means to bend or turn backwards (Hancock 1999). This infers that reflection is a process of going back over something after it has already occurred. This might include recalling thoughts and memories, in cognitive acts such as thinking or contemplation, as a way of making sense of the situation so that necessary changes may be identified or made (Taylor 2000). We all reflect on what goes on around us to some extent. If you think about it, we do not generally just walk around in the world without noticing things or thinking about what has happened and how it has impacted on us. Similarly, we all reflect at some level on our practice, but it may only involve thinking about what happened rather than theorising about what happened and looking for ways to improve it in the future.

Thus the type of reflection to be discussed in this chapter is actually a much more purposeful activity that leads to action that is better informed than that which occurred before the reflection took place (Francis 1995). Rolfe et al (2001) argue that not all knowledge for practice comes from textbooks, research journals and lectures, or other classroom activities. Rather, they claim that, in addition to what they call scientific knowledge, practitioners actually 'pick up' practical knowledge from their everyday experience, and reflection is the process of *theorising* about that knowledge. As a result, they claim that reflection provides practitioners with access to the processes by which they make clinical judgments, which can then be used to justify actions to others or pass on expertise to less experienced colleagues.

Taylor (2000) sees it as necessary to alert clinicians to the intricacies of nursing practice and the knowledge embedded in it. However, Johns (1998) claims that being a reflective practitioner is more than just noticing things by chance in a situation. He suggests that it involves a deep sensitivity to what is happening around us, or 'a constant monitoring of self within the situation that ripples along the surface of conscious thought' (Johns 1998:14). It is also important not to assume that improved skill in reflective thinking equals learning, which equals improved nursing practice. A study of reflective thinking in nursing by Teekman (2000) demonstrated that learning from reflection is not something that happens automatically. He identified the importance of coaching by a mentor, and a supportive environment, as ways to reduce the uncritical reinforcement of existing patterns of practice.

Much of the contemporary emphasis on reflective practice in nursing can be attributed to the work of the American educationalist Donald Schön (1983, 1987). Even though he was not the first to write about it, he actually coined the term 'reflective practice' (Teekman 2000), and has been very influential in the way nursing has embraced the notion. Schön (1983) argued that reflection is a strategy whereby professionals become aware of their implicit knowledge base. While he did not attempt to define reflection or reflective practice, he advocated two distinct types of reflection: *reflection-on-action* and *reflection-in-action*. The former, reflection-on-action, occurs after the event or action where details are recalled and analysed in some way with the aim of reviewing practice. It has been referred to as a type of cognitive 'postmortem' or an act of looking back at practice (Burton 2000).

Reflection-in-action occurs simultaneously or at the same time as practice. That is, reflection-in-action is said to occur when the practitioner engages in practice and makes adjustments as a result of relevant feedback. Rolfe (2001) claims that reflection-in-action is a more advanced form of reflection and leads to more advanced practice. He describes it as a process whereby the nurse is constantly testing theories and hypotheses in a cyclical process while simultaneously engaged in practice—what he termed 'nursing praxis' in an earlier paper (Rolfe 1993).

Boud et al (1985), however, noted an additional step in the reflective process, that of *pre-reflection*. In other words, they recognised the importance of reflection in anticipation of events. Greenwood (1998:1049) explains how preparing for experience involves the learner becoming aware of what they bring to the event and what they want from it (the personal), the constraints and opportunities the event provides (the context) and how they may acquire what they need from the event (the learning strategies).

THE ROOTS OF REFLECTIVE PRACTICE

The ancient Greek philosopher Plato declared that the unreflective life was a life not worth living. Plato was drawing attention to the view that reflection is a distinctively human activity and without it we would be no more than unthinking automatons, our lives governed by our biological instincts, and forever subject to those forces, human and natural, exerting power over us. Plato saw reflection, in other words, as vital to our identity as human beings, and to our having minds of our own, and thus to our personal freedom. We are free only to the extent that we are a reflective being.

This idea resurfaced and drove the huge change of thinking that occurred in seventeenth and eighteenth century Europe, which became known as the Enlightenment. Enlightenment philosophers such as John Locke in England, and Jean-Jacques Rousseau in France, argued that human beings were free to think and decide for themselves, rather than simply accept the prevailing norms, largely imposed by those in power, and notably by the Christian churches. Today, we just accept this as natural, and probably do not think twice about it, but in those days it was a radical and rather dangerous claim.

This history reminds us of several important principles concerning reflection. First, reflection is not an artificial technique that is being imposed by regulatory authorities or universities; rather, it is the refinement of a natural process that is part of being human, and which needs to be nurtured and encouraged. Second, we should always reflect upon, and if necessary challenge, prevailing ways of thinking and acting, even if it occasionally means being unpopular or thought foolish. When it involves 'big issues', this may be hard to do, but reflection and action working together (i.e. 'praxis') is the impetus for change, and ultimately for improvement. This applies in all arenas of human activity, including your local healthcare setting.

Although there are many ways of conceiving reflective processes, even within the same discipline, reflection as we refer to it here is not simply thinking, but rather thinking deeply, systematically, logically and deliberately. Political theorists have emphasised the role of reflection in challenging the status quo, and it plays an important part in the teachings of some political radicals and revolutionaries. Educationalists, such as the American John Dewey, have emphasised the role of reflection in learning and problem solving, and have explored how reflection is related to experience. Dewey observed that 'we learn by doing and realising what came of what we did'; this 'realising' is the result of reflection.

Reflection also played an important part in the development of psychology as a discipline during the nineteenth century, in the form of 'introspection'—that is, reflection focused upon oneself. Until the rise of scientific psychology in the 1880s, introspection was the primary source of data for the elucidation of human psychology. An especially important figure, who brings the political and educational aspects together, is the Brazilian Marxist, Paulo Friere. His work is widely cited as the basis for the development of reflective processes in nursing, although nurses have mostly avoided acknowledging the political revolutionary aspects of his work. Friere's concept of reflection was developed as part of a strategy for educating and politicising the impoverished and largely illiterate peasants of Brazil, and has an explicit emancipatory intent. The key idea, which makes it 'emancipatory', is that reflection and action should work together (as praxis), in order to generate new, enlightened and empowering ways of thinking and behaving.

This is an important way for you to think about reflection because, as a nurse, you will work in complex systems where you may feel powerless and unable to express your concerns and opinions; in this sense, you too may feel 'illiterate'. In order to create a sense of control and of having a worthwhile part to play, you can begin by engaging in reflective processes, and out of these should arise constructive courses of action, which constitute 'praxis', an idea discussed further by Holmes and Warelow (2000).

Nursing's descriptions and adaptations of reflective processes have been clearly explored in a series of chapters in the classic Australian text edited by Gray and Pratt (1991), and you should read these as part of your continuing education as a nurse (Cox et al 1991, Crane 1991, Emden 1991, Gray & Forsstrom 1991, Lumby 1991). The authors explain how reflective processes bring theory and practice together, what forms they can take, and how they can be used by nurses in clinical, educational and research contexts.

The opening remark in Carolyn Emden's brilliant contribution nicely captures the spirit behind these chapters: 'Reflective practice is of pre-eminent interest to nurses', she says, and '[t]o be a *reflective practitioner* suggests professional maturity and a strong commitment to improving practice—a reasonable aspiration for every registered nurse' (Emden 1991:335). The work of Boud and his colleagues (1985), which was mentioned earlier, plays an important role here. Emden (1991) explains how his three phases of reflective learning—preparatory, experiential and processing—can be undertaken by you, in your workplace, and provides actual examples of nurses' 'field notes', or written reflections. For Emden (1991), as for most nurse authors, reflective processes are inextricably tied to the 'critical social science paradigm'—that is, the politically informed approach we have noted above, which is interested in identifying and changing irrational, oppressive or counterproductive beliefs and practices (Kemmis 1985).

Historically, the most important exemplars of this approach in Australian nursing were the School of Nursing at Deakin University, where reflective processes and critical social theory were used as the basis for the undergraduate nursing curriculum from 1988, and subsequently formed part of the Master of Nursing Studies degree, and the Flinders University of South Australia, where they formed part of the Master of Nursing degree from 1991. Most Australian nurse scholars who have written about these topics are in some way linked to these two schools.

Emden (1991) summarises the ways in which reflective processes have the effect of 'educating the emotions'. Reflective processes should be mutually encouraged, and there is an educative element, as you help others by recognising and responding to their needs and sensitivities, as well as your own; reflective processes also help you come to terms with the uncertainty of clinical practice and with its inevitable injustices and inadequacies. Clinical practice is never perfect; it is always constrained by resource shortages and by the failings of the system and those who work in it. It is part of the human condition that we cannot do everything right all the time, and that things sometimes go wrong. Reflective processes enable us to face up to this reality, but at the same time challenge us to overcome the obstacles and aspire to the best possible standards of practice. They contribute to our development as thinkers, practitioners and as people; that is why Emden (1991) referred at the outset to them being the hallmark of the mature professional.

THE BENEFITS OF REFLECTION

We have referred already to some of the benefits that derive from reflective processes, but let us now discuss these in more detail. Freire (1972) insisted that action and reflection must work together, and we can agree with Emden when she describes action as a 'key outcome' of reflection. 'Action' can take many forms. For example, when you reflect upon your practice world and become sensitive to its inadequacies and injustices, you are most likely to want to do something about them, especially as you consider them in relation to individuals' rights. In contrast, action might involve improving your own clinical skills; your reflections having alerted you to shortcomings in your attitudes or skills, and you take action to bring them to a higher standard.

Another benefit of reflection is that it can help you elucidate the theory–practice relationship. Critical social theory insists that this relationship is 'reflexive'; in other words, theory feeds into your practice, and practice informs your theory. This supports the suggestion by nurse theorists Walker and Avant (1983) that reflective processes can be used to help develop clinical practice by helping you to recognise, evaluate and refine your personal nursing theories (i.e. your beliefs about nursing and clinical practice). Indeed, much of Emden's (1991) chapter is about how to use reflection to help elucidate and develop your own theory of nursing. Since critical social theory is closely tied to these conceptions of reflection, it is widely argued that any theory of nursing developed in this way should be consistent with critical social theory, and many nursing scholars have attempted to show how this can work (good places to begin exploring this topic are Holter (1988) and Crane (1991)). This link has become more difficult to sustain, however, as critical social theory has been the subject of criticism in light of alternative ways of thinking about social structures and processes, including 'poststructuralism' and 'postmodernism' (Holmes 1995).

Another positive outcome of reflection, which follows on from its role in the 'education of the emotions' noted above, is that it sensitises us to the plight of the less fortunate and marginalised people in society. We become more sensitive to the suffering, courage and determination of people who are faced with serious illness, and to the problems faced by those who are oppressed, such as mentally disordered and intellectually disabled people, and people who belong to ethnic and religious minorities. This increased sensitivity impels you towards greater engagement with such people, and a willingness to become involved in their problems. Not only are you aiming to improve your clinical performance with all your patients, but also to act as their support and advocate. You are not only motivated to question inadequate practices, but also to generate possible strategies for improvement. Even though it may be challenging, you will find that you cannot do otherwise, and you will enjoy increased levels of job satisfaction because this heightened level of engagement is intrinsically rewarding.

Once again, it is Carolyn Emden who sums up this aspect so accurately. She says:

The outcomes of reflection are so profound, and so personally enlightening, that you are unable to let them go, or to return to former unquestioning ways. Increasingly, you are likely to recognise, and challenge, those political, social, and historical forces which are unjust, irrational, and oppressive in your professional life: together with colleagues and clients, you will wish to create and implement strategies of empowerment that lead to informed choice and fulfilling forms of action (Emden 1991:352).

We might add that these benefits accrue not just in the context of your work, but also in your life generally. The big claim being made here is that reflection, because it educates your emotions and impels you to action, helps make you a better person and not just a better nurse. Let us now turn to consider the 'how' of reflection.

STRATEGIES FOR REFLECTION

Many strategies can be used for reflection, including writing (e.g. journalling and critical incident analysis), and photography, drawing and other forms of creative expression.

Writing

Reflective writing has been advocated as a technique to aid reflection (Jasper 2006, Johns 2006, Rolfe et al 2001, Usher et al 1999). It involves the use of writing as a strategy to assist us to learn from experiences and involves engaging in the reflective process using writing as an instrument. It differs from other forms of writing in that it is undertaken primarily for the purpose of learning and to assist us to develop a deeper understanding of the subject of our reflection (Rolfe et al 2001). Van Manen (1990) says that writing is a reflective activity where we come to know and understand the way in which we know what we know. This can be achieved by writing and rewriting, so that we come to understand something in greater depth, in ways not previously open to us, and in new or more intimate ways. Further, the 'act of writing forces a coherence and anchors thinking in a way that permits revisiting and reworking' (Usher et al 1999).

Journalling and critical incident analysis are two well-known types of reflective writing, but clinical supervision, poetry, letter, story and group writing activities are also examples of reflective writing.

Journalling

Journal writing has been advocated as a strategy for the development of reflective practice (e.g. Boud et al 1985, Cox et al 1991, Heath 1998, Holly 1984, Usher et al 1999). By the term journal we mean what is commonly referred to as a diary or log. Writing a journal involves the writing of accounts of practice experiences after they occur and allows the writer to take ownership of the content—for example, using the first person and writing about themselves. A simple format for writing a reflective journal in conjunction with a professional diary is available in a pocketsized, spiral-bound format (Baillière Tindall 2008).

However, journal writing offers the practitioner more than the opportunity to recount an experience; it provides an opportunity to return to the experience in its written form and then theorise about the experience from which conclusions are drawn. This type of reflective writing provides for many returns for analysis (Owens et al 1997), and the writer can add, delete or change entries as often as they wish. As a result, it becomes an ongoing critique of the practitioner's thoughts about an experience. Journals have also been described as cathartic because they offer an opportunity to 'work through' problems or difficult situations (Davies & Sharp 2000). The box below lists some journalling techniques, which are taken from Owens et al (1997).

> **JOURNALLING TECHNIQUES**
> - Write a short biography to begin your reflective journey.
> - Select a quiet environment where you will not be interrupted.
> - Write vividly and as close to the event as possible.
> - Include your initial thoughts, but leave space where you can add comments at a later time.
> - Where possible, make use of diagrams, illustrations, photographs and drawings to aid your memory.
> - Make use of a book and use one side for writing and leave the other for later reflections.

Some students find starting a reflective journal a difficult task, but you should remember that there is no right or wrong way to do it. Cox et al (1991:380–381) identify three challenges that face the newcomer to journalling:

1. valuing journalling so that time and effort are allocated appropriately
2. removing the 'censor' that inhibits us from writing honestly and accurately, and
3. reviewing the journal critically in order to identify areas of strength and weakness, and new ways of thinking and acting.

The use of a framework or model as a prompt for reflection has been advocated (Heath 1998, Jasper 2006, Johns 1998, Rolfe et al 2001) and you may find this useful. Have a look at the model proposed by Rolfe et al (2001) in Figure 8.1, and think about how you might use it to aid your reflection.

Taylor (2000:67–68) offers a number of hints that may also be helpful: be spontaneous; express yourself freely; remain open to ideas; choose a time to suit you; be prepared personally; and choose a reflective method. It is also important to avoid the use of abbreviations, and resist the temptation to censor your writing, as this is more likely to assist with the exposure of the 'isms' we hold as an individual.

A further strategy that may also be helpful is the notion of a *critical friend*. Sharing with others opens reflective journal entries to a different perspective. The other person may offer alternative actions that could have been taken or might challenge you to think more deeply about a particular issue (Heath 1998). It is important that the critical friend is someone you trust, as they will be reading your entries and discussing them with you. The role of a critical friend is to support and guide you in your reflection, while posing questions and offering alternatives in a non-judgmental way (Taylor 2000). Duke describes how critical friends have:

> … acted as a sounding board for my ideas and thoughts, sometimes they have given me an 'expert' view of an area of knowledge new to me, and sometimes they have stimulated a thought that I have then gone on to explore (Duke 2000:152).

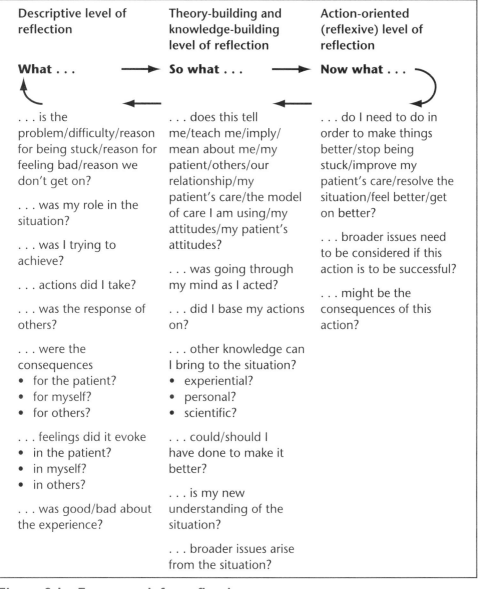

Figure 8.1 Framework for reflection
Source: Rolfe G, Freshwater D, Jasper M 2001 Critical reflection for nursing and the helping professions: a user's guide. Palgrave, New York, p 35.

Ethical and legal issues related to journalling

One aspect of journalling that became a problem in the early 1990s, when reflective processes were still considered strange and dangerous by those in authority in health services, concerns their ethical and legal status. In short, these concerns were:

- whether journalling required the consent of institutions and individuals to whom they refer

- whether journalling was appropriately conducted in work time or in the clinician's own time
- who owned the journals, and who had a right of access to them, and
- what status the journals had in law—whether they could, for example, be used as evidence in the court room.

With the formal recognition that clinicians generally, and registered nurses in particular, are required to be 'reflective practitioners', it is now widely accepted that they should be journalling, and that this is part of their clinical work. Intellectual property is a vexed issue in law, and there does not appear to be any precedent set in Australian law as to the obligations of clinicians in relation to journals, but there does appear to be general acceptance that they belong to their authors, and that employers therefore normally have no right of access. You should, however, be able to reassure managers that your reflective journal conforms to the usual ethical standards that apply in healthcare situations—namely, that they are securely stored and accessible only to authorised individuals (such as your supervisors or educators), that you use pseudonyms when referring to particular patients or colleagues, and that they are strictly for your private professional use.

Like all documents, journals may be ordered to be submitted as evidence in courts of law. Although this is extremely unlikely, and most of what appears in a journal may only have the status of 'hearsay evidence', it is wise to bear this possibility in mind. Another principle you should adopt, therefore, is that your journal should always refer to your colleagues and patients in a professional and respectful manner, even though it may express criticism. Your journal is, after all, not a vehicle for catharsis—that is, unrestricted emotional expression—rather, it is the professional documentation of your deeply and carefully considered thoughts.

Critical incident analysis

A critical incident is usually an event that is remembered as important to an individual or one that is provided to a learner for the purpose of reflection. The notion of a critical incident is discussed by Rolfe et al (2001) who outline how the term is negative because it brings to mind something unfortunate or life threatening, something we certainly found in a study that utilised critical incident analysis with nursing students (Usher et al 1999).

Critical incidents, however, should be thought of as events that are meaningful or significant in some way; they need not necessarily be large or major occurrences (Rolfe et al 2001), and they can be negative or positive experiences (Davies & Sharp 2000). Critical incident analysis is thought to lead to:

> … a deeper and more profound level of reflection because it goes beyond detailed description of an event that attracted attention, to analysis of and reflection on the meaning of the event (Griffin 2003:208).

A study by Usher et al (1999) found that writing critical incident analyses offered undergraduate nursing students an opportunity to distance themselves from an event and, as a result, come to understand it in new ways.

The box below provides a framework for a critical incident analysis, which has been taken from Davies and Sharp (2000:67–68).

FRAMEWORK FOR CRITICAL INCIDENT ANALYSIS

1 Give a concise description of the incident (which relates to the learning outcomes).

2 Outline the rationale for choice of incident and its significance and relevance to you.

3 Identify pertinent issues related to the incident.

4 Reflect on and analyse the key issues, focusing on: your own involvement; feelings and decision making; the involvement and role of others; identification of any dilemmas or ethical elements; and the rationale for action, drawing on relevant theory evaluation of the situation and the implications for practice and personal learning.

5 Conclusion.

Photography, drawing and other forms of creative expression

Taylor (2000) describes how reflection can be facilitated by creative expression. She explains that it is unclear whether the awareness of the creative expression precedes or follows the reflection, but that it occurs sufficiently to include it as a way of reflective thinking. Some have been inspired to draw or write poetically as a result of events they have experienced, while others have used art forms, such as photography, drawing, painting or music in an attempt to express their reactions. Rolfe et al (2001) explain that these techniques are described as creative because they involve using the imagination to transform experience away from the more accepted ways of analysis to the use of metaphor as a way of creating insight and facilitating learning.

SELF-AWARENESS AND CLINICAL SUPERVISION

In essence, self-awareness is the foundation skill upon which reflective practice is based. It offers individuals the opportunity to see themselves in certain situations and to observe how they affected the situation and the situation affected them (Atkins 2000). In fact, this is what differentiates reflection from other types of mental activity such as logical thinking or problem solving (Boud et al 1985). Reflection is also a very personal experience, as it opens the self up to scrutiny (Johns 1998, Johns 2006). As a result, reflection can be disconcerting to the individual, as taken for granted competence and ways of coping are exposed as inadequate.

Self-awareness is also an essential skill for professional monitoring. As a professional you are required to be aware of yourself, and the influence you have on patients and the healthcare context. Consequently, constant and vigilant self-monitoring is an important skill that every nurse needs to develop. Registered nurses need to come to an understanding of their racist, sexist and ageist attitudes, for example, and identify how these impact on their practice. An awareness of your own frailties and susceptibilities is crucial to maintaining high standards of practice.

There may be times when nurses may not care adequately for their own psychological and physical wellbeing, and yet are under pressure from their work and their domestic lives. This is becoming all too common in many professional work settings, and is not just confined to nursing. It is important to consider whether you are going to work tired and distracted; whether you are overanxious, depressed or angry; whether you are going to work with a hangover and suffering the effects of too much alcohol. Many nurses find that the stress of their lives leads them to overuse medications, smoke heavily, or resort to illicit drugs. The reflective practitioner is aware of these tendencies and will take remedial action, seeking appropriate advice and support.

A similar argument applies to any tendency that may ultimately lead to professional misconduct, including inappropriate sexual thoughts, feelings of aggression, and racist, sexist, ageist or other prejudiced attitudes. A reflective practitioner becomes aware of these possibilities, takes action, and thus maintains high standards of practice. This self-monitoring role leads us almost seamlessly into the issue of clinical supervision.

Reflective processes have been linked by many authors to the process of clinical supervision. Marrow et al (1997), for example, outlined ways in which supervision could help develop reflective nursing practice among both supervisors and supervisees, through group supervision sessions, diary writing and so on. Severinsson (2001) has described how clinical supervision in nursing can be based on a 'reflective practitioner model', citing the work of Schön and Johns, both authors we have mentioned in this chapter. She sees reflective processes as integral to the analysis and understanding of the theory–practice relationship, which is one of the goals of the supervisee, and the consequent development of 'know-how'. She also sees reflection as essential to self-awareness, emotional education, and the development of 'know-what'. Supervision should be 'centred on enhancing the practitioner's ability to "reflect-in-action"' (Severinsson 2001:40)—that is, on the care being provided. She explains that:

> Clinical supervision demands reflection on what care is being provided. Reflection can result in a better understanding of oneself. There is a difference between concentrating on the dissatisfaction within oneself and striving not to repeat what caused it (e.g. feelings of guilt). It is important to find answers to questions such as: Why did I make this mistake? Why did I fail to observe factors of relevance in caring for this patient? A deeper insight into patient needs may thereby be developed (Severinsson 2001:43).

When you think about Severinsson's statement, it is not difficult to see how reflection could become a powerful tool in the supervisory process, and lead to real improvements in patient care.

PROBLEMS, CRITICISMS AND RESPONSES

Despite their endorsement by regulatory authorities and encouragement by educators, the use of reflective processes in nursing is not without critics. Some have argued that the evidence for their effectiveness, in increasing critical thinking, promoting learning and improving practice, remains weak (e.g. Burton 2000). However, there are several counterarguments:

- although little research has been conducted on its value to nursing, the concept of reflective practice is supported by empirical research conducted and elaborated over many years, notably in education, and the accumulated evidence as to its value in a variety of disciplines (e.g. science, social work, medicine, law, education) cannot be ignored

- the research results, although limited, are favourable, and there is no evidence that clinicians taking time to engage in critical reflection has any detrimental effects
- there are strong arguments in its favour, which precede any consideration of the value or experience of reflection itself, such as the argument that a problem is unlikely to be acted upon unless it is recognised as a problem, and that learning entails reflection, and not merely experience or the absorption of facts
- reflective processes acknowledge the value of the experiences and beliefs of all members of a discipline in contributing to its knowledge base and practice development; the alternative is that the views of a privileged group are allowed to dominate, and
- reflective processes happen naturally, and one cannot simply stop them without denying an integral part of one's personal identity; the alternative is to be robotic.

Oncology nurses reported reflective practice to be an important aspect of their work and of their support structures (Loftus & McDowell 2000), while the study by Johns (2001) showed that reflective practice serves to reveal the ways in which nurses care.

Finally, for the sake of balance, we should add that there are also a number of theoretical arguments that can be levelled at reflective processes in nursing. Cotton (2001) has brought attention to some of these, notably:

- despite its championship by many nursing authorities, reflection remains ill-defined and elusive; she notes Johns' (1998:2) observation that 'it seems an academic pastime to try and define exactly what [reflective practice] is'
- reflection is a strategy for scrutinising private thoughts, a form of policing or surveillance by oneself on behalf of others; this complaint derives from the work of the French philosopher Michel Foucault (1972)
- reflection only masquerades as radical; in reality it is aimed at imposing a standardised way of thinking and acting, and
- not enough attention is paid to the negative effects of reflection and the problems that arise in trying to be a reflective practitioner.

We believe these are important issues that need to be considered by those who champion reflection, but we do not regard any as fatal to that cause. Our response to these criticisms is, in short, that:

- the meaning of words is a matter of convention, and agreement takes time
- self-scrutiny is a positive feature of professional life; indeed, 'profession' is often characterised by such self-regulation
- the aim is to open up the practitioner's mind to possibilities, not to impose rules, and reflective practitioners are therefore more likely to be creative, to challenge the status quo, and to be independent thinkers, and
- the problems of reflective practice may have been underestimated, but they are increasingly acknowledged; in any case, this means only that we need to be better at reflective processes, not that they should be abandoned.

You should consider carefully, and reflect upon, the claims we have made in this chapter, and come to a reasoned and practical personal arrangement for your own development as a reflective practitioner. To help you do this, consider the following questions, and undertake some further reading on the subject.

REFLECTIVE QUESTIONS

1 How would you use pre-reflection to prepare yourself for the challenge of clinical practice?

2 Write a paragraph about how you will use reflective processes during your clinical practice. In the paragraph, address the following:

   (a) the technique you think would be best suited to you and why

   (b) whether a framework would help you, and

   (c) the benefits you might receive.

3 How will you use reflective processes to enhance your self-awareness and ensure you practise at the highest possible standard?

4 Why is it important for you as a reflective practitioner to understand the theoretical background of reflection?

RECOMMENDED READINGS

Emden C 1991 Becoming a reflective practitioner. In: Gray G, Pratt R (eds) Towards a discipline of nursing. Churchill Livingstone, Melbourne, pp 335–54

Freshwater D 2002 Therapeutic nursing: improving patient care through self-awareness and reflection. Sage, Thousand Oaks, California

Heath H 1998 Keeping a reflective practice diary: a practical guide. Nurse Education Today 18:592–598

Johns C 2006 Engaging reflection in practice: a narrative approach. Blackwell, Oxford

Johns C, Freshwater D (eds) 1998 Transforming nursing through reflective practice. Blackwell Science, London

Rolfe G, Freshwater D, Jasper M 2001 Critical reflection for nursing and the helping professions: a user's guide. Palgrave, New York

Taylor BJ 2000 Reflective practice: a guide for nurses and midwives. Allen & Unwin, Sydney

REFERENCES

Atkins S 2000 Developing underlying skills in the move towards reflective practice. In: Burns S, Bulman C (eds) Reflective practice in nursing: the growth of the professional practitioner, 2nd edn. Blackwell Science, Oxford, pp 28–51

Australian Nursing and Midwifery Council (ANMC) 2005 National competency standards for the registered nurse. ANMC, Canberra

Australian Nursing and Midwifery Council (ANMC) 2006 National competency standards for the midwife. ANMC, Canberra

Australian Nursing and Midwifery Council (ANMC) 2008a Code of professional conduct for midwives in Australia. ANMC, Canberra

Australian Nursing and Midwifery Council (ANMC) 2008b Code of professional conduct for registered nurses in Australia. ANMC, Canberra

Baillière Tindall 2008 Nursing diary and reflective journal. Baillière Tindall, Oxford

Boud D, Keogh R, Walker D 1985 Reflection: turning experience into learning. Kogan Page, London

Burton AJ 2000 Reflection: nursing's practice and education panacea? Journal of Advanced Nursing 31(5):1009–1017

Cotton A 2001 Private thoughts in public spheres: issues in reflection and reflective practices in nursing. Journal of Advanced Nursing 36(4):512–519

Cox H, Hickson P, Taylor B 1991 Exploring reflection: knowing and constructing practice. In: Gray G, Pratt R (eds) Towards a discipline of nursing. Churchill Livingstone, Melbourne, pp 373–89

Crane S 1991 Implications of the critical paradigm. In: Gray G, Pratt R (eds) Towards a discipline of nursing. Churchill Livingstone, Melbourne, pp 391–411

Davies C, Sharp P 2000 The assessment and evaluation of reflection. In: Burns S, Bulman C (eds) Reflective practice in nursing: the growth of the professional practitioner, 2nd edn. Blackwell Science, Oxford, pp 52–78

Department of Employment, Education, Training and Youth Affairs (DEETYA) 1998 Review of higher education financing and policy (final report): learning for life. DEETYA Publication No. 6055HERE 98A. Australian Government Publishing Service, Canberra

Duke S 2000 The experience of becoming reflective. In: Burns S, Bulman C (eds) Reflective practice in nursing: the growth of the professional practitioner, 2nd edn. Blackwell Science, Oxford, pp 137–55

Emden C 1991 Becoming a reflective practitioner. In: Gray G, Pratt R (eds) Towards a discipline of nursing. Churchill Livingstone, Melbourne, pp 335–54

Foucault M 1972 The archaeology of knowledge (transl. by Sheridan Smith AM). Tavistock, London

Francis D 1995 The reflective journal: a window to pre-service teachers' practical knowledge. Teaching and Teacher Education 11(3):229–241

Freire P 1972 Pedagogy of the oppressed (transl. by Myra Bergamn Ramos). Penguin, Harmondsworth

Gray G, Forsstrom S 1991 Generating theory from practice: the reflective technique. In: Gray G, Pratt R (eds) Towards a discipline of nursing. Churchill Livingstone, Melbourne

Gray G, Pratt R (eds) 1991 Towards a discipline of nursing. Churchill Livingstone, Melbourne

Greenwood J 1998 The role of reflection in single and double loop learning. Journal of Advanced Nursing 27:1048–1053

Griffin ML 2003 Using critical incidents to promote and assess reflective thinking in preservice teachers. Reflective Practice 4(2):207–220

Hancock P 1999 Reflective practice: using a learning journal. Nursing Standard 13(17):37–40

Heath H 1998 Keeping a reflective practice diary: a practical guide. Nurse Education Today 18:592–598

Holly ML 1984 Keeping a personal professional journal. Deakin University Press, Geelong

Holmes CA 1995 Postmodernism and nursing. In: Gray G, Pratt R (eds) Scholarship in the discipline of nursing. Churchill Livingstone, Melbourne, pp 351–70

Holmes CA, Warelow PJ 2000 Nursing as normative praxis. Nursing Inquiry 7(3):175–181. Reprinted with comments in Reed P (ed.) 2003 Nicoll's perspectives on nursing theory, 4th edn. Lippincott, Williams & Wilkins, Philadelphia

Holter JM 1988 Critical theory: a foundation for the development of nursing theories. Scholarly Inquiry for Nursing Practice: An International Journal 2(3):223–232

Jasper M 2006 Reflection, decision-making and professional development. Blackwell, Oxford

Johns C 1998 Opening the doors of perception. In: Johns C, Freshwater D (eds) Transforming nursing through reflective practice. Blackwell Science, London, pp 1–20

Johns C 2001 Reflective practice: revealing the [he]art of caring. International Journal of Nursing Practice 7:237–245

Johns C 2004 Becoming a reflective practitioner, 2nd edn. Blackwell, Oxford

Johns C 2006 Engaging reflection in practice: a narrative approach. Blackwell, Oxford

Kemmis S 1985 Action research and the politics of reflection. In: Boud D, Keogh R, Walker D (eds) Reflection: turning experience into learning. Kogan Page, London

Lauder W, Meehan T, Moxham L 2004 Preface: changing the face of mental health nursing. Journal of Psychiatric and Mental Health Nursing 11:1–2

Loftus LA, McDowell J 2000 The lived experience of the oncology clinical nurse specialist. International Journal of Nursing Studies 37:513–521

Lumby J 1991 Threads of an emerging discipline: praxis, reflection, rhetoric and research. In: Gray G, Pratt R (eds) Towards a discipline of nursing. Churchill Livingstone, Melbourne, pp 461–83

Lumby J 2000 Theory generation through reflective practice. In: Greenwood J (ed.) Nursing theory in Australia: development and application, 2nd edn. Pearson Education Australia, Sydney, pp 330–48

Marrow CE, Macauley DM, Crumbie A 1997 Promoting reflective practice through structured clinical supervision. Journal of Nursing Management 5:77–82

Nursing Council of New Zealand 2007 Competencies for the registered nurse. Nursing Council of New Zealand, Wellington

Owens J, Francis D, Usher K, Tollefson J 1997 Risks and rewards of reflective thinking. James Cook University, Townsville

Parker S, Clare J 2000 Becoming a critical thinker. In: Daly J, Speedy S, Jackson D (eds) Contexts of nursing: an introduction. MacLennan & Petty, Sydney, pp 249–64

Rolfe G 1993 Closing the theory–practice gap: a model of nursing praxis. Journal of Clinical Nursing 2:173–177

Rolfe G 2001 Reflective practice: where now? Nurse Education in Practice 2(21):21–29

Rolfe G, Freshwater D, Jasper M 2001 Critical reflection for nursing and the helping professions: a user's guide. Palgrave, New York

Schön DA 1983 The reflective practitioner: how practitioners think in action. Basic Books, New York

Schön DA 1987 Educating the reflective practitioner: towards a new design for teaching and learning in the professions. Jossey-Bass, San Francisco

Severinsson EI 2001 Confirmation, meaning and self-awareness as core concepts of the nursing supervision model. Nursing Ethics 8(1):36–44

Taylor BJ 2000 Reflective practice: a guide for nurses and midwives. Allen & Unwin, Sydney

Teekman B 2000 Exploring reflective thinking in nursing practice. Journal of Advanced Nursing 31(5):1125–1135

Usher K, Foster K, Stewart L 2008 Reflective practice for the graduate nurse. In: Chang EM, Daly J (eds) Transitions in nursing, 2nd edn. Churchill Livingstone, Sydney, pp 275–89

Usher K, Francis D, Owens J, Tollefson J 1999 Reflective writing: a strategy to foster critical inquiry in undergraduate nursing students. Australian Journal of Advanced Nursing 17(1):7–12

Usher K, Tollefson J, Francis D 2001 Moving from technical to critical reflection in journaling: an investigation of students' ability to incorporate three levels of reflective writing. Australian Journal of Advanced Nursing 19(1):15–19

van Manen M 1990 Researching lived experience. State University of New York Press, New York

Walker L, Avant K 1983 Strategies for theory construction in nursing. Appleton Century Crofts, Norwalk, Connecticut

CHAPTER 9

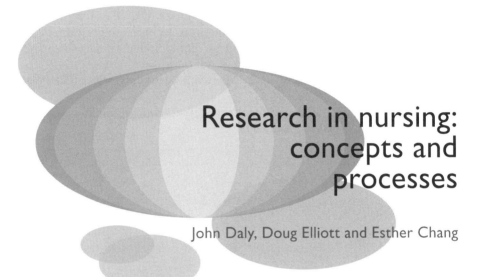

Research in nursing: concepts and processes

John Daly, Doug Elliott and Esther Chang

LEARNING OBJECTIVES

Upon completion of this chapter, readers should have gained:

- an understanding of the role of research in the development of contemporary nursing
- an appreciation of the need for a range of approaches to research in nursing
- basic knowledge and understanding of research processes in nursing
- an appreciation of the contribution of research to the development of knowledge and clinical practice standards in nursing, and
- a beginning understanding of research critique and research dissemination processes in nursing.

KEY WORDS

Quantitative research, qualitative research, dissemination, critique, evidence

RESEARCH IN NURSING

This chapter introduces you to basic concepts and processes of research in nursing. Research has assumed a position of significance in Australian nursing, and there continue to be advances in knowledge development and the sophistication of research approaches.

The concept of research in nursing is not new in the Western world (D'Antonio 1997, Mulhall 1995). In Britain, Florence Nightingale was active in research in nursing in the nineteenth century, though it was not until 1940 that further progress occurred and it was 1963 before the first government-funded post to facilitate research in nursing was established in the Ministry of Health (Mulhall 1995). Nursing research and educational centres were established in some universities in the 1970s. In the United States, government support for research in nursing was initiated in the 1950s (D'Antonio 1997). By that time, many universities had nursing degree courses at undergraduate and postgraduate level, as well as a significant number of nurse researchers with doctorates who were able to provide research leadership for the profession.

In Australia and New Zealand, it was in the late 1980s when nursing was established as an academic discipline with a significant presence in universities. There continues to be growth in appropriately prepared nurse researchers who can provide research leadership, disciplinary scholarship and contribute to the ongoing professionalisation of nursing throughout Australasia. The discipline of nursing, through various professional bodies, has highlighted the important role of research in the continued development of nursing as a practice discipline with a research-based body of knowledge (e.g. Australian Nursing and Midwifery Council 2006, Council of Deans of Nursing and Midwifery (ANZ), Royal College of Nursing Australia 2003). The Australian Nursing and Midwifery Council (ANMC) competency standards for the registered nurse (Australian Nursing and Midwifery Council 2006) clearly identify the importance of research to the registered nurse role. This is given expression in competency standards 3.1 to 3.4 in particular:

- 3.1 Identifies the relevance of research to improving individual/group health outcomes,
- 3.2 Uses best available evidence, nursing expertise and respect for the values and beliefs of individuals/groups in the provision of care,
- 3.3 Demonstrates analytical skills in accessing and evaluating health information and research evidence, and
- 3.4 Supports and contributes to nursing and health care research (Australian Nursing and Midwifery Council 2006:4).

WHAT IS RESEARCH?

Research is a rigorous process of inquiry designed to provide answers to questions about phenomena of concern within an academic discipline or profession. It is defined as 'the systematic study of materials and sources to establish facts and reach new conclusions' (*Compact Oxford English Dictionary* 2004:1). Research is a complex subject and field comprised of a number of well-established but diverse traditions. In a chapter such as this, it is possible to present only broad brushstrokes to familiarise the reader with key underpinnings of research processes in nursing. To develop in-depth knowledge and understanding of any one or a range of research traditions, processes and/or methods, further study and reading from a variety of sources will be necessary.

Research traditions can be investigated in relation to their philosophical underpinnings, and in the course of your reading of research you will encounter a number of essentially different paradigms. A research paradigm is an overarching framework that is based on values, beliefs and assumptions (Parse 1987). This framework contains theory about the nature of reality and guidelines for the methods to be used in carrying out research using (or within) the paradigm (Parse 2001). In addition, the ideas within the paradigm have implications for the type of knowledge being sought in a research study, the way in which the study will be carried out and the way in which outcomes from the work will be used.

As nursing is a complex field, researchers access a range of approaches, including positivist, feminist and interpretive paradigms. Quality research is labour, skill and resource intensive; therefore, a number of important decisions need to be made before embarking upon a research project. Not least, all research must be ethical, requiring adherence to strict guidelines (National Health and Medical Research Council 2007) and obtaining the necessary approval from institutional human research ethics committees.

Research has the potential to serve a number of purposes in a practice-based discipline such as nursing. Research is necessary to:

- test commonly held knowledge or assumptions
- widen understanding of a subject
- stimulate self-action/study
- develop best practice (i.e. research-based practice)
- explain behaviours
- allow predictions, and
- assist in the formation of a body of nursing knowledge.

The use of research knowledge in practice is the most common contact professional and student nurses have with research. This contact will be through reading, reviewing and critiquing research studies published in the literature. Constructing a review of the relevant literature is often called 'secondary research', while developing and conducting an original study is called 'primary research'. Levels of research use and understanding can be described by the '4 As of research' (Crookes & Davies 2004:xiii). These are:

1. **Awareness** of and access to the research literature
2. **Appreciation** or the ability to understand and critique the language of research
3. **Application** of research findings to local practice settings, and
4. **Ability** to conduct original (primary) research independently or in a team.

The aim of the first three As of research is not to produce research workers, but to cultivate and nurture nurses to:

- accept research as a normal and integral aspect of nursing practice
- read and understand research reports
- apply research findings to clinical practice (i.e. evidence-based practice)
- influence colleagues on the use of research data, and
- accept responsibility for their own professional development (Crookes & Davies 2004:xii).

That is, not all nurses need to undertake research, but *all nurses* should *use research* in their practice. Some nurses will also undertake original research (the fourth 'A').

WHERE DO WE FIND RESEARCH?

Literally hundreds of research journals, dissertations, reports and books are published each year. One of the most important steps in the research process is conducting a thorough literature review. Students are often faced with the dilemma of how extensive a review is necessary. There is no formula to determine that 20 or 120 articles will provide the necessary background for the study. The number of references will depend on how familiar you are with the area under investigation, and the scope of the review will depend on how much research is available for that topic. Checking the reference list at the end of recent articles can often assist in the process. Experienced researchers know that maintaining an up-to-date review of the literature is an ongoing process throughout any research activity.

To begin with, it is important to differentiate between primary and secondary sources (this is equivalent to primary and secondary research approaches). A primary source is a report written by the study author/s themselves. A primary source includes information on the rationale of the study, its participants, design, methods of collecting data, procedure, results, outcomes, limitations, recommendations and references. Most research articles published in professional journals are primary sources. A secondary source is one that summarises information from primary sources presented by other authors (see Table 9.1). When an author cites a previous study in the review of literature section, it is a secondary source.

Term	Meaning
Construct validity	The extent to which a measuring instrument measures a theoretical construct or characteristic
Descriptive statistics	Description of characteristics (e.g. frequency, percentages), but no inference of relationships between variables
Exclusion criteria	A list of characteristics that exclude an individual from being in a study (e.g. less than 24 hours admission in hospital, presence of other illnesses that may influence patient outcomes)
Explanatory variable	Independent variable; the intervention being manipulated to exhibit a change in the outcome variable
Inclusion criteria	A list of the characteristics required for a subject to be included in a study (e.g. patients admitted for cardiac surgery, 16 years or older, English language skills (reading and writing) sufficient to complete the study questionnaires)
Inferential statistics	Statistical procedures used to test an hypothesis about the relationships between two or more variables (e.g. t-tests, analysis of variance, regression modelling) and the application of study findings to the population being studied (generalisability)
Integrative review	A style of literature review that combines findings from quantitative and qualitative studies, theoretical and methodological literature using narrative analysis

➡

➡

Term	Meaning
Measuring instrument	The tool used to measure the concept of interest (e.g. questionnaire, biochemical test)
Normal distribution	Distribution of scores for a particular variable follow a bell-shape pattern around the mean score for the sample; required to use inferential statistics
Outcome variable	Dependent variable; measurement of the concept being studied
Primary research	Original research conducted with participants (e.g. patients, health professionals, students)
Primary source	A report of original research written by the study author/s that includes information on the study rationale, participants, design, methods of collecting data, procedure, findings, discussion, limitations, and recommendations for practice and further research
Reliability	The consistency or stability of a measure or instrument on repeated uses
Responsiveness	The ability of a measuring instrument to detect small but important differences of a dynamic characteristic
Sample	A selected group of participants who have similar characteristics to the population from which they were drawn (i.e. representative); allows for generalisation of results from the study sample to the wider population
Secondary research	A process where data from previous primary research studies are reinvestigated (e.g. literature review, systematic review)
Secondary source	A source of literature that summarises information from original research (primary source) presented by other authors
Systematic review	A style of literature review combining findings from quantitative studies with similar hypotheses and methods, to inform research and practice using narrative and/or statistical analysis

Table 9.1 Glossary of common research terms

Both primary and secondary sources are important in different circumstances. Secondary sources such as systematic reviews (SRs) are becoming increasingly common as the best available evidence when reviewing clinical practice issues. However, secondary sources should be limited when undertaking your own secondary research (i.e. a literature review), while every effort to obtain relevant primary sources should be an aim of the activity.

Indexes, abstracts and databases

Most libraries now provide reference sources via computer databases to assist students in locating references on a specific topic and to undertake their own computer searches. A computer search will generate complete bibliographic citations, often including abstracts of many articles published in a particular area of interest. An abstract is a concise summary of a study. A variety of indexes and databases are available, providing bibliographic listings of articles, abstracts, conference proceedings and books. All indexes provide bibliography citations, giving the authors' names, publication date, article title, journal volume and issue number, and pages. Each academic discipline has an index to its collection of journals.

A valuable index and database in the health science literature is the Cumulative Index to Nursing and Allied Health Literature (CINAHL), which has journals from nursing and allied health disciplines listed. Another important index and database is Medline, a bibliography of medical studies (Elliott 2007c). The related database, Pubmed, provides free public access to Medline studies (see www.ncbi.nlm.nih.gov/entrez). Other important abstract indexes that may be relevant to your topic are: Education Resources Information Centre (ERIC); Psychology Abstracts, Sociological Abstracts, Cancer Therapy Abstracts (CANCERLIT); and Dissertation Abstracts International.

Most indexes and databases use key words or medical subject (MeSH) headings. When a topic is not found in the subject headings, you can search key words that have been adopted by most of the journal publishers. Many journals also publish key words with an article. Most university libraries hold extensive collections of refereed journals across a range of disciplines. Many databases now provide full-text papers online, although this function may be restricted to journal subscribers (check with your professional library for access rights to journals).

Peer-reviewed journals

Peer-reviewed journals serve many important functions, including facilitation of expert review of manuscripts, reporting the findings of research studies or theoretical papers, dissemination of papers that have been approved for publication following peer review, and serving as a resource for scholars and researchers involved in compiling and/or developing knowledge in an area of nursing research or practice. Criteria that must be met before a paper is approved for publication in a refereed journal vary, but all editors will be concerned with maintaining a standard of excellence in regard to scientific merit and the literary standard of the work, and the relevance of the paper in terms of its potential to contribute to knowledge development in the topic area.

There are many peer-reviewed journals in nursing internationally. Each has its own aims, purposes and requirements, which must be followed by nurses wishing to submit their work for peer review with a view to being published in the journal. Most journals have a related website that provides further details for readers and authors.

DEVELOPING RESEARCH QUESTIONS

Research ideas come from many sources. Some ideas are derived from theoretical considerations, while others arise from the need to solve practical problems or to improve the quality of care. Having a good idea is often not enough—you need to translate that idea into research questions. This section briefly discusses how to develop research questions based on the amount of knowledge and/or theory about the topic, and describes the importance of a thorough review of the literature to identify relevant theory and research.

A research question is usually developed to direct a study. It needs to be a concise inquiring statement about a problem or issue that can be challenged to generate new knowledge. Although there are no specific rules and procedures for asking research questions, the way research questions are worded can have an effect on the research design and methods that follow.

When formulating a research question, it is important that you discuss your topic and question with your colleagues or experts in the field, as this will assist you with the development and refinement of the question. Often the initial research question is structured too broadly to provide a feasible project in terms of timeframe and resources. Consider the following example: Do undergraduate students taught in a supportive environment increase their learning capabilities as graduates? Before this can be answered, a number of issues have to be clarified. What exactly is a supportive environment? What does it mean to increase their learning capabilities? How do we measure learning capabilities? How do we determine learning capabilities in graduates? Until you can define the terms and determine how to measure the variables they represent, you cannot answer the original question. Frequently, researchers have to narrow the topic area or, in some cases, the types and number of settings or the number of participants they include in the study. This process of narrowing the topic ultimately must also be consistent with the research design and methods of the study.

Research questions can be classified based on the amount of knowledge and/or theory about the topic area. Questions may be exploratory and descriptive, through to testing or confirmatory. Once the question has been formulated, the type of study design becomes clear. Exploratory studies are used when there is little or no literature on either the topic or the population to be researched. Questions at this level are designed to explore the topic or a single population. For example, 'What is ...?' or 'What are ...?' the phenomena or concepts of interest.

Studies that build on exploratory studies have some existing knowledge and theory about the topic and population. Questions at this level often examine relationships between phenomena or measurable variables. For example, 'What is the relationship ...?' between two or more concepts. These questions lead to correlation designs, where statistical analysis is used to determine the significance of the relationship between the variables. Questions at a testing or confirmatory level require considerable knowledge about the topic. Research at this level begins at knowing the relationships between variables; therefore, questions at this level are designed to examine why this relationship exists, with a rationale and with an explanation. These questions lead to experimental designs. Healthcare professionals should constantly evaluate their practice. A questioning approach to healthcare is important in the care of patients.

Reviewing the literature

Whether you begin with a vague idea of a study or a well-developed research plan, every project needs to be considered an extension of previous knowledge. An appropriate review of the literature, in which students will draw on evidence from multiple sources, is therefore a common beginning stage of a study. First, your research question may have been addressed and answered, or a review can be the initial source of ideas for a research question. Searches of the literature will be more successful if they have well-formulated questions. Librarians will often help to focus your question, to assist you in the search and to select databases appropriate to your topic.

By being familiar with the literature and understanding what is already known and not known with existing research and theory in an area, you can devise your research study to explore any newly identified questions. A review will also assist you to establish a theoretical context and rationale for your study. From a practical (methodological) perspective, the review can also reveal appropriate research strategies, measuring instruments, techniques and analysis. The review allows you to learn from the strengths and limitations of other researchers' work in regard to successful outcomes and assumptions, and keeps you current with the research work being undertaken in your area of interest.

NURSING RESEARCH PROCESSES

Research can be either quantitative or qualitative (see Table 9.2 for examples of different types of research approaches). In addition, some research studies incorporate quantitative and qualitative methods. Not all researchers agree that 'mixed methods research' (Burke Johnson & Onwuegbuzie 2004:14) is appropriate because of differing philosophical positions. The issues inherent in this debate are well summarised by Burke Johnson and Onwuegbuzie (2004).

Design	Purpose
Descriptive	Examines characteristics of a single sample; clarifies concepts; generates questions about potential relationships between variables (e.g. case study, cross-sectional analysis)
Correlation	Examines (describes, predicts or tests) relationships between two or more variables, but does not infer a cause-and-effect relationship
Quasi-experiment	Tests a cause-and-effect relationship, but without control or randomisation (e.g. case control, intervention only)
Experiment	Tests a cause-and-effect relationship using randomisation, manipulation of an intervention and control of other variables (e.g. randomised controlled trial (RCT), laboratory experiment)

Table 9.2 Common research designs

Quantitative research

The term 'quantitative research' refers to studies that seek to measure some concept or phenomenon of interest (e.g. blood pressure, pain, or student attitudes to learning about research). The quantitative research paradigm is also called positivist, reductionist or empirical. Quantitative reasoning is termed deductive, which means the thinking leads from a known principle to an unknown, and is used to test a particular research hypothesis.

Quantitative research encompasses a range of research designs and associated methods; the most common designs used in healthcare research are listed in Table 9.2. Selection of an appropriate design relates to the research question being posed (Sackett & Wennberg 1997). The topic of interest may be framed as a question, objective or research hypothesis. Each design incorporates a number of variations; readers are directed to any number of nursing research texts for amplification of these designs (e.g. Burns & Grove 2005, Crookes & Davies 2004, Schneider et al 2007).

Quantitative studies rely on sampling a smaller group of individuals who have similar (representative) characteristics to the overall population of interest. Inclusion and/or exclusion criteria (defined in Table 9.1) are developed, which guide the selection of participants. In experimental studies, the explanatory (independent) variable (an intervention) is manipulated by randomly assigning subjects to a treatment or control group, while the outcome (dependent) variable of interest is measured and other related variables are controlled (e.g. randomised controlled trial or RCT).

Measurement of the concepts of interest is conducted using single or multiple 'measuring instruments' (also called tools). These can be physiological (e.g. heart rate monitor, blood glucometer) or psychological/psychometric (e.g. anxiety scales, functional status, quality of life). Ideally, an instrument should exhibit characteristics that are valid, reliable and responsive. Development of new instruments is time-consuming and resource-intensive, as the validity, reliability and responsiveness must be tested, and modification of items (questions) may be required to improve the performance of the instrument. Established instruments generally have had their validity and reliability rigorously tested over time, and have been accepted as useful research tools.

Instrument (measurement) validity refers to whether the instrument actually measures what it is intended to measure. The aim is for an instrument to have appropriate construct validity—that is, the extent that an instrument accurately measures a theoretical construct or trait that is established over time, following repeated use and testing of the instrument in various studies. With any instrument there is the possibility of measurement error. The aim of a good study or instrument is to minimise the chance of that error. There are numerous subforms of construct validity that have been used to describe increasing rigour for testing an instrument's performance (Elliott 2007a:214). For example:

- **Content**. This appears to include all major elements of the concept. It is often assessed by an expert panel of relevant professionals and includes face validity (i.e. on the face of it, the instrument appears to measure the concept).
- **Relationship**. The relationship to other variables or measures (e.g. criterion-related, which examines the instrument against another or the 'gold-standard' criteria).
- **Hypothesis testing**. This uses theory to test the relationships between concepts.

Reliability relates to the accuracy with which the instrument measures the concept being investigated, and which can be tested in terms of stability (test–retest: similar scores on repeated testing for a stable trait), homogeneity (internal consistency: all parts of the instrument measure the same characteristics), and equivalence (interrater reliability: consistency between observers using the same instrument with the same study participants). There are a number of statistical tests for reliability, which are commonly expressed as a correlation coefficient, ranging from 0.0 to 1.0. A reliability of 0.80 is considered the minimal acceptable coefficient for a developed instrument.

Responsiveness is the ability of an instrument to detect clinically important changes in the variable of interest with a participant (Elliott 2007a:217). This is the opposite characteristic to stability, and relates to the precision of measurement for the instrument. Unfortunately, assessment of this performance characteristic has been minimal when compared to reliability and validity testing.

In addition to the 'Glossary' at the end of this book, Table 9.1 explains some common quantitative research terms used in this chapter. More detailed glossaries are available in specific nursing research texts (e.g. Burns & Grove 2005, Schneider et al 2007).

Quantitative studies collect numerical data to answer the questions or objectives posed. All information is therefore transformed to numbers prior to data management and analysis. Data analysis procedures can be descriptive or inferential, depending on the design and the levels of measurement for each variable (i.e. nominal, ordinal, interval, ratio). The categories must be mutually exclusive and collectively exhaustive:

- **Nominal**. Nominal measurement assigns values to classify characteristics into non-ordered categories (e.g. sex, religion, diagnosis). The assigned numbers do not convey any relative order or weight between the values (e.g. 1 = male, 2 = female; in this instance, there is no implication that '1' is ordered higher than '2', or that '2' is twice the score of '1').
- **Ordinal**. Values are ordered in a logical way in providing a relative ranking (e.g. pain, levels of mobility, self-care, use of Likert scales—'strongly agree', 'agree', 'undecided', 'disagree', 'strongly disagree').
- **Interval**. Values exhibit a rank ordering with equal distance between values (e.g. temperature, scores on a linear analogue scale (from 1 to 10)).
- **Ratio**. Values have the above characteristics plus a meaningful baseline or absolute zero (e.g. weight, height, heart rate).

Data management and analysis are commonly undertaken using software packages (e.g. MS Excel spreadsheet software can undertake certain statistical analysis procedures or Statistical Package for the Social Sciences (SPSS) is a comprehensive analysis package). Study designs and methods that provide findings using inferential statistics allow the researcher to 'infer' that the results from a sample of participants (e.g. patients) can be applied to the wider population being investigated. Inferential statistics are further categorised into parametric or non-parametric procedures. Parametric tests are used when the following assumptions are met: the sample was drawn from a normal distribution; random sampling was used; and data were measured at least at interval level.

As beginning research consumers, students must consider the objectives of the study and the related purposes for the statistical tests performed. Table 9.3 can be used to critique papers for consistency between the purpose, the level of measurement, and actual tests that are appropriate to answer those questions. More in-depth information regarding the actual statistical tests is beyond the scope of this chapter, but can be found in comprehensive research texts.

Qualitative research

The term 'qualitative research' spans a range of research designs and approaches. This field of research has its origins in the humanities disciplines, such as philosophy, anthropology, history and sociology (Denzin & Lincoln 2005). Qualitative research focuses on human experiences, including accounts of subjective realities, and is conducted in naturalistic settings involving close, often sustained, contact between the researcher and research participants (Denzin & Lincoln 2005, Sarantakos 2005). Naturalistic research is often referred to as field research (Polit et al 2001), because it is conducted in the 'field'. This label may be applied to a range of contexts—for example, a community health centre, an intensive care unit or a participant's home.

The purely qualitative researcher approaches a study with a particular set of values and beliefs, which is different from the purely quantitative researcher. These differences relate to the world view (ontology) of the researcher, notions about epistemology (ways of knowing) and research methodology (Parse 2001, Sarantakos 2005). For example, in the qualitative or interpretive paradigm, value is placed on individual

Statistical purpose	Parametric test	Non-parametric test
Compares *mean scores* for two independent samples	Two sample (unpaired) *t*-test (*interval/ratio data*)	Mann-Whitney U test (*ordinal data*)
Compares *mean scores* for two sets of observations from the same sample	Paired *t*-test (*interval/ratio data*)	Wilcoxon matched pairs test (*ordinal data*)
Compares *mean scores* for three or more sets of observations	One-way analysis of variance (ANOVA)	Kruskall-Wallis ANOVA by ranks
Compares *proportions* from two samples	Chi-square (χ^2) test	Fisher's exact test
Compares *proportions* from a paired sample	No equivalent	McNemar's test
Assesses strength of straight line *association* between two variables	Product moment correlation coefficient (Pearson's *r*)	Spearman's rank correlation coefficient (r^s)
Describes *relationship* between two variables, allowing one to be *predicted* from the other	Simple linear regression	Non-parametric regression
Describes *relationship* between a dependent variable and several predictor variables	Multiple regression	Non-parametric regression

Table 9.3 Statistical purposes and related parametric and non-parametric tests
Source: Adapted from Burns N, Grove SK 2005 The practice of nursing research: conduct, critique and utilization, 5th edn, Elsevier/Saunders, St Louis; Greenhalgh T 1997 How to read a paper: the basics of evidence based medicine, BMJ Publishing, London; and Schneider Z, Elliott D, LoBiondo-Wood G, Haber J (eds) 2003 Nursing research: methods, critical appraisal and utilisation, 2nd edn, Mosby, Sydney.

subjectivity, multiple truths are accommodated and individuals who participate in the study are regarded as active participants and partners in the research (Sarantakos 2005). In the positivist paradigm, the opposite applies and concepts such as control, precision, objectivity, testing, one truth, prediction and cause–effect are valued, while individual perceptions are not considered or trusted.

Qualitative research methods are richly descriptive in nature (Sarantakos 2005) and allow exploration of a range of human experiences, which are of interest in a discipline such as nursing—for example, the experience of suffering for people living with terminal cancer, the characteristics of cultural groups, including their health beliefs, or the question: 'What is comfort for recipients of nursing?' It may be possible to study these phenomena using a quantitative approach, but this could be very limiting. Human interaction and intrapersonal and interpersonal communication processes may influence the experience of comfort for recipients of care. Qualitative research approaches would therefore produce richer, more in-depth accounts of this phenomenon.

Sampling approaches in qualitative research deliberately seek people who have lived the experience under investigation. Reasoning in qualitative research is inductive, but may involve a process of induction–deduction. The advantage of using a qualitative approach is that the phenomenon may be studied more holistically, taking account of individual and group perspectives (Nieswiadomy 2002), with a focus on the human experience; this is sometimes referred to as 'lived experience' (Parse 2001). In qualitative studies, the researcher's aim is development of a thick description of the experience under investigation—that is, 'a rich and thorough description of the research context' (Polit et al 2001:472).

Qualitative studies are commonly carried out with small numbers of research participants and involve in-depth inquiry into the phenomenon of concern. The data in qualitative research are presented in the form of words rather than numbers. The researcher may interview participants and audio-tape the conversation, which is later transcribed for data analysis. In this way, narrative text is often assembled by the researcher in working with the research participants. The text of the interview can be analysed and developed into themes to reflect core ideas or recurring features in the data (Miles & Huberman 1994). This process involves intensive reflection on the part of the researcher. The qualitative paradigm is often referred to as interpretive because:

> … social interaction is a process of interpretation; social reality is constructed through interpretation of the actors; social relations are the result of a process of interaction based on interpretation; and theory building is a process of interpretation (Sarantakos 1993:50).

A range of research approaches are available, depending on the aims or purposes of the study. Each approach incorporates a way of structuring the study, selecting the research participants, and collecting and analysing the data. Some examples are provided below. Readers are also directed to nursing and social science research texts for amplification of the approaches to qualitative research described below (Denzin & Lincoln 2005, Munhall & Oiler Boyd 1993, Parse 2001, Sarantakos 2005, Schneider et al 2007).

Phenomenology is a philosophy and a descriptive research method designed to uncover the essence and meaning of lived experiences—for example, suffering or grieving (Parse 2001). 'The phenomenologist investigates subjective phenomena in the belief that critical truths about reality are grounded in people's lived experiences' (Polit et al 2001:214).

Ethnography is a qualitative, theory-building, holistic research approach that is applied to study of the culture of a group (Nieswiadomy 2002, Polit et al 2001).

> In ethnographic research, the researcher frequently lives with the people [being studied] and becomes a part of their culture. The researcher explores with the people their rituals and customs. An entire cultural group may be studied or a subgroup in the culture. The term *culture* may be used in a broad sense to mean an entire tribe of Indians, for example, or in the more narrow sense to mean one nursing care unit (Nieswiadomy 2002:153).

The ethnographer sets out to uncover the insiders' (emic) view of the culture under study as opposed to the outsiders' (etic) view (Polit et al 2001).

Grounded theory is a research process designed to lead to generation of theory through study of a particular human context. In grounded theory research studies, 'data are collected and analyzed and then a theory is developed that is "grounded" in the data' (Nieswiadomy 2002:360).

HOW NURSES CAN USE RESEARCH

Nursing and other health professionals are concerned with improving the quality of patient care and establishing standards for best clinical practice, by examining the current knowledge base of the discipline. Findings from research studies are disseminated at conferences and in professional journals. Some studies are designed to inform practice development by describing a clinical practice, or comparing two (or more) different ways of performing a practice. Other types of studies may shed light on patients' experiences of phenomena that are poorly understood, such as hope or suffering.

The ability to critique studies is therefore a fundamental skill for undergraduate nurses to master in preparation for professional practice as registered nurses. Current registered nurses also need these skills in terms of continuing professional development. However, the skill is not easily attained, and does not magically appear at the end of a single university research course. Rather, the ability is additive and experiential, as it is related to experience, practice and reflection over time. In fact, it is an ability that relates to 'lifelong learning' where we can always learn and improve our skills.

Evidence-based practice

Evidence-based practice has major currency in contemporary healthcare. One of the movement's major aims is promotion of best practice in healthcare based on the best available evidence.

> The evidence-based practice movement currently focuses on the effectiveness of interventions and activities and the term 'systematic review' is now interpreted as a process that summarises and synthesizes the result of experimental and other quantitative studies. The results of descriptive, observational and interpretive studies are therefore afforded little, if any, status in most systematic reviews (Joanna Briggs Institute 2008:1).

The systematic review (SR) is an adaptation of the narrative literature review, which addresses a well-defined question, and provides specific information on the processes undertaken to minimise bias in the review process; it uses a systematic approach to assess the quality of each study (Droogan & Cullum 1998). The question for an SR has a specific clinical focus, with four components forming the acronym PICO:

P   Problem (patient-related or a health issue)
I   Intervention
C   Comparison of interventions and/or control practice
O   Outcome (that is measurable) (Elliott 2007b:53).

When conducting an SR, the search strategy describes the databases (e.g. CINAHL, Medline) used and any journals searched by hand. Selection of articles is by key words in the article title or abstract, as well as any other filters (e.g. English language, study design). A preliminary review of the abstract enables identification of the papers for inclusion in the SR. The excluded papers may also be noted, including the reasons for exclusion. Included studies are then assessed according to structured and explicit criteria. An SR may also include the pooling and analysis of data from the studies investigated; this process is called a meta-analysis.

A number of organisations are now developing repositories of SRs to appropriately guide clinical practice (Cochrane 1972).The Cochrane Collaboration was one of the first to develop as an international multidisciplinary collaborative group to systematically review clinical research, and is now represented in many countries including Australia (see www.cochrane.org.au). The Cochrane Collaboration aims to develop, maintain and disseminate SRs of healthcare interventions, and includes a database of completed and in-progress reviews, a bibliography of SR abstracts and methodological articles.

The majority of the current SRs are related to medicine. This is not surprising, given the number of studies and journals devoted to topics in the various medical subspecialties. The most powerful and rigorous design (the 'gold standard') for examining cause-and-effect questions in clinical practice is the randomised controlled trial (RCT). Thus, the classification developed for rating the levels of evidence (National Health and Medical Research Council 1999) regard the RCT as providing the best evidence to answer these types of clinical practice questions:

Level I: a systematic review of all relevant randomised controlled trials (RCTs)
Level II: at least one properly designed RCT
Level III—1: well-designed controlled trials without randomisation
Level III—2: well-designed comparative studies with concurrent controls
    (e.g. cohort, case-control)
Level III—3: well-designed time-series studies with historical controls
    (before–after)
Level IV: post-test, pretest/post-test

If there is no rigorous scientific evidence available, then the opinions of respected authorities, clinical experience, descriptive studies, or reports of expert committees, can be used to support clinical practice (National Health and Medical Research Council 2000).

The Joanna Briggs Institute for Evidence-Based Nursing and Midwifery (see www.joannabriggs.edu.au) and the Centre for Evidence-Based Nursing in the UK (see www.york.ac.uk/healthsciences/centres/evidence/cebn.htm) conduct SRs of specific clinical practices, which are of importance to nurses.

It should be noted, however, that nursing uses a variety of research paradigms and methods to answer questions that cannot be appropriately investigated by RCTs. We therefore need to consider how to evaluate non-RCT observational studies of nursing practice so that these findings can also guide nursing care. Further, how do we incorporate findings from qualitative studies, which have no generalisability to the patient group in question, but which may provide valuable insights of patient experiences in guiding quality nursing practice? One approach has included explicit assessment of the study description, methodological rigour (including documentation, procedure, confirmability of data collection and analysis), analytical preciseness and theoretical connectedness (Cesario et al 2002).

The development of these necessary frameworks continues to evolve, but they are not yet formed or developed to an adequate level nationally or internationally. The goal remains to foster SRs of relevant studies on clinical nursing so that quality nursing practice will be informed by the best available evidence, regardless of the research design.

CONCLUSION

An understanding of basic concepts and processes in research is central to professional nursing practice. Ideally, quality nursing care is based on the outcomes of quality research processes. It is envisaged that, in time, one of the hallmarks of the profession of nursing will be the utilisation of research evidence to inform the best, safest and most appropriate care for patients and their families. All nurses engaged in nursing practice require research utilisation skills in order to make judgments about how relevant and applicable research findings are to practice. Nursing is a complex, practice-based discipline in which researchable questions will always require answers in order to extend knowledge. A range of research paradigms and approaches are available to appropriately answer these questions.

In the course of your reading and learning about research processes in nursing, you will discover that in some instances researchers use 'triangulation' of both quantitative and qualitative research processes to study a particular area of interest. The evaluative criteria for establishing the scientific validity of qualitative research are the subject of continuing development and debate (e.g. Cesario et al 2002). As the content of this chapter is introductory, you can also expect to learn of other research traditions, paradigms and methods during your undergraduate education.

REFLECTIVE QUESTIONS

1 What processes could be followed in formulating a research problem in nursing?

2 What are the critical features of a comprehensive review of the literature?

3 What are the factors that would guide you in using a particular research approach?

RECOMMENDED READINGS

Bowling A 2002 Research methods in health: investigating health and health services, 2nd edn. Open University Press, Philadelphia

Burke Johnson R, Onwuegbuzie AJ 2004 Mixed methods research: a research paradigm whose time has come. Educational Researcher 7:14–26

Burns N, Grove SK 2005 The practice of nursing research: conduct, critique and utilization, 5th edn. Elsevier/Saunders, St Louis

Carper B 1978 Fundamental patterns of knowing in nursing. Advances in Nursing Science 1(1):13–23

Schneider Z, Whitehead D, Elliott D, LoBiondo-Wood G, Haber J (eds) 2007 Nursing and midwifery research: methods and critical appraisal for evidence-based practice, 3rd edn. Mosby, Sydney

REFERENCES

Australian Nursing and Midwifery Council (ANMC) 2006 National competency standards for the registered nurse, 4th edn. ANMC, Canberra

Burke Johnson R, Onwuegbuzie AJ 2004 Mixed methods research: a research paradigm whose time has come. Educational Researcher 7:14–26

Burns N, Grove SK 2005 The practice of nursing research: conduct, critique and utilization, 5th edn. Elsevier/Saunders, St Louis

Cesario S, Morin K, Santa-Donato A 2002 Evaluating the level of evidence of qualitative research. Journal of Obstetrics, Gynecology and Neonatal Nursing 31:531–537

Cochrane AL 1972 Effectiveness and efficiency: random reflections on health services. Nuffield Provincial Hospitals Trust, London

Compact Oxford English dictionary 2004 Online. Available: www.askoxford.com/concise_oed/research

Council of Deans of Nursing and Midwifery (ANZ). See www.cdnm.edu.au

Crookes PA, Davies S (eds) 2004 Research into practice: essential skills for reading and applying research in nursing and health care. Baillière Tindall, Edinburgh

D'Antonio P 1997 Toward a history of research in nursing. Nursing Research 46: 105–110

Denzin NK, Lincoln YS 2005 (eds) Handbook of qualitative research, 3rd edn. Sage, Thousand Oaks, California

Droogan J, Cullum N 1998 Systematic reviews in nursing. International Journal of Nursing Studies 35:13–22

Elliott D 2007a Assessing measuring instruments. In: Schneider Z, Elliott D, LoBiondo-Wood G, Haber J (eds) Nursing research: methods and appraisal for evidence-based practice, 3rd edn. Mosby, Sydney

Elliott D 2007b Reviewing the literature. In: Schneider Z, Elliott D, LoBiondo-Wood G, Haber J (eds) Nursing research: methods and appraisal for evidence-based practice, 3rd edn. Mosby, Sydney

Elliott D 2007c Searching the literature. In: Schneider Z, Elliott D, LoBiondo-Wood G, Haber J (eds) Nursing research: methods and appraisal for evidence-based practice, 3rd edn. Mosby, Sydney, pp 91–107

Joanna Briggs Institute 2008 The JBI approach to evidence-based practice. Online. Available: www.joannabriggs.edu.au/pdf/about/Approach.pdf

Miles MB, Huberman M 1994 Qualitative data analysis: an expanded sourcebook, 2nd edn. Sage, Thousand Oaks, California

Mulhall A 1995 Nursing research:what difference does it make? Journal of Advanced Nursing 21:576–583

Munhall PL, Oiler Boyd C 1993 Nursing research: a qualitative perspective. National League for Nursing Press, New York

National Health and Medical Research Council (NHMRC) 1999 A guide to the development, implementation and evaluation of clinical practice guidelines. NHMRC, Canberra

National Health and Medical Research Council (NHMRC) 2000 How to use the evidence: assessment and application of scientific evidence. NHMRC, Canberra

National Health and Medical Research Council (NHMRC) 2007 Joint NHMRC/ARC/AVCC national statement on ethical conduct in human research. NHMRC, Canberra. Online. Available: www.nhmrc.gov.au/publications/synopses/_files/e72.pdf

Nieswiadomy R 2002 (ed.) Foundations of nursing research, 4th edn. Prentice Hall, New Jersey

Parse RR 1987 (ed.) Nursing science: major paradigms, theories and critiques. WB Saunders, Philadelphia

Parse RR 2001 Qualitative inquiry: the path of sciencing. Jones & Bartlett, Boston

Polit DF, Beck CT, Hungler BP 2001 Essentials of nursing research: methods, appraisal and utilisation, 5th edn. Lippincott, Philadelphia

Royal College of Nursing Australia 2003 Position statement: nursing research. Online. Available: www.rcna.org.au/content/

Sackett DL, Wennberg JE 1997 Choosing the best research design for each question: it's time to stop squabbling over the 'best' methods (editorial). British Medical Journal 317(7123):1636

Sarantakos S 1993 Social research. Macmillan Education Australia, Melbourne

Sarantakos S 2005 Social research, 3rd edn. Palgrave Macmillan, London

Schneider Z, Whitehead D, Elliott D, LoBiondo-Wood G, Haber J (eds) 2007 Nursing and midwifery research: methods and critical appraisal for evidence-based practice, 3rd edn. Mosby, Sydney

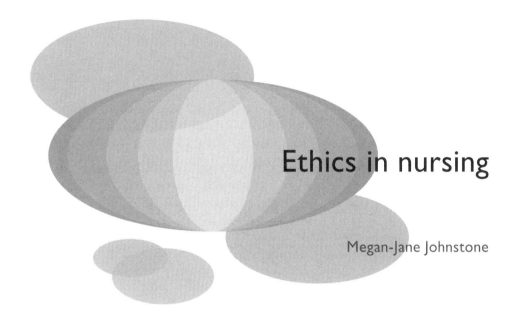

CHAPTER 10

Ethics in nursing

Megan-Jane Johnstone

LEARNING OBJECTIVES

This chapter will:
- define nursing ethics
- outline the development of Western-based bioethics
- discuss the relationship between nursing ethics and Western-based bioethics
- explore a range of 'everyday' ethical issues that nurses might face in the course of providing nursing care to clients/patients, and
- discuss five areas in which a reexamination of the ethical issues faced by the nursing profession is warranted.

KEY WORDS

Morality, ethics, nursing ethics, bioethics, everyday ethics

NURSING AND ETHICS

Nurses at all levels and in all areas of practice are confronted every day with having to make morally relevant choices and to take action on the basis of these choices during the course of their work. This 'everyday' occurrence should not be taken to mean, however, that deciding and acting morally in nursing care contexts is simply a matter of habit or 'daily routine', and therefore as something trivial requiring little knowledge, skill or attention. As can be readily demonstrated, dealing with everyday ethical problems requires of decision makers an exquisite moral sensibility, 'moral knowing', moral imagination, life experience, virtue (e.g. compassion, empathy, kindness, integrity, care, 'decency'), general 'informedness' (e.g. about law, social and cultural processes, human psychology and behaviour, politics), and a deep personal commitment to 'doing what is right'. In some instances 'being moral' also requires political savvy and an ability (personal and professional) to overcome the many obstacles that may obstruct or prevent morally just outcomes from being achieved.

Although it should be otherwise, there are times when deciding to act morally can require enormous courage and even 'moral heroism' on the part of those choosing to take a moral course of action. This is especially so in the case of nurses who, despite an apparent increase in professional status over the past several decades, continue to lack authority in their own realm of practice, continue to be burdened with enormous responsibilities without the lawful authority to fulfil them, and continue to be forced into silence when what they have to say on important ethical issues may threaten the status quo (Johnstone 1994, 2009).

All aspects of nursing (e.g. education, practice, management, leadership and research) have a profound ethical dimension. The ethical dimension of nursing (to be distinguished from the legal and clinical dimensions of nursing) has as its focus the inherent moral demands to:

- promote human wellbeing and welfare
- balance the needs and significant moral interests of different people
- make reliable judgments on what constitutes morally 'right' and 'wrong'conduct, and
- provide sound justifications for the decisions and actions taken on the basis of these judgments.

Members of the nursing profession cannot escape these demands or the stringent responsibilities they impose. One reason for this is that no nursing decision or action (however small or trivial) occurs in a moral vacuum, or is free of moral risk or consequence—even the most 'ordinary' of nursing actions can affect significantly the wellbeing, welfare and moral interests of others. This is so whether in a nursing education, practice, management, leadership or research setting.

Nursing codes of ethics around the world make clear that nurses have a stringent moral responsibility to promote and safeguard the wellbeing, welfare and moral interests of people needing and/or receiving nursing care (Fry & Johnstone 2008). These codes also variously recognise the responsibility of nurses to balance equally the needs and interests of different people in healthcare contexts. What is often not stated, however, is how nurses ought to fulfil their moral responsibilities to deal effectively with the many ethical issues they encounter on a day-to-day basis. 'Dealing effectively' with ethical issues in this instance includes being able to:

- identify correctly the most pertinent ethical issues facing nurses (locally and globally) at any given time

- recognise both the short-term and long-term implications of these issues for the nursing profession generally, and
- develop strategies for responding effectively to these issues, once identified.

Dealing effectively with ethical issues in nursing also requires at least a rudimentary understanding of what nursing ethics is and its relationship to the broader field of Western-based bioethics.

WHAT IS NURSING ETHICS?

In advancing this discussion, it is important to first provide a brief definition of the notion of 'nursing ethics'. Nursing ethics can be defined broadly as 'the examination of all kinds of ethical and bioethical issues from the perspective of nursing theory and practice' (Johnstone 2009:16). In turn, these issues rest on the agreed core concepts of nursing: person, culture, care, health, healing, environment, and nursing itself (i.e. what is it and what is its end or *telos*). In this regard then, nursing ethics is 'not synonymous with (and indeed is much greater than) an ethic of care, although an ethic of care has an important place in the overall moral scheme of nursing and nursing ethics' (Johnstone 2009:16).

Unlike other approaches to ethics, nursing ethics recognises the 'distinctive voices' that are nurses', and emphasises the importance of collecting and recording nursing narratives and 'stories from the field' (Benner 1991, 1994, Bishop & Scudder 1990, Parker 1990). Collecting and collating stories from the field are regarded as important, since issues invariably emerge from these stories that extend far beyond the 'paramount' issues otherwise espoused by mainstream bioethics (to be identified shortly). Analyses of these stories tend to reveal not only a range of issues that are nurses' 'own', but also a whole different configuration of language, concepts and metaphors for expressing them. As well, these stories often reveal issues that may have been overlooked or marginalised by broader bioethics discourse.

Given this, nursing ethics can also be described as 'methodologically and substantively, inquiry from the point of view of nurses' experiences', with nurses' experiences being taken as a more reliable starting point than other bioethics discourses (texts, practices and processes) from which to advance meaningful discussions on nursing ethics and the development of helpful processes for addressing ethical issues in nursing and related healthcare contexts (Johnstone 2009).

NURSING ETHICS AND ITS RELATIONSHIP WITH BIOETHICS

Contemporary nursing ethics has been profoundly influenced by the Western-based bioethics movement. Whether this influence has been advantageous to the development of nursing ethics, however, remains open to question.

In the English-speaking world,* the term 'bioethics' first found its way into public usage in 1970–71 in the United States (Reich 1994). Although originally only cautiously accepted by a few influential North American academics, the new term quickly

---

* A German conceptualisation and usage of the term 'bio-ethics' (*bio-ethik*) dating back to 1927 has also recently been identified (Sass 2007). The German concept, like the first US conceptualisation of the field, 'closely related nineteenth-century progress with the life sciences' and, proposing a 'bioethical imperative', had as its focus the relationship of humans to animals and plants (Sass 2007).

'symbolized and influenced the rise and shaping of the field itself' (Reich 1994:320). Significantly, within three years of its emergence, the new term was accepted and used widely at a public level (Reich 1994:328). Today, both in lay and professional circles, bioethics (and all the issues commonly associated with it) has become the subject of major interest and debate.

Initially, the term 'bioethics' was used in two different ways. The first (and later marginalised) sense had an 'environmental and evolutionary significance' (Reich 1994:320). The other, competing sense in which the word 'bioethics' was used referred more narrowly to the ethics of medicine and biomedical research. Significantly, it was this latter sense that 'came to dominate the emerging field of bioethics in academic circles and in the mind of the public', and which remains dominant today (Reich 1994:320).

The primary focus of contemporary bioethical debate tends to be on 'the big' issues such as abortion, euthanasia and assisted suicide, organ transplantation and reproductive technology. Other issues such as informed consent, privacy and confidentiality, the economic rationalisation of healthcare and research ethics have also all been comprehensibly debated in the bioethics literature since its inception in the 1970s. Not only has bioethics come to refer to and represent these and similar issues but, controversially, has positioned them as the most pressing (or 'paramount') bioethical concerns of contemporary healthcare in the Western world.

The nursing profession, like other healthcare professions, has responded proactively to the modern bioethics movement. Since the late 1970s, there has been a plethora of texts and journal articles published specifically on the topic of 'nursing ethics', in which a full range of the popular bioethical issues have been raised and explored. These works have made an important contribution to knowledge of the field, and have assisted many nurses in their quest to competently and confidently fulfil the many moral responsibilities associated with their professional practice. Nevertheless, the apparent and possibly obvious practical importance of bioethics to nurses, while recognised, is not without controversy.

One reason for this controversy relates to the dominance of the so-called 'big' ethical issues in the nursing ethics literature—a dominance that has sometimes resulted in other issues of greater relevance to the profession and practice of nursing being overlooked. For example, although a great deal has been written on the subject of promoting patients' rights in healthcare contexts (e.g. the right to confidentiality, the right to give an informed consent to treatment, the right to die), comparatively little has been written on the subject of the role of nurses in promoting patients' genuine wellbeing and welfare—which are sometimes compromised, paradoxically, in the interests of upholding their rights (Johnstone 2009). To cite another example, while much has been written on patients' rights to refuse medical treatment at the end stage of life, comparatively little has been written on patients' rights to request and receive healthcare at the end stage of life, including (and perhaps especially) the provision of high quality nursing care from appropriately qualified registered nurses.

IDENTIFYING AND RESPONDING EFFECTIVELY TO ETHICAL ISSUES IN NURSING

It is important to understand that ethical issues in nursing and healthcare contexts do not only involve the so-called 'big' or 'exotic' issues (e.g. abortion, euthanasia); they also involve fundamental questions about the nature and quality of professional–client relationships. This includes examining the more fundamental day-to-day practical ethical concerns relating to the precise impact that nurses' decisions and actions (or non-actions) have on the lives and welfare of other human beings, and the capacity of nurses 'to do harm to others while claiming scientific and professional legitimacy' (adapted from Lifton 1990:xiii).

The kinds of ethical issues faced by nurses today are as complex as they are varied. While in the past attention has tended to be focused on the better known bioethical issues already identified, over the past decade there has been a significant shift in attention towards examining the other kinds of ethical issues faced by nurses today. These issues include:

- 'everyday' practical ethical issues faced by nurses
- a genuine *nursing* perspective on common mainstream bioethical issues, and
- (the otherwise neglected) broader social justice issues associated with promoting the welfare, wellbeing and significant moral interests of highly vulnerable, stigmatised and marginalised groups of people.

'Everyday' ethical issues faced by nurses

As stated earlier, nurses have to deal with ethical issues everyday. The nursing ethics literature does not, however, always represent or reflect the reality of these 'everyday' problems for nurses. Instead, this literature has borrowed heavily from bioethics to shape nursing ethics discourse, and that has sometimes been at the expense of nurses' own experiential knowledge and wisdom.

There is room to suggest that the actual lived experiences of nurses would (and do) provide a far more reliable methodological starting point to nursing ethics inquiry than do the 'top-down' theories of Western-based moral philosophy and the field of Western-based bioethics that derives from it (Johnstone 2009:16). An examination of nurses' lived experiences would, for example, yield important insights into such areas as:

- *moral boundaries of nursing* (e.g. nurses as carers being 'in relationship' with others, as opposed to being what the North American philosopher John Rawls (1971) describes famously as, 'detached observers choosing from behind a veil of ignorance')
- *catalysts to moral action* (e.g. 'experiential triggers' such as 'the look of suffering in a patient's eyes', as opposed to abstract moral rules and principles)
- *operating moral values* (e.g. sympathy, empathy, compassion, kindness, human understanding, and a desire 'to do the best we can', rather than an obsession to 'do one's duty')
- *ethical decision-making processes* (which tend to be collaborative, communicative, communal and contextualised, rather than independent, private, individual, solo and decontextualised)
- *barriers to ethical practice* (which tend to be structural rather than knowledge-based—for example, the power and authority of doctors to determine patient care, organisational norms forcing compliance with the status quo, and negative attitudes and a lack of support from co-workers and managers), and
- *need for catharctic moral talking* (e.g. 'talking through' moral concerns in a safe and supportive environment to help relieve the distress that so often arises as a result of trying to be moral in a world that appears to be growing increasingly amoral) (Johnstone (2009:127).

What talking with nurses often reveals is that it is not the so-called paramount ('exotic') bioethical issues that trouble them, but the more fundamental issues of:

- how to help a patient in distress in the 'here and now'
- how to stop 'things going bad for a patient'
- how to best support a relative or chosen carer during times of distress and when the 'system' appears to be against them
- how to make things 'less traumatic' for someone who is suffering
- how to reduce the anxiety and vulnerability of the people being cared for
- where nurses can get help for their own moral distress, and
- how to make a difference in contexts where indifference to the moral interests of others is manifest (Johnstone 2009:128).

The above and other related concerns are all issues worthy of attention and consideration within and outside of the nursing profession. They are also issues that deserve to be recognised as being an integral part of a sound moral framework and approach that might be appropriately described as nursing ethics.

A nursing perspective on Western-based bioethics

When first emerging as a field of inquiry in the 1970s, Western-based bioethics had as its principal concern the ethics of medicine and biomedical research. This emphasis on biomedical concerns, however, was at the expense of consideration being given to the ethical issues faced by other healthcare professions, including nursing (Reich 1995). One major consequence of this was that the viewpoints of nurses on the ethics of certain medical and healthcare practices were invalidated, marginalised, trivialised or ignored altogether (Johnstone 2009). From the mid-1990s onwards, however, this situation began to change, with the 'special' ethical issues faced by nurses receiving increased attention in mainstream bioethics discourse. An important example of the changes that occurred can be found in the 1995 revised edition of the internationally acclaimed *Encyclopedia of Bioethics* (discussed at length in Johnstone 1999:31–36), and other works (too numerous to list here), which are now much more inclusive of a nursing point of view.

It is also evident by the plethora of nursing literature on the topic of ethical issues in nursing that, for all its past neglect of the ethical issues faced by nurses, since its inception in the early 1970s, bioethics has made an enormous contribution to the development of nursing ethics and will continue to do so. Indeed, as nurses have frequently commented informally over the years, the study of bioethics has enabled them to make sense of their moral experiences and has helped them to feel more confident in dealing with ethical issues in their practice—especially those involving the rights and interests of patients.

Broader bioethical issues

Earlier, it was explained that the word 'bioethics' has come to refer narrowly to the ethics of medicine and biomedical research. This has not only resulted in the marginalisation of the ethics of other professions (e.g. nursing) (Reich 1995), but in the marginalisation of other important issues that do not 'fit' with the mainstream ethical concerns of medicine and biomedical research. For example, a cursory glance at the bioethics literature will reveal a troubling neglect of the ethical issues associated with providing healthcare to highly vulnerable and stigmatised populations—for example, people with mental health problems, the poor, the homeless, the unemployed, people who are drug and alcohol dependent, prisoners, people living with severe disabilities, the aged, adult survivors of child abuse, people from different ethno-cultural and language backgrounds, Aboriginal and Torres Strait Islander peoples, refugees and asylum seekers, sex workers, and gay, lesbian and transgendered people.

As long as nurses interact with and care for people from these stigmatised, often marginalised and highly vulnerable groups, they will be faced with having to make morally relevant choices associated with their care. Given this, it is morally imperative that the many special and complex ethical issues inherent in caring for people within these populations are identified and addressed as a matter of priority, and that nurses working in the field are educationally prepared to respond effectively to these special problems when they arise.

ISSUES AND RECOMMENDATIONS

It is timely to raise important questions about the nature and future directions of contemporary nursing ethics. I do not suggest that the better known issues of abortion, euthanasia, organ transplantation, reproductive technology, patients' rights to informed consent, confidentiality, and so forth, are not important. Clearly, they are important, and will continue to be as long as people are confronted with having to make morally relevant choices related to these issues. There is room to suggest, however, that these more 'mainstream' issues might not have the same priority in different healthcare contexts, nor necessarily be the most important ethical issues that nurses, and indeed other health professionals and the community at large, need to be grappling with at this present time (disparities in attitudes, practices and public policy in regard to end-of-life decision making across different countries is an important example of this (see Blank & Merrick 2005)).

A reexamination of the kinds of ethical issues faced by nurses today is warranted, as is the need to make visible the experiences of nurses in trying to be moral in contexts which can be—and for the most part are—extremely demanding at both a personal and a professional level, and which are likely to become even more so in our rapidly changing and highly unpredictable world (see, for example, Johnstone 2008a, 2008b). While it has not been possible to identify or do justice to all the 'new' ethical issues that nurses face, perhaps the brief discussion given here will provide a catalyst for further discussion and reflection on the nursing profession's global task of making visible and, through this, giving legitimacy to what might be appropriately described as the distinctive field of 'nursing ethics'.

In particular, attention needs to be given to identifying, considering and responding effectively (at local, national and global levels) to issues relevant to the following key areas:

- **Nursing education**. This includes, for example, the ethics of ethics education for nurses (what to teach, how to teach, when to teach, whether teaching ethics is possible, cross-cultural considerations); designing curricula to prepare nurses in 'preventive ethics'; devising and teaching an 'ethics of personality' (e.g. What does it mean to be a virtuous or 'decent' human being? Are nurses as 'decent' as they could be? Is virtue enough to fulfil the task of ethics? Can virtue/decency be taught? How should nurses deal with the problem of evil and 'evil doers'?); preparing nurses to take a stand (e.g. against unscrupulous practices, conscientious objection, action lobbying on local policy issues, broader public policy issues, professional ethical issues, law reforms relevant to nursing ethics); global ethics (e.g. environmental, cultural and political concerns); climate change ethics (including the ethics of refusals to care in emerging situations and 'climate change euthanasia' (see Johnstone 2008a, 2008b, 2009); and ethical issues in nursing education itself.

- **Nursing practice**. This includes, for example, the ingredients of and the processes which facilitate the ethical practice of nursing; 'everyday' issues versus large philosophical issues; the nature and implications of the moral boundaries of nursing and nursing relationships; catalysts to moral action; guiding moral values; ethical decision-making processes; barriers to ethical practice; moral distress; institutional/management support of nurses dealing with moral quandaries; formulation of position statements by professional nursing organisations; the unacceptable moral consequences of the economic rationalisation of nursing care provided by appropriately qualified and skilled nurses; and the increasing use by healthcare agencies of lower paid, unqualified carers.

- **Nursing management**. This includes, for example, how best to prepare nurse managers not just to manage ethically (e.g. treat employees fairly), but also to manage ethical problems effectively in the workplace (e.g. using their positions to develop an ethical culture within the workplace, supporting staff, providing a 'safe place' for cathartic moral talking, institutional/unit policy development, resource mobilisation).

- **Nursing leadership**. This includes, for example, advancing inquiry into the relatively new field of leadership ethics and how best to prepare nurse leaders to *lead ethically* (see also Johnstone 2004).

- **Nursing research**. This includes, for example, improving recognition of philosophic inquiry (of which ethics inquiry is a form) as a legitimate and important form of research within nursing; developing an ethics research agenda (involving all research approaches); facilitation of research into ethical issues in nursing; keeping visible the nursing profession's experience of ethical issues; developing nursing ethics theory; and ethical issues in nursing research itself.

CONCLUSION

Nurses in all areas and levels of practice are confronted with ethical issues on a daily basis. In order to deal effectively with these issues, nurses must be able to identify correctly the ethical issues facing them, recognise the short-term and long-term implications of these issues for the broader nursing profession, and develop strategies for ensuring moral outcomes to the ethical issues encountered in work-related contexts. Achieving these outcomes, however, requires a constant reappraisal of nursing ethics education, ethical nursing practice, ethical nursing management, nursing leadership ethics and nursing ethics research. By undertaking such a reappraisal, members of the nursing profession will be able to ensure that they are well situated to meet the complex challenges and responsibilities of ethical nursing practice that inevitably lie ahead.

REFLECTIVE QUESTIONS

1 Nurses are faced with ethical issues every day. In your view, what are the most pertinent and pressing ethical issues facing nurses today? What are some of the professional implications of these ethical issues for the nursing profession generally, and how might nurses best deal with these issues both locally and globally?

2 How, if at all, might the study of nursing ethics assist nurses to practise nursing in an ethically just, effective and responsible manner?

3 What is the future of nursing ethics, and what influence, if any, do you envisage it will have on the broader field of healthcare ethics generally?

4 Is nursing ethics 'up to the task' of guiding sound ethical decision making in crisis situations?

RECOMMENDED READINGS

Beauchamp T, Childress J 2008 Principles of biomedical ethics, 6th edn. Oxford University Press, New York

Johnstone M 2009 Bioethics: a nursing perspective, 5th edn. Churchill Livingstone/ Elsevier, Sydney

LaFollette H (ed.) 2007 Ethics in practice: an anthology, 3rd edn. Blackwell Publishing, Oxford

REFERENCES

Benner P 1991 The role of experience, narrative, and community in skilled ethical comportment. Advances in Nursing Science 14(2):1–21

Benner P (ed.) 1994 Interpretive phenomenology: embodiment, caring, and ethics in health and illness. Sage, Thousand Oaks, California

Bishop A, Scudder J 1990 The practical, moral, and personal sense of nursing: a phenomenological philosophy of practice. State University of New York Press, Albany

Blank R, Merrick J 2005 End-of-life decision making: a cross-national study. MIT Press, Cambridge, Massachusetts

Fry S, Johnstone M 2008 Ethics in nursing practice: a guide to ethical decision making, 3rd revised edn. Blackwell Science/International Council of Nurses, London UK/Geneva

Johnstone M 1994 Nursing and the injustices of the law. WB Saunders/Baillière Tindall, Sydney

Johnstone M 1999 Bioethics: a nursing perspective, 3rd edn. WB Saunders/Baillière Tindall, Sydney

Johnstone M 2004 Leadership ethics in nursing and health care. In: Daly J, Speedy S, Jackson D (eds) Nursing leadership. Churchill Livingstone, Sydney, pp 89–102

Johnstone M 2008a Emergency situations and refusals to care. Australian Nursing Journal 15(9):21

Johnstone M 2008b Questioning nursing ethics. Australian Nursing Journal 15(7):19

Johnstone M 2009 Bioethics: a nursing perspective, 5th edn. Churchill Livingstone/ Elsevier, Sydney

Lifton R 1990 Foreword to HM Weinstein. Psychiatry and the CIA: victims of mind control. American Psychiatric Press, Washington DC and London, pp ix–xiv

Parker R 1990 Nurses stories: the search for a relational ethic of care. Advances in Nursing Science 13(1):31–40

Rawls J 1971 A theory of justice. Oxford University Press, Oxford

Reich W 1994 The word 'bioethics': its birth and the legacies of those who shaped its meaning. Kennedy Institute of Ethics Journal 4:319–335

Reich W 1995 The word 'bioethics': the struggle over its earliest meanings. Kennedy Institute of Ethics Journal 5:19–34

Sass H-M 2007 Fritz Jahr's 1927 concept of bioethics. Kennedy Institute of Ethics Journal 17(4):279–295

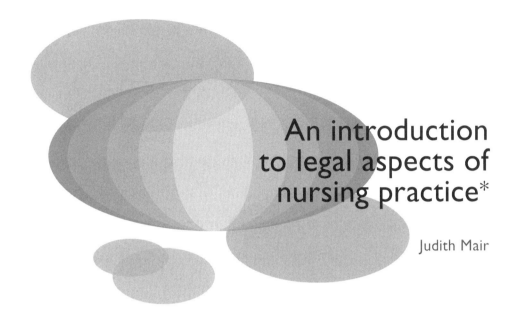

CHAPTER II

An introduction to legal aspects of nursing practice*

Judith Mair

LEARNING OBJECTIVES

Upon completion of this chapter, the reader will have gained insights into:

- the basics of the Australian legal system
- basic principles of law applicable to nursing practice
- the legal rights of patients
- the role of the criminal law in nursing practice, and
- legal rules governing the registration and discipline of nursing.

KEY WORDS

Litigation, common law, precedents, legislation, assault, safety, negligence, duty of care, consent

---

*The author acknowledges that material for this chapter was drawn from a previously published work: Mair J, Blackmore K 1992. In: Cuthbert M, Duffield C, Hope J (eds) Management in nursing. WB Saunders/ Baillière Tindall, Sydney.

INTRODUCTION

Today, more than ever, nurses have to consider the legal implications of their practice. Litigation against healthcare professionals has increased as healthcare consumers become more aware of their legal rights and, as the law develops, to recognise more factual circumstances that can give rise to a legal action. Operating alongside these changes is a higher patient expectation of a good outcome from the delivery of healthcare services.

This chapter serves as an introduction to law relevant to nursing practice. This introduction is necessarily brief, and does not cover all aspects of the law that affect nursing practice. Nurses should develop a deeper understanding of the legal system in which they practice, and the laws that govern clinical practice, through lectures and further reading.

THE COMMON LAW BASIS

The common law developed in England from the fourteenth century and became the basis of the legal systems of countries that were colonised by England. Thus the English common law forms the basis of the legal systems of, among others, Australia, New Zealand, Canada and the United States. It is within these jurisdictions, as well as in England, that law relevant to nursing practice has developed.

The primary source of law in common law countries is a combination of common law and legislation. Common law consists of the application of legal principles developed in past cases to determine the outcome of present cases. Common law is based upon the doctrine of precedent (i.e. by looking at how cases have been decided in the past and applying the principles developed in those cases to the present). Cases that have an important impact on the common law are reported in law reports relevant to particular courts. Less important cases are unreported but can still be accessed.

Precedents are either binding or authoritative. *Binding precedents* are those laid down by a high court in a hierarchy of courts, which a lower court must follow. In the absence of a binding local precedent, a court may apply *authoritative precedents*, which are binding principles developed in courts of other jurisdictions, and which appear to be good law applicable to the local jurisdiction.

The common law remains the major source of law covering clinical practice. For example, the law relating to assault, false imprisonment, negligence and negligent advice is found within cases in which relevant principles of law recognising the right of a person to individual autonomy and bodily integrity have been developed. A court exercising equity can provide an alternate remedy where a common law remedy is insufficient to redress the wrong complained of. A court exercising equitable jurisdiction can issue an injunction to require another to desist from doing something, or can make an order for specific performance to a defaulting party under a valid contract to perform their part of the contract.

The second type of law is *legislation*, or statutory law, which is law developed by parliamentarians through the parliamentary process. An individual piece of legislation is referred to as a statute or an Act of parliament. Legislation is important in that legislative provisions prevail where there is any inconsistency with the common law. Thus parliamentary law can be used to change the law where it is considered that the common law is deficient.

Legislation can create new law that is not known at common law. An example of this is the statutory definition of brain death, which has enabled the removal of organs from a person whose brain has ceased to function but whose heart and lung activity is being sustained artificially.

Nurses practising in Australia need to be aware that, under the Australian system of Federation, the law can and often does differ from state to state or territory. As well as state-by-state and territory differences, the federal government has power, by virtue of the Constitution, to make laws that are binding on all states and territories (i.e. the *Commonwealth of Australia Constitution Act*). In some cases, this law-making power is exclusive to the federal government (e.g. the defence power). In other cases, the states and territories have a concurrent power to make law (e.g. taxation). However, in the latter case, a federal law will override a state/territory law where the federal law is intended to cover the field or there is an inconsistency between a valid federal law and a state/territory law (section 109 of the Constitution). The states and territories have residual power to make laws in all cases where the federal government has no power under the Constitution, express or implied, to do so. Most health law, such as the regulation of hospitals and nursing practice, falls within state/territory law.

Differences in law from state to state and territory are less obvious in common law cases. In the absence of any binding judgment from the High Court of Australia, judges in the superior courts of each state and territory are free to interpret and apply the common law as cases come before them for adjudication. However, judges generally adhere to the principles developed in previous common law cases heard locally, or from other respected common law courts.

It is within parliamentary law that significant differences can arise. Legislation in one jurisdiction (state/territory) does not bind people in another jurisdiction unless the legislation has valid extraterritorial application. Even in this latter case, there must be some connection with the state/territory promulgating (proclaiming) the law. Thus a criminal offence which is found in one state/territory statute cannot serve to convict a person where the offence occurs in a state/territory which does not have such an offence embodied within its legislation. Individual states/territories may enact parliamentary law to govern particular matters, while other states/territories may leave such matters to be covered by common law. For example, not all states/territories have legislated to control the reproductive technologies and those that have are not identical.

Law is divided into civil and criminal. *Civil law* involves legal actions taken by complainants against another or others seeking a civil remedy for a legally recognised wrong—for example, a complainant (the plaintiff) seeking compensation for pain and suffering as a result of a nurse giving an injection incorrectly. The negligent practitioner is normally referred to as the defendant in the case. The task (onus) of proving the case rests with the plaintiff on the balance of probabilities.

The *criminal law* consists of prosecutions brought on behalf of the state/territory to punish breaches of criminal offences, and a guilty verdict results in a fine and/or custodial sentence. The onus of proving a criminal offence lies with the prosecution, which must prove its case beyond a reasonable doubt. The criminal law of murder and manslaughter, criminal assault and criminal negligence are some of the major criminal offences that can apply to nursing practice.

Legislation in all jurisdictions provides for limitation periods to apply for civil claims in the courts (e.g. *Limitation Act 1969* (NSW)). An aggrieved party must commence an action within the specified limitation period; otherwise the claim will become statute barred. Limitation periods vary from jurisdiction to jurisdiction, but most are around three to seven years after the cause of action arises, or, in some cases, when the plaintiff first becomes aware that a cause of action exists. Notwithstanding that a limitation period has lapsed, it is usually possible to apply to a court to extend a limitation period in prescribed circumstances (e.g. a person who contracts HIV through a blood transfusion may not be aware that they have contracted the disease until sometime after the expiration of a limitation period).

Whatever limitation period applies, most jurisdictions suspend the limitation period while an injured party is a minor. Therefore, a child who suffers an injury as a result of alleged negligence is not affected by a limitation period until reaching majority. A person acting as 'tutor' for the child may take action on behalf of the child in the child's name prior to majority. If this is done, the evidence necessary to prove the case is more easily available sooner after the event than later.

Unless specifically stated, no limitation periods apply to most criminal offences. Thus a nurse who causes the death of a patient intentionally or recklessly could be charged with murder or manslaughter many years after the event should evidence to support such a charge arise.

CIVIL LAW

As noted above, civil law involves legal actions taken by complainants against another, or others, seeking a civil remedy for a legally recognised wrong. Nurses need to work within the context of civil law, as it relates to: patient safety; negligent advice; patient consent; patient freedom of movement; and patients' property.

Patient safety

By the very nature of their practice, nurses are engaged in close physical contact with patients. Some of the procedures performed by nursing staff pose risks to patients should the procedures be performed without due care and skill. If a patient suffers harm as a result of a nurse's failure to perform nursing duties at the standard to be expected of the nurse in the circumstances, then the patient has a right to sue in negligence to recover compensation.

Negligence is a *tort*, which means a civil wrong. The tort of negligence arises from the common law and is a means by which a person who suffers injury through a negligent act or omission can obtain compensation from the person responsible for the injury. The onus of proving the negligence lies upon the plaintiff, the person alleging the negligence. To succeed in an action of negligence against a nurse, the plaintiff must prove, on the balance of probabilities, that the nurse was negligent. The plaintiff must prove that the nurse owed the patient a legal duty of care, that the nurse breached this duty of care, and that the patient suffered harm as a result of that breach. The plaintiff must prove each and every one of these elements. Any act or omission that is not found to be negligent is referred to as an unavoidable accident.

In determining whether or not a legal duty of care exists, the courts resort to a test of foreseeability. Thus a duty of care can be shown to exist when a person can reasonably foresee that his or her acts or omissions are likely to place another at risk (see the case of *Donoghue versus Stevenson* [1932] AC 562). This is an objective test and the defendant's conduct is measured by a 'reasonable person' test. The fact that something is foreseeable is not sufficient—the test is 'reasonable foreseeability'. Thus it is reasonably foreseeable that a patient may suffer harm, such as nerve damage, if an injection is given incorrectly. On the other hand, it may not be reasonably foreseeable if the patient suffers some reaction to a drug which is idiopathic that could not have been anticipated with all proper care and history taking. Some risks are unknown and are therefore unknowable until such time as research and experience reveal them (e.g. the fact that giving Thalidomide to pregnant women to treat morning sickness can cause phocomelia in the unborn). Once known, the question arises as to whether the newly discovered 'foreseeable' risk is an 'unreasonable risk'.

The duty of care is to avoid unreasonable risk of harm to another. All people living in a society are expected to take some care for themselves and cannot complain if they suffer loss or injury from an accepted risk of harm. The law will often determine an unreasonable risk of harm by looking at the harm that is likely to be caused and/or the frequency of its occurrence. For example, if a particular harm is known to occur frequently as a result of particular acts or omissions, then the law is likely to hold that these will give rise to a duty of care. Likewise, the law will hold that a duty of care exists in any case where the foreseeable risk can result in serious disability or death, however infrequently such harm is likely to occur.

In some cases the law will hold that a particular risk, which may normally be considered 'unreasonable', may be taken to avoid a greater risk of harm. This is sometimes referred to as 'balancing the risks'. Thus it may be reasonable to do something that clearly poses a risk of harm to another, where the act is intended to avert a greater risk of harm. In one American case it was held that burns resulting from the application of hot water bottles in an emergency were not caused by negligence, as they arose from a calculated risk to avoid a grave risk of harm to the patient. The patient was suffering from severe shock caused by severe postpartum haemorrhage and the hot water bottles had been applied as a part of emergency treatment (*McDermott versus St Mary's Hospital* 133 A 2d 608 (1957)).

Clearly, a duty of care will exist to avoid unreasonable risk of harm to patients receiving nursing care. However, the law does not require that there be an identified person in existence at the time that a negligent act or omission occurs. The law can impose a duty of care in circumstances where a class of persons is likely to be affected now or in the future. Thus, a duty of care can arise to avoid harm to an unborn child, as well as to one that is not even conceived at the time of the negligent act or omission. In such a case, the child must be born alive and prove that any injury present at birth resulted from a breach of duty to take care not to injure it while it was unborn (*X & Y (by her tutor) versus Pal and Ors* (1991) 23 NSWLR 27).

Whether or not a breach of the duty of care has occurred requires consideration of the standard of care required in the circumstances. The standard of care is not perfect care, but reasonable care. It is an objective test and therefore is not dependent upon the particular skills and knowledge of the practitioner. The standard expected of the healthcare worker is that which is attributed to the class of healthcare workers to which the defendant belongs. Thus the conduct of a nurse will be measured against that of the 'hypothetical reasonably competent nurse'.

Nurses who claim to have special skills will be required to exhibit a higher standard of care. Thus the clinical nurse specialist will be measured against the standard of the reasonably competent clinical nurse specialist, while the general ward staff will be measured against the standard expected of the reasonably proficient general ward nurse. An enrolled nurse's practice will be measured against that of the reasonably competent enrolled nurse.

The standard of care required can vary according to the condition of the patient and the patient's capacity for self-care. In considering the standard of care required, the nurse must take into account characteristics of the patient that may pose an additional risk for that person. Thus a higher standard of care will be required for a patient recovering from a general anaesthetic following surgery than for a patient who is fully conscious and has been returned to the ward.

The circumstances in which care is being provided can also be a relevant consideration in determining the standard of care required. A nurse involved in resuscitating a person at an accident site away from a well-equipped hospital with trained staff at hand can only be expected to provide the standard of care that is reasonable in the circumstances. Provided the nurse exercises reasonable care and skill in the circumstances, there would be no breach of the duty of care.

Damage is the gist of the case in an action of negligence; a plaintiff must prove that foreseeable damage resulted from a breach of duty by the nurse. Damage may be physical, mental, financial, or a combination of these. Once the plaintiff has proved that the nurse's breach of duty caused damage that was reasonably foreseeable, the defendant will be held liable to compensate for that damage and any further loss that flows reasonably and naturally upon the initial injury. Pain and suffering, loss of enjoyment of life, loss of expectation of life, loss of opportunity in life, and financial consequences are examples of accepted heads of damage (categories of damage recognised by the courts) for which compensation can be sought in a negligence action.

There is a principle in law that a person must take his victim as he finds him. This is called the 'egg-shell skull rule'. What it means is that if the victim suffers greater harm because they have a particular disability, disorder or trait that renders them vulnerable to greater harm, then the tortfeasor must compensate for the full cost of the harm even though it is greater than that for other victims (*Smith versus Leech Brain* [1962] 2 QB 405). An example would be harm caused by increased blood loss where the victim is a haemophiliac. In such cases it is irrelevant whether the tortfeasor was aware that the victim was particularly vulnerable.

If death occurs as a result of negligence, legislation provides that prescribed persons, usually close relatives, can bring an action against the person whose negligence caused the death (e.g. *Compensation to Relatives Act 1897* (NSW)), provided the deceased would have been entitled to make a claim had they lived. For example, a man and his children may commence an action to be compensated for nervous shock suffered as a result of the death of the wife and mother caused by a negligent nursing act or omission.

Finally, the plaintiff must prove causation—that is, that the breach of duty caused the alleged harm. To prove a direct causal connection, the 'but for' test can be applied. But for the act or omission of the defendant, would the plaintiff have suffered the alleged harm? Even when an act or omission can be shown to have been negligent, a claim for damages will fail if the plaintiff cannot prove that the alleged harm was caused or materially contributed to by the defendant's negligent conduct.

There are three main defences to an action in negligence. These are contributory negligence, *novus actus interveniens* and *volenti non fit injuria*. A defendant can claim contributory negligence where the plaintiff can be shown to have been partially responsible for what happened. The court will award damages in proportion to the extent it accepts that the plaintiff was negligent (*Kalokerinos versus Burnett* CA 40243/95).

Novus actus interveniens is applicable when a second negligent act results in increased harm to a person who has suffered harm from a prior negligent act. However, the second negligent act must be such that the chain of causation flowing from the first negligent act is broken. For example, if a nurse's negligence caused brain damage to a child, necessitating intensive care, and the negligence of a second nurse in the intensive care unit exacerbated the harm to the child, then the first nurse could still be held liable for the increased harm as it was the original tortfeasor's act or omission which exposed the child to a subsequent risk of harm. However, if the child were discharged from hospital following the maximum care that could be given, and then dies from other injuries sustained in a motor vehicle accident caused through another's negligence, then the first nurse is unlikely to be held responsible for the death.

Volenti non fit injuria applies when a plaintiff can be shown to have knowledge of risks and voluntarily undertakes those risks. As such, this defence has not been a major factor in cases involving the provision of healthcare services. Its main application is to cases involving sports and dangerous occupations. It cannot be argued that a patient voluntarily agrees to accept all known risks in healthcare.

When a plaintiff has suffered harm as a result of another's negligence, the plaintiff is required by law to minimise (mitigate) any loss. Thus an injured person is required to take reasonable steps to reduce the effects of (ameliorate) the harm caused. To the extent that there is an unreasonable failure to mitigate, a court will discount the amount of compensation that the plaintiff would have received.

In 2002, the New South Wales Parliament enacted the *Civil Liability Act*, which modifies the law of negligence for New South Wales. In addition to statutorily providing the principles upon which claims for negligence may be made, which reflects the common law, the Act modifies the criteria for the awarding of damages in civil negligence cases. Insofar as professional negligence is concerned, the Act provides that, subject to exceptions:

A person practising a profession ('a professional') does not incur a liability in negligence arising from the provision of a professional service if it is established that the professional acted in a manner that (at the time the service was provided) was widely accepted in Australia by peer professional opinion as competent practice (section 5O).

Section 57 of the *Civil Liability Act* protects 'good samaritans' from personal civil liability in respect of their acts or omissions in providing emergency assistance to an injured person or a person at risk of being injured. This protection from liability does not extend to where the good samaritan's ability to exercise reasonable care and skill was impaired due to being under the influence of drugs or alcohol or when the good samaritan is impersonating a healthcare or emergency services worker or a police officer. The New South Wales *Health Care Liability Act* 2001 makes provision with respect to the recovery of damages for injury or death caused by medical practitioners and other healthcare providers and makes professional indemnity compulsory for medical practitioners.

All other states and territories have introduced similar legislation to New South Wales. These Acts enhancing or modifying the common law, to a greater or lesser degree, are variously called civil liability (Queensland, South Australia, Tasmania and Western Australia), wrongs (Victoria), or personal injuries (Northern Territory) Acts. Some also provide protection from liability for persons rendering healthcare in emergency situations. Given that each of these Acts varies from state to state, nurses should source the relevant statute in the state in which they are practising.

Negligent advice

During the course of professional practice, patients ask nurses for advice on a whole range of matters such as diet and how to care for themselves after discharge from hospital. In giving advice, nurses must exercise a reasonable standard of care where the patient could suffer harm as a result of following the advice. Failure to exercise reasonable care in giving advice could leave a nurse open to an action of negligent advice.

The tort of negligent advice is a negligence action that is brought for damage caused by the giving of advice rather than by a defendant's act or omission. Liability for the tort is also applicable to the giving of information where the defendant has a sufficient interest to see that the information given is correct (e.g. providing an information sheet outlining dietary requirements).

For an action in negligent advice to be successful, the plaintiff must prove that the advisor is a professional (or claiming to have equivalent skills) and that the advisor was willing to use those skills to advise the plaintiff, in the knowledge that the plaintiff intended to make a decision in reliance upon that advice. It must be reasonable for the plaintiff to do so.

The plaintiff cannot succeed simply because the advice was wrong. The plaintiff must prove that the nurse owed a duty of care, failed to exercise reasonable care in the giving of the advice—according to the standards of a reasonably competent nurse—and that the plaintiff suffered harm following the advice (*Hills versus Potter* [1983] 3 All ER 716). It must be reasonable for the patient to rely upon the nurse's advice. A disclaimer of responsibility is effective; however, disclaiming responsibility for any advice given in the context of nursing care would be inappropriate given that a nurse's role involves giving advice to patients.

In order to avoid being sued for negligent advice, nurses should ensure that their nursing knowledge remains up to date and never give an impression that they have particular skills when they lack the capacity to give advice. When asked to give advice on a matter about which they lack knowledge, a nurse should either make it clear to a patient that they are not skilled in giving particular advice and consult with someone who can give appropriate advice, or not give the advice and refer the patient to another experienced and competent practitioner. In so doing, a nurse will be exercising an appropriate standard of care.

Patient consent

Most nursing practice involves touching patients. In accordance with common law principles, all persons have the right to determine what treatments or diagnostic tests they will be subjected to, unless there is some overriding law which allows treatment without consent. When a competent adult patient is treated without consent, that patient has a right to sue for assault. If a patient claims that treatment was carried out without sufficient information being given, then the patient must 'sue in negligence'.

Assault is a tort, which serves to protect an individual's right to autonomy and self-determination. Assault consists of intentionally creating in another person an apprehension of imminent unwanted and unlawful contact. Although the actual touching of another without lawful authority is technically known as battery, the term assault is now in use to represent both the apprehension of and the unlawful contact itself.

Touching in anger, even if slight, is an assault. However, an assault may also be committed where a person is touched without consent and the touching is not an accepted incident of everyday life, for which a person is deemed to have given consent. Touching which occurs during medical examinations and diagnosis is not regarded in law as an incidental touching in society; therefore, for such touching to be lawful, it must be with the patient's consent or other lawful justification.

An assault is complete once touching has occurred without lawful justification; therefore, there is no need for a patient to prove that damage occurred as a result of the touching. It is not a defence to assault that treatment was carried out in good faith for the benefit of the patient when the patient is capable of giving consent and has not done so. A nurse may have intended to benefit the patient, but this issue will only go to mitigation and does not negative an assault if treatment was carried out without consent.

The law acknowledges that there are a number of ways in which consent can be sought. Consent may be obtained orally by asking the patient's permission before commencing treatment, and receiving an affirmative response. Consent may also be implied by the patient's overt physical response to suggested treatments. For example, the patient turns over and exposes a buttock when the nurse approaches with an expected injection. Consent in writing, and witnessed, is usually sought for major intrusions of the body, such as surgery. However, consent in writing cannot be taken to be absolute evidence of consent. A written and signed consent form comes under the best evidence rule but is not conclusive of a valid consent. In an emergency where a person is unable to give consent, a nurse is entitled to proceed to carry out measures that are aimed at saving life or avoiding severe injury while the emergency exists.

A patient's consent must be valid. A valid consent is one that is voluntarily given, covers the treatment to be carried out, and is given by a legally competent person who has been given sufficient information about the procedure to be performed. A voluntary consent is one that is given freely by the patient in the absence of fraud or duress (see *Beausoleil versus Sisters of Charity* (1966) 53 DLR 2d 65). The consent must cover the treatment to be carried out, and any treatment that is related to the initial treatment. Any procedures carried out beyond that for which the patient consented can result in a complaint of assault.

In order to give an informed consent, the patient must have a good understanding of what is to be done and the risks involved. Once the patient has been advised in broad terms of the nature of the procedure to be performed and agrees to it being performed, then there is no assault. However, any issue relating to the degree of information given regarding risks involved is a matter for the general law of negligence and is determined by what a patient should be told. In short, all patients should be told all 'material risks' inherent in a procedure, together with any risks that are of particular importance to the patient. What is a material risk is one, if in the circumstances of the particular case, a reasonable person in the patient's position, or the practitioner is or should be reasonably aware that the particular patient, if warned of the risk, would be likely to attach significance to it (*Rogers v Whitaker* (1992) 175 CLR 479). The concept of therapeutic privilege (withholding information from a patient) may still be applicable in very limited circumstances.

Legal capacity covers mental capacity and children. Mental health patients have issues involving consent to treatment covered by legislation in the various states/ territories. Where a patient is unconscious or otherwise mentally incompetent, the defence of necessity applies and treatment may be carried out that is necessary to avoid a severe risk to the life of the patient or others (e.g. sedating a psychotic patient who is a risk to self and others). Legislation (e.g. the *Guardianship Act 1987* (NSW) and its equivalent in other states) may provide for a guardian to be appointed to give consent for medical procedures on behalf of a person who is mentally disabled, or a court may make such an appointment.

A combination of common law principles and legislation applies when treating children. At common law a child may consent to treatment that is therapeutic, provided he or she has sufficient mental capacity to understand the nature and consequences of the proposed treatment. The application of this principle requires a balance between the intellectual and emotional maturity of the minor and the complexity and seriousness of the proposed treatment (see *Gillick versus West Norfolk and Wisbech Area Health Authority* [1985] 3 All ER 402, approved by the High Court in the case of *Department of Health and Community Services (NT) versus JWB and SMB* [1992] HCA 15). Presumably, a child of a quite young age could give a valid consent to a simple procedure that does not involve a great risk of harm. For example, a child who falls over and suffers a graze in school grounds could be expected to have the capacity to consent to the wound being treated. In all other cases, parental or guardian consent should be obtained. A court authorisation must be sought if consent is sought to carry out an elective procedure that will lead to an intellectually disabled person being made infertile.

Legislation can modify the common law. For example, legislation in New South Wales provides that consent to medical and dental treatment given by a parent or guardian of a minor aged less than 16 years, or by a minor aged 14 years or upwards, is a defence to an action for assault and battery in respect of that treatment. Below the age of 14 years, the consent of the parent or guardian is required (except in an emergency to save the life of the child). The definition of medical treatment includes treatment carried out by persons following the orders of a medical practitioner, and this would apply to nurses when they are carrying out a doctor's orders (see section 49 of the *Minors (Property and Contracts) Act 1970 (NSW)*).

When a parent or guardian has not given consent, or is refusing to consent to treatment that is for a child's benefit, most states/territories have legislation that enables doctors to perform life-saving treatments on children without parental consent (e.g. section 174 of the *Children and Young Persons (Care and Protection) Act 1998 (NSW)*). The matter may be referred to the Supreme Court of a state/territory in its *parens patriae* jurisdiction, or the family law courts can make a decision consistent with the best interests of the child where parents or guardians refuse consent to non-urgent treatment for a child, or there is any dispute regarding consent. Children who are wards of the state/territory have issues relating to consent to medical treatment covered by relevant child welfare legislation in each state/territory.

There are a number of defences against an action in assault that are relevant to the provision of healthcare. The defence of necessity permits a health professional to carry out treatment without consent, provided the treatment is intended to avoid a greater risk of harm to the person. The defence operates in those circumstances when patients are unable to give consent and the treatment is necessary to preserve them from a serious danger to their life. An example would be a patient who has suffered head injuries in a car accident and is unconscious.

Legislation may authorise particular acts without consent. For example, mental health legislation provides the rules for non-consensual treatment of mentally ill patients.

Finally, the defence of self-defence is applicable in the event that a patient or others assault a healthcare worker in anger, or vice versa. People who are assaulted are legally entitled to defend themselves, but the force used must not exceed what reasonably appears to be necessary to repel the attack.

Patient freedom of movement

During the course of clinical practice, a nurse will encounter patients who wish to leave a healthcare institution against advice. Unless there is some law that allows for the detention of patients without consent, then patients do have the right to leave.

The tort of false imprisonment compensates a person who has been subjected to an intentional and total restraint of movement without lawful justification. Restraint is either by total confinement or by preventing the person from lawfully leaving the place in which he or she is. The tort can be committed where a patient is too ill to move, or is unaware of the fact that he or she was imprisoned by reason that he or she is in a state of drunkenness, while asleep or while they were a lunatic (see *Meering versus Grahame-White Aviation Co Ltd* (1920) 122 LT 44).

The plaintiff must prove the confinement was total. If the person can leave by some reasonable alternative exit, there is no false imprisonment. To lock a patient in a room with no reasonable avenue of escape, or barring a patient from lawfully leaving a healthcare institution, could amount to false imprisonment in the absence of lawful justification.

Using bed rails, manacles and chemical restraints can also be regarded as false imprisonment if they are used without lawful justification and totally confine the patient. It can also amount to false imprisonment if a patient reasonably believes that any attempt to leave a healthcare institution will be prevented by a nurse, even if there are no physical restraints. However, the patient would have to prove the submission to the nurse was complete and was reasonable.

Hospitals develop policies requesting patients to see a doctor and to sign a release form in the event that a patient wishes to leave hospital against medical advice. There is no problem if a patient voluntarily agrees to the request. Some doubt exists as to whether hospital staff could detain a patient without consent in order to fulfil the hospital requirements. In the event that a patient leaves without advising staff, or refuses to stay to sign a release form and see a doctor, the patient should not be prevented from leaving and the events should be clearly documented in the nursing notes.

The fact that a patient wishes to leave hospital against medical advice does not relieve the staff from advising the patient of any deleterious effects a premature departure from hospital could entail if the patient will remain to accept such advice. Wherever possible, staff should ensure that the patient fully appreciates the risks involved in leaving against medical advice.

Defences that can be raised against an allegation of false imprisonment include the common law defence of necessity, which permits the restraint of persons who are a danger to themselves or others. However, restraint is not justified if it is merely for the convenience of staff; there must be a real necessity to protect the patient. The restraint of a patient attempting to jump off the roof of a hospital, or threatening staff and other patients with violence, would be justified on this basis.

A second defence exists where legislation authorises the detention of persons (e.g. mental and public health Acts). A third lawful means of detaining patients is where a court authorises the detention of a person for treatment. Such orders are usually reserved for the detention of children when parents wish to remove a child in need of care from a healthcare institution. Finally, detention without consent is permissible to affect a lawful arrest.

Patients' property

During the course of clinical practice, nurses will be faced with the prospect of taking charge of a patient's valuables, particularly when the patient is to be temporarily away from the ward to undergo surgery. When a patient's valuables are handed to a hospital for safekeeping, the law of bailment governs the relationship. The law of bailment is a contract and applies when one person (the bailor) delivers goods to another (the bailee) so that they may be used or stored until they are to be delivered back to the bailor.

Bailment may be for reward or gratuitous (free). When bailment is for reward, the bailee will be held liable to compensate for the loss of the goods according to the ordinary rules of negligence, whereas the bailee is only liable if gross negligence is shown in cases of gratuitous bailment. With respect to patients' valuables handed over to a hospital for safekeeping, the hospital is legally regarded as a bailee for reward and therefore has an obligation to exercise reasonable care in securing the safety of the valuables.

A hospital can become an involuntary bailee for patients' property. A hospital in New Zealand was held liable to compensate the estate of a deceased woman for a ring that disappeared from a woman's hand at the time of her death (*Southland Hospital Board versus Perkins Estate* [1986] 1 NZLR 373). The woman's personal control over her property ended with her death, and the hospital was held to be involuntary bailee for the ring.

Where a patient dies in hospital, any valuable property should be removed and kept in safekeeping to be handed over to the deceased patient's legal personal representative. Non-valuable items such as clothing and toiletries can be sent home with a relative or friend. Police usually deal with the property of a person who is brought in dead on arrival.

Healthcare institutions draw up policies and procedures in order to fulfil the duty of care to protect a patient's valuables and nursing staff should follow these. The valuables should be recorded in a document that is signed by the patient. When the patient is unable to sign, the valuables should be recorded by one nurse and witnessed by another.

The valuables must then be stored in a safe place. For short-term care the valuables may be stored in a locked cupboard at ward level (not the dangerous drugs cupboard). If the valuables are to be cared for on a long-term basis, they should be stored in a hospital safe. Patients are generally required to sign for the goods upon return to them. In the case of a deceased patient, the person legally entitled to deal with the patient's property after death would sign for receipt of the valuables.

In the event that the goods are lost, the patient has the onus of proving negligence and the value of the property. Nurses are not trained in evaluating the quality of valuable goods such as jewellery, and should not attempt to describe such goods as being of any particular kind and value. For example, a sapphire and diamond ring in a gold setting should be described as a ring with blue and clear stones set in a yellow coloured band, even if the patient states that the stones are a sapphire and diamonds, and the metal is gold.

Where theft of valuables is suspected, the police should be notified. The police can undertake an investigation and lay criminal charges where they reasonably suspect a member of the nursing staff or other person is responsible.

CRIMINAL LAW

During the course of practice, a nurse may cause serious bodily harm or death to patients. As well as providing facts that may be the subject of a civil action, such events may result in charges of criminal negligence, manslaughter or homicide.

Criminal negligence

Nurses can be charged with criminal negligence where an act causing serious bodily harm or death shows such a disregard for the life and safety of another that it goes beyond a mere matter of compensation at civil law. The death of a patient resulting from treatment by a nurse would amount to manslaughter where the nurse's negligence was gross and the nurse did something no reasonably skilled person would have done. A charge of murder could be laid where the nurse intended the patient to die or was grossly reckless as to whether the patient died. Criminal charges may result from a referral by a coroner to the relevant Crown law authorities following a coronial inquiry into the death of a patient.

Charges of criminal negligence against healthcare workers are rare and are difficult to prove to the requisite standard required in criminal law (i.e. 'beyond a reasonable doubt'). The prosecutor must prove both *mens rea* (guilty mind) as well as *actus reus* (an unlawful act). The *mens rea* element can be satisfied by proving that the accused committed an unlawful act, either with intent or could have foreseen that someone could suffer harm but nevertheless proceeded to commit the act.

A further issue is causation. The prosecutor must prove that the act led to the serious injury or death of the victim—a 'but for' test. This is not always easy to do. For example, if a person suffers brain damage as a result of an act (e.g. negligently given an overdose of a drug) and is placed on a life support system, then it cannot be said that the act has caused the death of the person. If the life support system is disconnected because the victim is brain dead, the question arises as to whether the defendant caused the death of the victim. When the initial act was the operative factor in causing the brain damage, then turning off the life support system does not break the chain of causation. But if the patient dies as a result of some other event, then it cannot be said that the act causing brain damage was the cause of the death. In the latter case a charge of murder or manslaughter could not be made out. A charge of criminal negligence may still be made out.

Criminal assault

Assault can be the subject of a criminal charge as well as a tort. In addition to the elements required to prove civil assault, there must be proof of a forcible or hostile act of the accused, without the consent of the victim. If a patient is criminally assaulted, the matter should be reported to administration and to the police, who can charge the responsible party with criminal assault. The same legal redress is available to nurses who are assaulted by others. When an assault takes place, which is intended to cause harm, it is referred to as an aggravated assault.

An assault with consent may not be an assault as is the case with most contact sports. However, if an act is unlawful, it cannot be made lawful because of consent of the victim. Thus sexual relations with a minor remain unlawful even if the minor is consenting. Deceit as to the identity of a person or the nature of the act will vitiate consent. The consent of a patient to a diagnostic or therapeutic treatment obtained by a person impersonating a nurse is invalid in law. Should a nurse examine a patient extending the examination to breasts or sexual organs beyond what is required for a legitimate examination, the nurse can be found guilty of a sexual assault (see *Staats versus R* [1998] NTSC 13).

Two defences to a charge of assault are misadventure and self-defence. To constitute misadventure, an assault occurs by accident. For example, a nurse slips on a wet floor and accidentally strikes a patient. Self-defence involves the use of force by one person to repel an attack on him or her. A person may use reasonable force to repel attacks, but must not use more violence than is necessary to repel the attack. The right of self-defence only lasts as long as any danger exists. A nurse would be entitled to exercise the right of self-defence if attacked by a patient or other person provided the nurse used no more force than was necessary to repel the attack. The onus of proving the reasonableness of the self-defence lies with the person relying upon it.

VICARIOUS LIABILITY

When a nurse's act or omission has caused harm to a patient and the patient has successfully sued to recover compensation for that harm, the question arises as to who is responsible for providing the compensation. Under the law of vicarious liability, an employer can be held responsible for the acts of its employees carried out in the course of their employment.

An employer's responsibility is limited to an employee's acts performed during the 'course of employment'. However, this term is fairly broad and encompasses all acts, authorised or not, which are reasonably within the scope of the employee's duties. Thus a healthcare employer can be held legally responsible to compensate an injured patient whose injuries resulted from an employee's negligence. It is only when a nurse's actions are so far removed from anything that can reasonably be held to be part of a nurse's role, that an employer will escape responsibility. Mere failure to follow guidelines in a procedure manual would not be enough to excuse the employer.

Vicarious liability merely means that the healthcare employer will generally be the party that will be held responsible for compensating a successful plaintiff and does not negate the nurse's personal liability. The nurse may be joined as a co-defendant. Responsibility under vicarious liability applies with respect to civil wrongs, but normally does not apply to criminal acts. Thus a hospital may be found vicariously liable for a nurse who commits a civil assault by giving an injection without consent, but not if the nurse angrily punched a patient.

An independent nurse practitioner is solely liable for harm caused by that practitioner's practice. An independent practitioner in turn becomes vicariously liable for harm caused by a person employed by the practitioner to assist in the practice.

It is usual practice for a healthcare institution or an independent practitioner to secure insurance cover in the event of successful litigation by a patient. This cover should be sufficient to pay the highest amount that could be awarded from time to time.

Even when an employer cannot be found to be vicariously liable because a person committing a wrong is not an employee, the courts have been prepared to find that an institution such as a hospital has a personal duty of care towards patients and others which is non-delegable. A hospital can be found negligent for harm caused to a patient by reason of its personal liability, when the act or omission of a visiting medical officer caused the alleged harm. When a hospital's policies and procedures could expose a patient to an unreasonable risk of harm, a duty arises to avoid that harm.

PATIENT RECORDS

Patient records are legal documents; therefore, it is important to keep accurate and complete records of all treatment and care administered to patients. The documents record the progress of patients admitted to healthcare facilities for the period of time that they are in care. Accurate and complete documentation can provide a good defence for a nurse who is faced with an action by a patient when the patient's record discloses that adequate and reasonable nursing care was delivered.

Even when adequate treatment may have been administered, failure to keep adequate patient records can lead to a finding of liability on the part of a nurse. Failure to record treatment may be accepted as evidence that such treatment was not in fact given. Overall failure to keep complete and adequate records can be regarded as a negligent omission, since a reasonable nurse would be expected to keep all patient record notes in order and up to date. It is reasonably foreseeable that a patient may suffer harm from failure to record a treatment given (e.g. a patient may be given two doses of a drug because a first dose was not recorded).

Although it is important that a patient's records be complete and up to date, a nurse should not write more than is necessary since this can lead to excessive questioning in evidence. In circumstances where a nurse offers treatment or advice, and a patient refuses, it would be prudent to include a notation to this effect in the patient record.

Patient records should be objectively written, and those responsible for writing records should avoid making value judgments. 'Patient has a headache' is a subjective statement and should be recorded as 'patient complaining of headache'. A description of the nature of the headache, the nursing action taken and the outcome of that action should follow this statement.

Records should be as near as possible contemporaneous with the event if they are to be accepted as reliable evidence in a court action. Delays in recording make the record less reliable as a true description of an event. In fact, a record made days after an event can be made to look as though it was an afterthought. Interlineations and notes made in margins should also be avoided, as they can suggest that information has been added to a record at a later date. It is for this reason that nurses are advised not to leave lines between individual reports.

Errors in recording should not be completely erased since this can appear suspicious in the event that a patient is suing on the basis of delivery of healthcare. Mistakes should be ruled through in a manner that enables others to be able to read what was initially written. A notation that the recording was made in error, signed by the person making the error, should be added to the record.

Nurses should recognise the fact that personal information given by patients in the course of administering care is to be kept confidential. Patients are entitled to expect that nurses will maintain a high degree of confidentiality. Should a nurse breach a patient's confidentiality, the legal rights of the patient are limited; nevertheless, the nurse should aim to preserve confidentiality to the maximum extent possible. A patient may be able to sue in defamation for unlawful disclosure if their reputation has been harmed, in negligence if they suffer foreseeable nervous shock, or in breach of contract. Commonwealth and state privacy Acts provide for investigation of complaints of breaches of privacy.

Access to a record can be granted to third parties with the consent of the patient. For all other purposes, access should be denied to all others except other health professionals treating the patient on a 'need to know' basis (i.e. those who have a genuine need to access the information in order to provide adequate care). Confidentiality may be legally breached by virtue of legal process (discovery and subpoenas), statutory authority, necessity and the criminal law.

Despite the fact that patients have a right to expect that their records will be kept confidential, there is no legally enforceable right, in the absence of statutory authority, to access the records themselves (see *Breen versus Williams* HC FC 96/025). The Commonwealth government and various state governments have enacted freedom of information legislation that gives people a right to have access to various documents, including personal documents held by public authorities. These Acts also provide for requesting that the documents be amended if there is any material that is false or misleading. However, the legislation applies to government departments and agencies only, and is not applicable to private agencies. A presumption that arises from this limitation is that patients in public hospitals could seek access to their records, but patients in private hospitals presumably could not unless there is legislation mandating such access. In 2002, the New South Wales Government introduced the *Health Records and Information Privacy Act*, which gives patients the right to access their healthcare records held by private practitioners.

As a general policy, patients should be given access to their records as freely as possible. A healthcare practitioner should be available when a patient is accessing their record in order to ensure that the patient understands the nature of what has been written and why it was written. When a patient could suffer some foreseeable harm, such as nervous shock, when faced with a particular diagnosis or other information contained therein, the patient's practitioner could make a decision as to whether access should be granted.

REGULATION OF DRUGS

Each state and territory has specific legislation that regulates the supply and use of drugs and poisons within its jurisdiction (e.g. the *Poisons and Therapeutic Goods Act 1966* (NSW)). The rules and regulations in relation to the drugs that nurses routinely administer to patients can be found within each relevant state or territory Act. While an Act may specify in broad terms the rules regarding the control of drugs and poisons, regulations formulated under the power of the Act set out in greater detail the specifics of the obligations of individuals under the Act.

Drugs and poisons are usually classified in Schedules according to the manner in which they may be supplied. Changes in the Schedules take place when new drugs come into use or there are changes in the manner in which a particular drug may be supplied. For example, a drug that formerly required a doctor's prescription may be moved to a Schedule that permits the drug to be purchased over the counter from a chemist.

All nurses should become familiar with the relevant Act operating in the state or territory in which they work.

REGULATION OF NURSING PRACTICE

Legislation in each state and territory governs the registration of nurses within its jurisdiction. Each Act provides for a nursing board or council to regulate and control the profession. These boards and councils have a responsibility for promoting and maintaining professional standards of nursing practice. Federal legislation provides for mutual recognition of a nurse's state or territory registration upon application to the board of another state or territory when a nurse wishes to work in that other state or territory (*Mutual Recognition Act 1992* (Cwlth)). When a nurse's name is removed from the register after disciplinary proceedings, or conditions on registration are imposed, this is reported to other states and territory nurses' registration boards.

Each Act also provides for penalties for breaches of the Act, and for the discipline of nurses who have been reported for acts or omissions bringing into question their professional competence. Major failures to exercise appropriate standards of patient care can lead to deregistration. In other cases, a nurse may be suspended or have conditions placed on their practice. Other powers include a reprimand or caution. A nurse who suffers any physical or mental impairment, or alcohol or drug addiction which affects or is likely to affect the nurse's physical or mental capacity to practise nursing, may be dealt with as a disciplinary matter, or may be dealt with in a non-disciplinary manner by Impaired Nurses Panels depending upon provisions in state/ territory legislation (e.g. the *Nurses and Midwives Act 1991* (NSW)).

One issue that can face a nurse and which can give rise to a complaint is when a nurse enters into a financial, personal and/or sexual relationship with a patient or former patient. The fact that the nurse–patient relationship has ceased does not legitimate the relationship if the circumstances were such that the profession regards the relationship as unethical. The therapeutic relationship can continue after the nurse–patient relationship has ceased to exist. This is particularly so when the nurse has become privy to a great deal of sensitive personal information regarding the patient's past and present life and health issues. Such matters are regarded as 'crossing the boundaries'. Whether or not such a relationship falls within prohibited behaviour will be decided on its facts. Nurses are well advised to seek advice regarding such actual or potential relationships, as it could lead to deregistration (see *Jacobsen versus Nurses Tribunal & Anor*, unreported 1997, restored to the register in 1999 with conditions for three years; *HCC versus Sunjic* [2008] NSWNMT 11).

All Acts have provisions for a right of appeal against a decision of a disciplinary body to an appropriate judicial body as nominated in each Act. All nurses should familiarise themselves with the provisions of any Act applying in the state or territory in which they are practising as a nurse.

It is anticipated that a scheme for national registration of health professionals will commence from July 2010. To become fully operational, it is dependent upon each state and territory government enacting legislation to implement the scheme. A new national agency will be established to bring the scheme into operation with local offices in each state and territory. Each profession will have its own board (e.g. a medical board, a nursing and midwifery board, a psychologists board). There will be a register of nurses with divisions for registered nurses, midwives and enrolled nurses. Nurses can obtain more detailed information from the Council of Australian Governments (COAG) at www.coag.gov.au.

MAKING COMPLAINTS

During the course of their nursing practice, nurses may observe behavior, professional or personal, which they believe to be inappropriate or wrong. A nurse may feel obliged to report another professional for their actions. In so doing, a nurse runs the risk that they will be sued for defamation or otherwise be disadvantaged for being a 'whistleblower'.

A nurse who reasonably believes that another professional has exhibited inappropriate or risky behavior with patients can legally make a complaint to the relevant registering body (e.g. a nursing or medical registration board). The matter can be investigated and the board will take what it considers as being the appropriate action. In New South Wales, a complaint can be made to the Health Care Complaints Commission, which will investigate and, in conjunction with the relevant registering body, determine a course of action to take. Provided the nurse has acted in good faith and without malice, such reporting is in the public interest.

Should a nurse decide to report to the administration of the institution in which they work, they must do so confidentially and restrict their complaint or report to senior authorities. In such cases, nurses should not take it upon themselves to discuss the issue with colleagues as this may lead them to being sued for defamation.

Defamation Acts in the various states are now uniform and the same provisions apply across all states. The person complaining of being defamed must prove that what was said or written was capable of being defamatory of them, and that their reputation has been harmed. There are a number of defences available to a defendant in defamation proceedings, including 'qualified privilege'. This defence applies where the recipient has an interest, or apparent interest in having information on some subject; the matter is published to them in the course of giving them information on that subject, and the defendant's conduct in publishing that information is reasonable. The information must be substantially true. Thus it could be argued that a nurse who passes on potentially defamatory material to the authorities in adherence to the above specifications would be able to avail themselves of this defence. It should be noted that the defence of qualified privilege is defeated if actuated by malice.

Legislation protecting whistleblowers is unsatisfactory in its scope and the way in which it protects whistleblowers. Legislation has been introduced largely to protect employees who disclose information about corrupt behavior in the public sector. Nevertheless, employees who disclose such information may face the risk of being considered as breaching their duty of confidentiality to their employer, and suffer general censure or legal consequences from that employer.

The ways in which a whistleblower may report would also seem to be restricted. The Department of Parliamentary Services (2005) published a research note on whistleblowing, which commented that: 'Most Australian state jurisdictions provide that, for whistleblowers to be protected, the information is to be disclosed internally or to a "proper" or "investigating" authority'.

Certainly, it is accepted that reporting corrupt or risky behaviour of another practitioner through the proper channels is a matter of public interest. Nurses who consider taking this path would need to take reasonable steps to satisfy themselves that what they are wishing to report is substantially true and a matter of public interest, and that they adhere to appropriate steps when doing so to protect themselves and to ensure that no unjustifiable complaints are made.

CONCLUSION

Knowledge of the law and its application to nursing practice has become a necessary component of a nurse's knowledge base. Nurses must be aware of and respect the legal rights of patients and the corresponding obligations of nurses in nursing care. Through an interest and knowledge of the law, a nurse can most effectively act as an advocate of patients by being involved in committees charged with the responsibility of formulating policies for the delivery of healthcare.

Failure to appreciate the legal rights of patients can lead a nurse to face a legal action mounted by a patient, or some disciplinary action taken by a nursing board or council under a relevant state/territory Act. Acknowledgment of, and adherence to, the legal rights of patients also goes a long way in maintaining the quality of nursing care delivered and the respect to be accorded to the profession. It is a professional obligation of all nurses to acquaint themselves with current legal issues touching upon the profession, and to do so by remaining up to date with their legal knowledge.

The discussion of the law and legal issues in this chapter is necessarily brief and is not meant to represent legal advice. Nurses who are faced with legal issues should seek appropriate legal advice through their professional organisations or other legal avenues, should they either wish to take action themselves or to respond to a summons or subpoena that has been served on them.

REFLECTIVE QUESTIONS

1 To what extent do you believe that the common law adequately provides for the resolution of complaints by patients allegedly harmed by healthcare?

2 What resources could you draw on in preparing to face court proceedings in relation to your professional practice?

3 How can you ensure that you remain up to date with the legal issues associated with the practice of nursing?

RECOMMENDED READINGS

Chiarella M 2002 The legal and professional status of nursing. Churchill Livingstone, London

Edginton J 1995 Law for the nursing profession. CCH Australia, Sydney

Irving K 2002 Governing the conduct of conduct: are restraints inevitable? Journal of Advanced Nursing 40(4):405–412

Johnstone M-J 1994 Nursing and the injustices of the law. WB Saunders, Sydney

McIlwraith J, Madden B 2006 Health care and the law, 4th edn. Lawbook Company, Sydney

Staunton P, Chiarella M 2003 Nursing and the law, 5th edn. Churchill Livingstone, Sydney

Online resources

Council of Australian Governments (COAG): www.coag.gov.au

Law and Justice Foundation: www.lawfoundation.net.au

New South Wales Nurses and Midwives Tribunal: www.austlii.edu.au

REFERENCE

Department of Parliamentary Services 2005 Whistleblowing in Australia: transparency, accountability … but above all, the truth. Research Note, Parliament of Australia, 14 February 2005, No 31

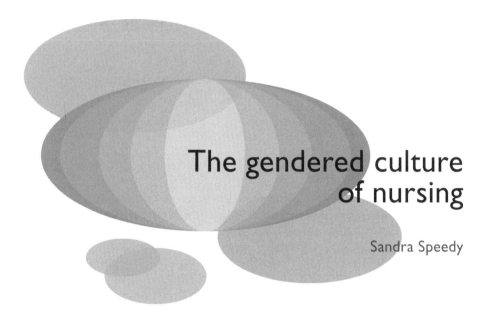

CHAPTER 12

The gendered culture of nursing

Sandra Speedy

LEARNING OBJECTIVES

On completion of this chapter, readers will have:

- understood and appreciated the historical development of feminist thinking on concepts such as nursing work and science
- examined the role that gender plays in defining the world of nursing work
- developed greater insight into how the healthcare system and health professionals are impacted upon by the issue of gender
- briefly explored the influence that feminisms have had on the discipline of nursing
- understood how feminist theory has influenced nursing research, and
- considered the debate about the relative advantages and disadvantages that gender provides for nurses.

KEY WORDS

Gender, nursing work, feminism, patriarchy, power, organisational culture

INTRODUCTION

In order to consider a range of gender issues—which are of interest and relevance to nurses all over the world—this chapter will consider the gendered nature of nursing work. This will involve discussion about the nature of women who provide the majority of the nursing workforce. It will also require some analysis of the nature of nursing work, as it is performed by women and men. Inherent in this discussion will be consideration of the role of science in determining views of the concept of 'woman', as well as the work women undertake. The chapter will also consider briefly the influence of the feminisms on nursing, and the influence of nurses and nursing on feminism. Finally, the chapter will examine the increasing role played by men in nursing, a gender issue of utmost importance for the future of nursing. It should be noted that there will be an extensive exploration of substantial volumes of literature that reflect classical thinking and debate over almost 20 years, but which remains relevant to the concepts presented here.

THE GENDERED NATURE OF NURSING WORK

A consideration of the gendered nature of nursing work must examine the concept of woman, since the majority of nurses are women. Whatever views are held regarding women will influence perception of women's work—in this case, nursing work. Perspectives on women are influenced by 'scientific' views about the nature of women, although it might also be argued that perspectives on women influence beliefs about the nature of science.

There is a considerable volume of literature that demonstrates a range of approaches and various viewpoints on woman as object and subject. Women can be examined from sociological, psychological, biological, philosophical or political perspectives—and other viewpoints as well. Many of these viewpoints feature devaluation of women, as any examination of the concepts of essentialism, biologism, naturalism or universalism will demonstrate. In an insightful work, Grosz (1990) suggests that all of these terms, which argue the nature of women (and men, incidentally), do fix and define the limits, because they 'are commonly used in patriarchal discourses to justify women's social subordination and their secondary positions relative to men in patriarchal society' (Grosz 1990:333). In their work, both David (2000) and Gherardi (1994:591) argue the similar point that 'masculinity and femininity are symbolic universes of meaning socially and historically constructed'.

Gherardi suggests also that the way we 'do gender' in our work 'helps to diminish or increase the inequality of the sexes: we use ceremonial work to recognize the difference of gender, and remedial work socially to construct the "fairness" of gender relationships' (Gherardi 1994:592). Ceci (2004) asserts that genders are identified by specific traits, virtues and behaviours that place us as either feminine or masculine—that is, identifiable and named as such. There is no question that in nursing each gender experiences 'cross-over', necessitating the management of dual presence in what are essentially separate symbolic contexts.

There are problems with constructing a 'universal feminism', since allowance must be made for difference and diversity between women, just as there is between women and men. What is worthy of exploration are some of the views about women and nurses within a medical and health professions context, because these views are influenced by the concepts mentioned above. The issue of how women are constructed by science is also relevant here (Kane & Thomas 2000).

175

Feminist literature argues that the masculinity of science is an image that has been perpetuated for centuries. This image creation is affected by textbook representations, curriculum organisation, classroom behaviour, and stereotypical beliefs and attitudes. It distorts science, yet scientific method has not been successful in filtering out patriarchal bias in the scientific construction of women. In the early 1990s, Lather wrote with clarity regarding this. She says:

> The claim of positivistic researchers that their method is sufficient protection against ideological incursion is debunked by feminist critiques of the conceptual and methodological orientations that reflect and reinforce sex-based inequality. Hence the construction of women brings into question that which has passed for knowledge in the human sciences (Lather 1991:17).

The masculinity of science is only an illusion (albeit a powerful one), not an intrinsic part of its nature. Science is a social construct, and 'its development is inextricably linked with social relations, not least the relations between men and women' (Kelly 1985:76). This leads, of course, to using male as the norm and female as the referent, a strategy that has been exposed and rejected in a wide range of disciplines, including psychology, sociology, psychiatry, medicine, education and biology. As long ago as the 1970s, it was pointed out that 'male' medicine misunderstood the female body, and these debates have now extended to cover all aspects of women's health, not just those of childbirth and reproduction.

In nursing and medicine, the presence of increasing numbers of women at all levels of authority indicates a modicum of success in producing women-friendly services and conditions. This has come about only because women have been forced to reclaim their healing role, which was given a boost by the knowledge and insights in the classic treatise written by Ehrenreich and English (1979), documenting the exclusion of women-as-healers from professionalised, modern medicine. There has long been 'increasing institutional awareness of the deficiencies and sexism of specific institutional practices' (Evans 1997:42). This has had both positive and negative effects. For the latter, it has resulted in some feminists 'beating up' on nurses, thus earning the title of 'anti-nurse'. This is:

> ... predicated on the belief that nurses willingly capitulate to male (and/or medical dominance), thereby making it difficult for 'real feminists' to achieve their goals. This ... 'complicity hypothesis' ... sees nurses as compliant with patriarchal demands to remain oppressed (Buchanan 1997:82).

Using this argument, nurses can be viewed as either the embodiment of the 'ideal' or 'good woman' (David 2000, Fealy 2004:653), conforming to masculine desires, or as the 'bad mother', 'thwarting women in their endeavours and assisting the medical profession in torturing women patients' (Buchanan 1997:82). In some ways this analysis, awareness and critique could be viewed as hostile criticism; however, it provides us with alternative views and insights that can be growth enhancing for women and nurses should we objectively and critically consider all perspectives.

Published studies over the last decade or so indicate that we do not need feminists to 'beat up' on nurses—nurses do that very well to each other, whether they are feminists or not (Briles 1994, David 2000). Horizontal violence has long been recognised by a range of authors, who suggest that nurses' self-hate and dislike of other nurses (which is very common in oppressed groups) is demonstrated by the lack of cohesion in nursing groups, as well as the phenomenon of 'eating our young' (Bent 1993, Kitson 2004, Roberts 2000). This concept arose out of the original work of Freire (2007) in his now classical book *Pedagogy of the Oppressed* (first published in 1968), which highlighted the relationship between the coloniser and the colonised, its power and its powerlessness. From these insights, we can conjecture that the systematic oppression of women will assist nurses to recognise the oppressive structures in which they practise, which:

> … includes recognising that nurses are placed in a culture that does not value their attributes, rather than 'blaming' them for ranking lower on self-esteem and higher in submissiveness in job-trait studies than do people in other occupations. Nurses must no longer assume that they are inherently inferior to the systems that surround them (Bent 1993:298).

Awareness of the social construction of women and nursing and its oppressive nature may change the way nurses relate to each other, and even refrain from 'horizontal violence'. As David makes clear:

> Nurses will never be able to expunge gender politics without first developing an understanding of how many use self-deception and how that action perpetuates nursing's professional mediocrity, limits freedom of thought and action, and preserves nurses' borderline status (David 2000:85).

This brings us to the work of nursing.

THE WORK OF NURSING

The role and function of nursing cannot be separated from those who undertake this activity. Literature published in the last two decades indicates that there are particular views held about women and nursing that create the definitions of women's work and nursing work, and, by implication, men's work (David 2000, Fealy 2004, Meadus 2000). Cheek and Rudge point out that:

> … the low status of nursing and the way in which the work of nurses is devalued, especially when compared to other health professionals, can at least in part be explained by its gendered nature (Cheek & Rudge 1995:312).

Labelling nursing as 'women's work' creates a deterrent that 'inhibits recruitment of men into the profession and aids promotion of the sex imbalance in the nursing workforce' (Meadus 2000:9). Nursing is thus viewed as a natural extension of the female role, valuing nurturance, caring, support, care and concern (Bent 1993, Brykczynska 1997, Evans 1997). These characteristics have been described as encompassing a 'tyranny of niceness' (Street 1995). Nevertheless, researchers have found that these characteristics are selectively eliminated during the educational and socialisation process (Doering 1992). For example, Treacy noted that current 'nurse training' endorses 'compliance, passivity and ladylike behaviour, but it negatively sanctions other female traits such as intuition, empathy, and emotional expression' (Treacy 1989:88).

The descriptors 'compliance, passivity and ladylike behaviour' are words which, it could be argued, are suggestive of 'powerlessness' and 'intuitiveness, empathy and emotional expression', and are often viewed as unscientific and hence unacceptable in the world of science. The social construction of women as emotional beings is also used to undermine their credibility as nurses (Ceci 2004). As David (2000:86) also points out: 'the gender dialectic is still so fundamental to gender politics that it permeates the traditions of nursing, such as the belief that nursing is woman's work'.

Because of this, it could be argued that women and nurses steer towards nursing as a career, while men are relatively inhibited from entering the nursing profession. According to Evans (2004:321), the 'ideological designation of nursing as women's work has excluded, limited, and conversely, advanced the careers of men in nursing'. The issue of male advantage will be addressed later in this chapter.

Evans (1997) notes that nineteenth century science and rationality perceived the 'feminine' as an abstraction, which assisted in marginalising women within institutional practices. Women, as we have seen, were constructed as hysterical and intellectually inferior, while men were expected to conform to the stereotype of masculine behaviour. Thus, 'the "soft" feminine and the "hard" masculine then received institutional recognition and confirmation in particular practices' (Evans 1997:39). Feminists have sought to demonstrate the disjunction between supposed institutional objectivity and actual institutional practice. Specifically, the institution of medicine, for example, defines its values as non-gendered, while in practice they are deeply gendered (Evans 1997). This has been exposed in many areas—for example, in the management of childbirth and women's sexuality (Erturk 2004).

Because the values that dominate our health system are so pervasive and reflect the values of society at large, 'it is a struggle for nurses to remain aligned to the person rather than the institution' (Huntington 1996:170). This creates difficulties in nursing work, as the dominant discourses that shape health, illness and perceptions of what it is to be a woman (and a man, incidentally) can disadvantage the individual. As Huntington (1996:170) points out: 'we have been left with only male language to explain the fundamentally female practice of healing bodies'. The only solution to this problem is to develop an alternative discourse to that constructed and dominated by orthodox scientific discourse characteristics of the medical world.

Clearly too, the feminist literature has challenged the cultural code of organisations, designed around masculinity and femininity, which suggests that 'gender is deeply embedded in the design and functioning of organisations' (Davies 1995:44). These workplaces are socially constructed, as is the position of 'nurse' (David 2000), neither of which are gender-neutral, and operate on masculine values for their legitimation and affirmation (Gherardi 1994). Nurses therefore find it difficult to function within such gendered organisations, and frequently resort to 'blaming the victims', who are usually other nurses struggling with their day-to-day functioning within a hostile environment. Alternatively, they may adopt a victim mentality, rather than recognising the dysfunctionality of their workplaces (Kitson 2004). Thus:

> [W]omen, in a very important sense, cannot be 'at home' in the public world—it is constructed in such a way that assumes home is somewhere else, somewhere far away and different (Davies 1995:62).

However, Kane and Thomas (2000) remind us that nursing has historically provided a haven for women who seek to control their lives within a professional context, although there are significant limits to what can be achieved. In fact, David (2000) suggests that this is delusion, because power does not belong to women in a male-dominated system (see also Paliadelis 2005, 2008, Paliadelis et al 2007).

As we continue our searching of pertinent literature, we find a range of other historical scholarly work that demonstrates the further weakening of nursing's value.

For example, Gamarnikow (1978) linked nursing to domesticity; Treacy (1989) suggested that the invisibility of nurses' contribution to care reflected the invisibility of much of the work contribution of women in society. Other scholars have pointed out that the sexual division of labour in the home disadvantages women in the workplace, which creates enormous stress for working women, and, in this case, nurses. This taps into the work of feminist scientists who have 'identified "women's work" the "caring professions", "unpaid domestic labour", "the double shift" and other manifestations of the apparently "natural" social division of labour' (Evans 1997:59).

It has been pointed out by many scholars that caring itself is a gendered construct, since notions of professional caring are derived from traditional concepts of caring as a feminine obligation (Caffrey & Caffrey 1994, Ekstrom 1999, Falk Rafael 1996, Paliadelis et al 2007, Wuest 1997). Caring in nursing has in the past been constructed as an inherently feminine pastime, and traditionally has received little social or economic recognition; it has been perceived as women's work, as unintellectual, unskilled and emotional, and thus likely to perpetuate gender exploitation (Bubeck 1995, Ceci 2004, Henderson 2001). It was long believed that the work nurses undertake in order to provide care does not require any particular skill or knowledge; it has been viewed as a quality that women possess 'naturally' (Falk Rafael 1998, Henderson 2001, Zebroski 2001).

However, this view has been challenged. For example, Meadus (2000) cites research that demonstrates that men enter nursing because of their desire to care for others, thus challenging the stereotype that only women nurses care. He also notes that such men run the risk of being perceived as 'gay' because of this role violation. This viewpoint is challenged by Bubeck (1995:114), as she notes that 'part of the practice of care is to focus on the needs of the other, to become attentive, to be selfless'. By the construction of masculinity, caring is very difficult for men; they also escape from the care burden through the 'public/private' split in responsibilities of women and men (Tronto 1999).

Nursing's detractors have long promoted the idea that nurses are 'doers' rather than 'thinkers'; that is, nurses do not need to 'think' to do nursing, as long as they can 'do' certain tasks. This has resulted in an anti-intellectual bias, which creates the perception that the 'intelligent nurse was not a good practical nurse' (Fealy 2004:652), a myth that then threatens the academic preparation of nurses (Liaschenko & Peter 2004). This has, in no small measure, led to a significant devaluation of nursing, assisted by the unequal power relations that characterise the position of nursing vis-a-vis medicine (David 2000). For many years, this view was used to justify the low-level education provided to nurses prior to their entry into the higher education system.

That caring is assumed not to require knowledge is not without practical consequence. The replacement of registered nurses with less skilled personnel could be considered less of a reflection of economic rationalism than a reflection of the idea that caring is unskilled activity intrinsic to domesticity and womanhood. To engender nurse caring as feminine, therefore positioning it as innately instinctive to women, is to deny the advanced knowledge and skills that lie within the therapeutic caring acts of nurses. Despite the fact that 'emotional labour' is a vital and necessary part of the nursing labour process, it 'tends to be marginalized as a skill that a predominantly female nursing workforce would naturally possess' (Bolton 2000:580).

The concept of emotional labour is derived from the work of Hothschild (1983) who suggested that stress occurs to those involved, as they need to repeatedly suppress their felt emotions while they express contradictory feelings. This dissonance creates emotional deadening and distancing from authentic feeling. Emotional labour can be conceived as a 'gift in the form of authentic caring behaviour' (Bolton 2000:586), which truly reflects the state of 'being a nurse' or acting out the social construction of the 'ideal nurse' (Mazhindu 2003:249). The fact that it is under-theorised and not appreciated is of serious concern (Henderson 2001).

Emotion work can be hard labour, because it requires containment of emotions and/or denial of feelings. Relief measures are sought to cope with this continuous labouring. Relief can be found in 'backstage regions', such as the nurses' station, where profound irritation with patients or emotional anguish can be expressed, where nurses can 'drop their public mask' and express their true feelings (Weir & Waddington 2008). As Fineman (1993:21) indicates, 'off-stage settings are not emotion-free ports'. Here, implicit feeling rules can come into play; colleagues can express emotion to a degree that will be cathartic for them, but will also maintain organisational order.

Despite the fact that it is now acknowledged that emotional labour occurs in organisations, and that employers have expectations about what sort of emotion one should feel in particular contexts, emotion work tends to be privatised and moved out of the realm of organisational responsibility (Boyle 2002a, 2002b, Martinez-Indigo et al 2007). Emotional labour work involves remaining continually vigilant and sensitive to the environment, constantly noting and responding to others' emotional states, alleviating resultant distress, and assisting those who are 'inappropriately emotional' to regain their stability (Lupton 1998). The fact that this creates workplace stress for nurses is rarely acknowledged (McVicar 2003, Mann & Cowburn 2005).

Emotional labour work can be emotionally and physically demanding, but requires interpersonal and intrapersonal skills and competencies that are not acknowledged (McQueen 2004, Myerson 2000, Nicolson 1996). They assert that this lack of acknowledgment occurs for three reasons. First, emotion work remains largely invisible. Second, it requires the development of awareness and of a vocabulary to describe this work as a competency. Third, this work is predominantly done by women. Women tend to be more involved in the caring and service industries than men (as in nursing), and also perform much of the 'backstage' or behind-the-scenes work (Goffman 1959). While this work may be perceived as trivial, it is usually of a supportive nature, enhancing the intellectual capability or productivity of organisations (Lupton 1998).

This is not to say that men do not 'do' emotional labour; some do. However, management is still predominantly done by men, and their power to demand emotional labour from both women and men is maintained by management, although it is 'often constructed as (non)emotions' (Hearn 1993:161). As an antidote, Boyle's (2002a) research on emotional labour and masculinities, given that males are not viewed to have a primary 'caring' role, when what is defined as emotionally acceptable in the workplace, and how this impacts on views of masculinity, have a 'lose–lose' predicament.

It is important not to forget the value of relationships that nurses develop with their patients, with relatives and carers, all of whom remain part of using the self in caring mode, often critical to recovery, and which can be very demanding. Sandelowski makes the point that those who engender nursing as female:

> … inadvertently minimise or deny nursing its record of expertise and innovation within technology, the primary roles nurses have played in the deployment of technology and the power and remuneration that comes with technological knowledge and skills in a high-technology culture (Sandelowski 1997:172).

Traditional expectations that surround caring as a feminine and nursing activity involve subjugation of the self and selfless devotion to duty (Caffrey & Caffrey 1994). In some circumstances nurses may experience feelings of powerlessness and eventually burn out, as a result of suppression of their own feelings and needs (Demerouti et al 2000). Others suggest that emotional labour is an integral part of caring in nursing (Henderson 2001, Weir & Waddington 2008). For an excellent and comprehensive analysis of caring, refer to Chapter 6 of this text.

THE INFLUENCE OF FEMINISMS ON THE DISCIPLINE OF NURSING

'The feminisms' refers to the variety of theoretical approaches to the advocacy of equal rights for women, accompanied by a commitment to improving the position of women in society. They are informed by a range of theoretical propositions, which include liberal feminism, socialist feminism, postmodern feminism, postcolonial feminism (Rancine 2003), feminist ethics (Peter et al 2004) and other forms.

This chapter has developed the argument, derived from decades of literature, that women and nurses are devalued in general, notwithstanding that gains have been made in recent years. Feminist nurses, and others, have provided feminist analyses of their clinical practice, their educational understandings and their research. It is most notable that the feminisms have been promoted more by nursing scholars than practitioners, which has led to some uneasiness between the two groups. This may have arisen because the feminisms have an 'image' problem due to stereotypical views of what constitutes a feminist.

In reality, the feminisms are political perspectives, which seek to balance societal power, to gain equalities and autonomies for women of all races, classes, ethnicities, ages, disabilities, sexualities and professional status (Peter et al 2004). These feminisms offer the opportunity for nurses to recognise and analyse the unequal power relations that have been discussed earlier in this chapter, and to develop a raised consciousness about gender issues (Dendaas 2004, Meadus 2000, Valentine 2001). Feminist analyses have been extended to clinical practice to examine nursing and healthcare contexts, particularly 'managed care' from the 'feminist philosophical assumption that "the personal is political"' (Georges & McGuire 2004:11).

It is noteworthy that the feminisms have been eschewed by a large number of women, particularly younger women (Baumgardner & Richards 2003). This may be partly attributed to (mis)understandings of the meaning of feminism. Those who seek to denigrate feminism and what it can offer suggest that feminists are 'man-haters' and therefore separatists; a number of other jaundiced and inaccurate epithets are hurled at them. Nevertheless, the literature also suggests that Generation Y women may believe that feminism is passé 'because it worked' (Wynter 2006). The argument runs that the successes of feminism must sow the seeds of its failure to be seen as relevant for adults of the present generation. Jayatilaka (2001) likens feminism to fluoride, suggesting that 'feminism is like fluoride—we scarcely notice we have it—it is simply in the water'. And the new generation of women can take advantage of the gains of their fore-mothers, but 'do' their feminism in different ways.

In reality, one can espouse feminist philosophy or be driven from a feminist perspective while celebrating womanhood, whatever individualistic form it takes. Thus, women can enjoy male company and be interested in fashion, and enjoy their youth and femininity.

The key point is that feminism can be individually practised, which includes making choices about life. This can range, for example, from career choice and relationship definition, to shaving whatever parts of our body we wish, wearing nail polish and make-up, and even enjoying relationships with males. Feminism is thus about taking control of one's life, respecting one's womanhood as well as men; feminists can (and do) enjoy male company. The radical left of the 1970s view was that all men were rapists and perpetrators of violence. The reality is that some are, but the majority are not. So adopting a feminist perspective does not mean rejecting relationships with men; there can be (and often is) a natural and harmonious coexistence between women and men.

There is a strong view that women of Generation X and Y, in failing to identify with feminism, are rejecting the radical feminist notion of what it means to be a feminist. As Jayatilaka (2001) notes, such women might be identified as feminist if they were recognised as doing it in their own way. Rockler-Gladen (2007) suggests that this is 'third wave feminism', developed in the 1990s, which 'focuses more on the individual empowerment of women and less on activism'. Essentially, this means that there is greater emphasis on using personal empowerment as a way to begin social change. It is this approach that is criticised by other feminists who believe that personal empowerment is unlikely to foster social change. Third wave feminism has also been identified as 'postfeminism'—a concept explored in a study by Aronson (2003). She found that, while younger women are more ambivalent about supporting feminism, they are supporters, and may, under the right conditions, become the drivers for the next wave of the feminist movement.

So while it is true that the feminisms have not been adopted wholeheartedly by nurses, they certainly have had an impact. Some feminists have been hypercritical of nursing and nurses because of the latter's inability to embrace feminist theories: they believe that nursing as a women's field needs 'rescuing'—that it is a victim of patriarchy and needs help in recognising this. As previously noted, some feminists place the blame for the continuance of nursing oppression at the feet of nurses who collude with their oppressors to prevent change in the system (David 2000). In this way, nurses are viewed as weak and compliant with the dominant forces that seek to retain the status quo, or as deceiving themselves. This may be a deliberate act, but it is more likely that insight and awareness has not been developed, thus disadvantaging nurses and nursing.

Nursing has, however, provided fertile ground for the development of feminist theories, as these provide useful perspectives for nurses who work with disempowered and marginalised groups in their practice. Many nurses have recognised that they are also disempowered, marginalised and disadvantaged within the healthcare system (Ceci 2004), and are developing understandings of these processes in order to action change. But while this is an ongoing movement, it certainly is no easy task.

While feminist theories have focused on nursing and the development of nursing research, there is a significant 'halo effect' that works against the valuing of nursing research. In accepting the premise that women and nurses are devalued in general, by 'scientific' researchers in particular, nursing research itself is devalued, because it is done by women and nurses. The qualities that define a 'good nurse' are quite distinct from those defining a 'good researcher'. Hicks (1997, 1999) argues that 'research has fundamentally masculine connotations and nursing is quintessentially feminine' (Hicks 1999:130), which in itself contributes to the relative paucity of nursing research output. Clearly, two cultures are in collision: nursing and research (Neuman 1999, Valentine 2001).

There is a long history of males who, in the past, were the academics and intellectual and political gatekeepers of Western thought. They constructed and reproduced knowledge. But with the deconstruction and reconstruction of knowledge by feminists who have challenged the 'received view', nurses can take advantage of the liberalising approach inherent in the scholarly work published since the 1970s and 1980s in academic feminism and nursing. Since this time, feminist critics of science have exposed the history and assumptions of science and identified its masculinist practices.

Evans (1997:54) argues that 'women then had to fight and argue their way back into science—and a scientific epistemology and community that they had had little or no part in constructing'. Not only were they literally absent from science, there was also a wider absence of the 'feminine' and an absence from the findings and conclusions of science. This was not surprising because 'the *questions* that science identified as important were determined by the construction of the social world in which men occupied the public, and women the private, space' (Evans 1997:54).

According to Huntington (1996), this created an opportunity for scientific knowledge to maintain the control of women (primarily through their bodies), as men have constructed a knowledge base that is able to be extrapolated to women. She continues: 'nurses … have not addressed the issue of the place of science in nursing nor the impact this has had on nursing generally, and the nursing of women in particular' (Huntington 1996:168). This, of course, has implications for nursing work and nursing research, as it suggests that nurses may be instrumental in maintaining a medical ideology for women patients, calculated to be negative and oppressive (Buchanan 1997).

Part of the rejection of masculinist science was fostered by scholars, intellectuals and researchers who adopted the 'emancipatory science' perspective promulgated by the Frankfurt School of Sociology and Philosophy. The inaugural address given by Habermas in 1965, entitled 'Knowledge and interest', defined emancipatory science as 'one which reveals the relationship of knowledge and interests which the objectivist attitude conceals' (Hagell 1989:227). This included a rejection of logical positivism as the only or most appropriate approach to research; interpretive and other qualitative forms were deemed by many to be superior for the task at hand in a range of disciplines, including nursing.

In the 1960s, the nursing discipline was given opportunities for development by a nursing science that was driven by an empiricist or logical positivist philosophy. Edwards (1999) suggests that nursing was driven to claim its science base for reasons of prestige and status, as well as a need to be perceived as a 'successful' profession. He concludes that nursing does not qualify as a legitimate science, since it must be empirical (and is not). Nurse researchers and scholars have long acknowledged the inappropriateness for *all* nursing research to be undertaken using the empiricist model, because many of the questions framed were not valid for nursing knowledge development (Whittemore 1999). Winters and Ballou (2004:533) argue that 'legitimate science includes both empirical and non-empirical scientific methods'.

However, if we return to the argument that has been developed, given society's attitudes to women, and hence nurses, there may be more value in conforming to the dominant culture (i.e. 'scientific research' that is acceptable to masculinist science). This is not appropriate, however, because it will not answer many of the questions nursing asks. Thus, Winters and Ballou (2004:533) propose that nursing should work towards integrating 'all applicable modes of scientific inquiry into the discipline'.

An alternative approach for the development of nursing knowledge underpinned by feminist principles can provide nurses with understandings of what it is that they know, and what it is they experience, which involves reclaiming and renaming nursing's experiences and knowledge of the social world lived in and daily constructed. Rancine (2003:91) contends that there are other promising and more appropriate ways of developing knowledge that support social activism, including that deriving from nursing research. These include the use of critical and feminist approaches to explore 'health issues related to race, gender, and social classes'. This builds on the work of Doering (1992:25), who suggested that feminism and poststructuralism were particularly relevant to nursing because they incorporate the concepts of the female experience and of power. These concepts reflect the historical, social and political dynamics in which the discipline of nursing operates. They encompass a theme central to nursing—that of powerlessness, characterised by oppression, submission and male domination.

It is important to note that feminist research 'permits the recognition and exploration of socio-cultural factors that transcend gender' (Jackson 1997:87), which signals that, while the concept of oppression is central to feminism, it is clearly shared with other groups (Evans 1997). Thus:

> Accepting that experiences around oppression and struggle are not exclusive to women permits recognition that institutionalised patriarchy and androcentricity are oppressive to all but those of the dominant class, race and gender (Jackson 1997:87).

This insight attempts to deal with the charge by Allen et al (1991) that feminist research marginalises men. These authors raised the question of whether research involving only women simply 'supports a conceptual scheme that reinforces the material subjugation of women' and thus 'perpetuates problematic social categories' (Allen et al 1991:50). They concluded, somewhat controversially, that 'a better strategy is to deconstruct the dichotomy itself and to expand awareness of the diverse contemporary and historical forms of gendered existence' (Allen et al 1991:56), which has subsequently occurred.

It may be reasonable to support the view that the value of feminist research is that it 'empowers women and addresses issues that can make a difference to the quality of life for all humankind' (Parker & McFarland 1991:66). There are those who believe that nursing research should be approached from a much broader perspective and incorporate a range of paradigms. The method used is defined by the questions being asked. Unfortunately, too, the method may be driven by other motives, such as economic rationalism, and the need to obtain research funding, regardless of the ethical and moral imperatives that would normally guide research behaviour. But it is clear that the research approach must take into account the context in which it is conducted, and for nursing this has political and power implications. There is no question that gender is a critical and all-encompassing variable to be acknowledged. And it is feminist theory that has largely been responsible for raising nursing's consciousness in this domain.

MEN IN NURSING

It has long been noted that men are a minority in nursing, despite the fact that their numbers have increased over the decades. In 2005, the nursing workforce in the United States consisted of 5.9% men (Donley 2005, Janiszewski Goodin 2003), while in 1998 they comprised 4.4% of the Canadian workforce (Meadus 2000). Note that this has improved to 5.1% by 2008 (see Table 12.1). This compares to statistics from Britain, where male nurses constitute 10.1% of the qualified nursing workforce, while in Australia it is around 7.2%. The International Council of Nurses Nursing Profile (2004) provides an international snap-shot of the gender breakdown of nurses in a range of countries (see Table 12.1).

In the United States, male students comprised 8.6% in baccalaureate programs, 9.6% in masters' programs, and 6.7% in doctoral programs (American Association of Colleges of Nursing 2002). The proportion of male nursing undergraduate students in Australia increased from 11.9% in 1987–90, to 15.9% in 1995 (Brown 1998).

A study by Sharman et al (1996) concluded that women were supporting men in the workforce and the home, often at the expense of their own career advancement. A more recent study found that taking a career break, or working less than full time for women, significantly reduced women's chances of occupying senior positions (Brown & Jones 2004). The major conclusion from this study was that length of experience was not a predictor of seniority. Rather, it was whether or not any significant interruption of full-time work was the major variable.

	Female	Percentage	Male	Percentage
Australia[1]	169,800	92.8%	13,244	7.2%
Canada	219,161	94.9%	11,796	5.1%
Denmark	50,817	96.5%	1,850	3.5%
Germany	10,003	94.5%	582	5.5%
Iceland (2003)	3,112	98.7%	40	1.3%
Ireland[2]	35,990	92%	3,129	8%
New Zealand	29,782	93.5%	2,056	6.5%
Norway (2003)	50,691	92.5%	2,056	7.5%
Sweden	107,382	90%	11,983	10%
United Kingdom	580,000	89.9%	65,000	10.1%
United States[3]	N/A	95%	N/A	5%

Table 12.1 Registered nurses gender breakdown
[1]Labour Force, Australian, Detailed, Quarterly: www.abs.gov.au/ausstats/abs@nsf/mf/6291.0.55.003.
[2]Loughrey M 2008 Just how male are male nurses …? Journal of Clinical Nursing 17: 1327–1334. This article suggests that the ratio of female to male general nurses is approximately 20:1.
[3]Donley Sr R 2005 Challenges for nursing in the 21st century. Nursing Economic$ 23(6):312.
Source: International Council of Nurses Nursing Workforce Profile 2004.
Online. Available: www.icn.ch/Flash/SewDatasheet04.swf 8 Aug 2008.

This is a finding that has previously been highlighted in other traditionally female occupations, such as teaching, physiotherapy, occupational therapy, librarianship and social work (Williams 1992). What it demonstrates is that males move into powerful positions over the largest occupational group in the health workforce, nursing, an occupational group that has traditionally been 'managed, taught, disciplined and organised almost entirely by women' (MacGuire, cited in Sharman et al 1996). There is little doubt that 'the ideological climate, socialisation processes and women's family and domestic responsibilities underlie a glass ceiling for women and a glass elevator for men in non-traditional occupations' (Sharman 1998:56).

Nevertheless, males continue to be viewed as increasingly disadvantaged and reduced to 'lifting machines' (Shakespeare 2003:53). Loughrey's research (2008) indicates that male nurses view themselves as a source of strength and valued for their ability to deal with aggressive patients. The negative side of this was, however, that male nurses account for up to 60% of nurses who are deregistered, when accused of physical abuse.

While men in some numbers are relative newcomers to nursing, they are increasingly being promoted to higher levels than women, despite their disproportionate numbers; furthermore, they seem to have less experience and fewer qualifications (Evans 2004). This appears to have been due to a recruitment campaign, which attacks the negative stereotype of men in nursing, and highlights the fact that management positions were 'made ripe for male capture', thus positioning men with 'poor formal educational qualifications' (Evans 2004:326) for leadership positions.

Brown's study (1998) found that men were overrepresented in senior nursing administrative positions. Although men comprised only 8% of the registered nurse workforce, they held 22% of senior nursing positions. Poliafico (1998) indicates that this comparative figure is only 6% in the United States, and suggests that there is a common misconception that men hold a disproportionate number of administrative positions. Brown (1998:21) considers a range of explanations as to why this is happening in Australia. One of the most compelling is that women are seen to be invading the workplace, since workplaces are constructed by men. So it is that even in 'women's occupations', such as nursing, where it may be expected that men would be perceived as not fitting in, the overriding culture of the workplace turns this disjunction into a benefit for men.

Thus men who enter nursing are seen to be 'lowering themselves, losing status by undertaking "women's work"' (Brown 1998:21), yet are expected to be better workers than female nurses. They retain the benefits of their ascribed gender role: they are seen to be the 'breadwinner', to have leadership qualities, to be worth mentoring (since they are more likely to be serious about their career), and they are more likely to be assisted in accessing 'power networks' in nursing. Hicks (1999) argues that if men in these top positions behave consistently with the findings of research studies, then they are most likely to reproduce themselves at these top-level positions. This will then serve to widen the gender/power divisions in nursing.

Further evidence that men are being promoted to the highest levels of service in nursing, despite their numerical minority, is provided by Boughn (2001:23) who notes that 'men who go into nursing rise like cream in milk' because they expect practical rewards and set up their lives to achieve and retain these, whereas women fail to recognise their economic and political power.

A study which examined senior nursing administrative positions in the United Kingdom found that, in 1987, 8.6% of registered nurses were men, but 50.3% held chief nurse/advisor posts, and 57.8% were directors of nursing education (Gaze 1987). There has been a disproportionate increase of males in senior nursing positions in the United Kingdom, which has also occurred in the United States. It should be noted, however, that there was a concerted effort in the United Kingdom to 'defeminise' management within nursing, enabling men to be more easily promoted into these positions (Carpenter 1977).

Jenkins (1989) notes that Florence Nightingale had a vision that nursing would always be under the control of women; she saw no place in nursing for men, just as there was no place for men in controlling nursing. Mackintosh (1997) and Meadus (2000) believe that the contribution of men to nursing has not been recognised and that it is time for affirmative action in favour of men for nursing to survive the twenty-first century. This means 'that the Nightingale image must be counter-balanced by the entry and acceptance of larger numbers of men into the profession' (Meadus 2000:10).

This view is rejected by other researchers who suggest that nursing, rather than increasing male numbers, should introduce feminist strategies to enhance the power of women nurses, since their lower disproportionate voice in academic writing and actual power in practice requires improvement (Ryan & Porter 1993:43). Other research that focuses on the experience of male nurses suggests that attrition is a major issue, due to the treatment given to males (Kelly et al 1996, Morin 1999).

To counteract the inequities experienced by men in nursing, the American Assembly for Men in Nursing was formed in 1971 (Evans 2004). Its aims were 'to recruit more men into the profession, to provide support to those men who already are nurses, and to increase the visibility of men in nursing' (Poliafico 1998:43). Evans (2004) documents how nursing associations have acted as gatekeepers of change, limiting men's participation in nursing, including the refusal of approval to employ male nurse educators, on the grounds that it was inappropriate for men to teach women how to nurse. Nevertheless, gendered attitudes, which are 'reinforced and perpetuated by patriarchal societal institutions and processes' (Evans 1997:231), continue. The solution lies in challenging our stereotypes of femininity and masculinity, and in the latter case, of assisting male nurses to critically examine their 'gender curio status' (Loughrey 2008). The matter of addressing structural relations is also an obvious requirement for change.

CONCLUSION

The aim of this chapter is to bring into sharp focus the gendered culture of nursing. Quite clearly there are inequities at work that can be documented with respect to control, management and leadership in nursing. Additionally, there are more subtle ways that gender impacts on nursing. This chapter has argued that nursing work in all its forms (including clinical practice, education and research), mostly undertaken by women, is affected severely by gender because of its construction and the context in which nursing is carried out (Valentine 2001). Becoming aware of such systematic oppressions is the first step in changing paternalistic structures and systems that operate to disadvantage nurses, their patients, and the overall healthcare system.

David (2000:90) suggests that nurses 'must reframe the sociopolitical reality and give it back'; otherwise, they will continue to be 'shackled in servitude, denied freedom to acknowledge the full benefit of their health and healing practices'. Failure to challenge the stereotypes rife in nursing effectively results in collusion 'with nursing's power brokers in maintaining for the nurse the status of "trained worker" as opposed to that of "learned professional"' (Fealy 2004:654). And such challenges are part of that which the feminisms seek to contribute to the nursing profession.

REFLECTIVE QUESTIONS

1 What do you think the feminisms have to offer to the various generations of nurses, from 'baby boomer' to 'generation Y', and to the discipline of nursing, including its academic and clinical aspects?

2 Do you believe that the role and function of nursing cannot be separated from nurses who undertake it? If so, why is this? If you disagree, outline your arguments to support your position.

3 What do you think of the fact that men in nursing, despite their numerical minority, have the majority of leadership positions? Why do you think this is? What implications does this have for nursing as a profession?

RECOMMENDED READINGS

Barrett M, Phillips A (eds) 1992 Destabilizing theory: contemporary feminist debates. Polity Press, Cambridge

Caro J, Fox C 2008 The F word: how we learned to swear by feminism. University of New South Wales Press, Sydney

Davies C 1995 Gender and the professional predicament in nursing. Open University Press, Buckingham

Donley R 2005 Challenges for nursing in the 21st century. Nursing Economic$ 23(6):312–318

Dux M, Simic Z 2008 The great feminist denial. Melbourne University Press, Melbourne

Jayatilaka G 2001 Rebranding feminism? Geethika Jayatilaka's talk. Online. Available: www.thefword.org.uk/features/2001/12/rebranding_feminism_geethika_ jayatilakas_talk 6 Aug 2008

REFERENCES

Allen DG, Allman KKM, Powers P 1991 Feminist nursing research without gender. Advances in Nursing Science 13(3):49–58

American Association of Colleges of Nursing 2002 Annual state of the schools. Online. Available: www.aacn.nche.edu/media/annual report02.pdf 14 Feb 2003

Aronson P 2003 Feminists or postfeminists? Young women's attitudes toward feminism and gender relations. Gender and Society 17(6):903–922

Baumgardner J, Richards A 2003 The number one question about feminism. Feminist Studies 29(2):448–454

Bent KN 1993 Perspectives on critical and feminist theory in developing nursing praxis. Journal of Professional Nursing 9(5):296–303

Bolton SC 2000 Who cares? Offering emotion work as a 'gift' in the nursing labour process. Journal of Advanced Nursing 32(3):580–586

Boughn S 2001 Why women and men choose nursing. Nursing and Health Care
     Perspectives 22(1):14–24
Boyle MV 2002a Sailing twixt Scylla and Charybdis. Women in Management Review
     17(3/4):131–141
Boyle MV 2002b You wait until you get home: emotional regions, emotional process
     work and the role of off-stage support. Paper presented at the 'Third emotions in
     organisational life conference', Bond University, Gold Coast
Briles J 1994 The Briles report on women in healthcare: changing conflict to
     collaboration in a toxic workplace. Jossey-Bass, San Francisco
Brown CR 1998 Gender segmentation in the paid work force: the case of nursing.
     Unpublished PhD thesis. Griffith University, Brisbane
Brown C, Jones L 2004 The gender structure of the nursing hierarchy: the role of
     human capital. Gender, Work and Organization 11(1):1–25
Brykczynska G (ed.) 1997 Caring: the compassion and wisdom of nursing. Arnold,
     London
Bubeck PE 1995 Care, gender and justice. Clarendon Press, Oxford
Buchanan T 1997 Nursing our narratives: towards a dynamic understanding of
     nurses in literary texts. Nursing Inquiry 4(2):80–87
Caffrey R, Caffrey P 1994 Nursing: caring or codependent? Nursing Forum 29(1):
     12–17
Carpenter M 1977 The new managerialism and professionalism in nursing.
     In: Stacey N, Reid M, Heath C, Dingwall R (eds) Health and the division of labour.
     Croom Helm, London, pp 165–91
Ceci C 2004 Gender, power, nursing: a case analysis. Nursing Inquiry 11(2):72–81
Cheek J, Rudge T 1995 Only connect … feminism and nursing. In: Gray G, Pratt R (eds)
     Scholarship in the discipline of nursing. Churchill Livingstone, Melbourne
David BA 2000 Nursing's gender politics: reformulating the footnotes. Advances in
     Nursing Science 23(1):83–94
Davies C 1995 Gender and the professional predicament in nursing. Open University
     Press, Buckingham
Demerouti E, Bakker AB, Nachreiner F, Schaufeli WB 2000 A model of burnout and
     life satisfaction amongst nurses. Journal of Advanced Nursing 32(2):454–464
Dendaas N 2004 The scholarship related to nursing work environments: where do
     we go from here? Advances in Nursing Science 27(1):12–21
Doering L 1992 Power and knowledge in nursing: a feminist poststructuralist view.
     Advances in Nursing Science 14(4):24–33
Donley R 2005 Challenges for nursing in the 21st century. Nursing Economic$
     23(6):312–318
Edwards SD 1999 The idea of nursing science. Journal of Advanced Nursing
     29(3):563–569
Ehrenreich B, English D 1979 For her own good: 150 years of experts' advice to
     women. Pluto, London
Ekstrom DN 1999 Gender and perceived nurse caring in nurse–patient dyads. Journal
     of Advanced Nursing 29(6):1393–1401
Erturk Y 2004 Considering the role of men in gender agenda setting: conceptual and
     policy issues. Feminist Review 78(1):3–21
Evans J 2004 Men nurses: a historical and feminist perspective. Journal of Advanced
     Nursing 47(3):321–328

Evans M 1997 Introducing contemporary feminist thought. Blackwell Publishers, Oxford

Falk Rafael A 1996 Power and caring: a dialectic in nursing. Advances in Nursing Science 19(1):3–17

Falk Rafael A 1998 Nurses who run with the wolves: the power and caring dialectic revisited. Advances in Nursing Science 21(1):29–42

Fealy GM 2004 'The good nurse': visions and value in images of the nurse. Journal of Advanced Nursing 46(6):649–656

Fineman S 1993 (ed.) Emotion in organizations. Sage, London

Freire P 2007 Pedagogy of the oppressed. Continuum, New York

Gamarnikow E 1978 Sexual division of labour: the case of nursing. In: Kuhn A, Wolpe AM (eds) Feminism and materialism. Routledge & Kegan Paul, London

Gaze H 1987 Man appeal. Nursing Times 83(20):24–27

Georges JM, McGuire S 2004 Deconstructing clinical pathways: mapping the landscape of health care. Advances in Nursing Science 27(1):2–12

Gherardi S 1994 The gender we think, the gender we do in our everyday organizational lives. Human Relations 47(6):591–601

Goffman I 1959 Presentation of the self in everyday life. Overlook Press, New York

Grosz E 1990 Conclusion: a note on essentialism and difference. In: Gunew S (ed.) Feminist knowledge: critique and construct. Routledge, London

Hagell EI 1989 Nursing knowledge: women's knowledge. A sociological perspective. Journal of Advanced Nursing 14:226–233

Hearn J 1993 Emotive subjects: organizational men, organizational masculinities and the (de)construction of 'emotions'. In: Fineman S (ed.) Emotion in organizations. Sage, London

Henderson A 2001 Emotional labour and nursing: an under-appreciated aspect of caring work. Nursing Inquiry 8(2):130–138

Hicks C 1997 The research–practice gap: individual responsibility or corporate culture? Nursing Times 93(39):38–39

Hicks C 1999 Incompatible skills and ideologies: the impediment of gender attributions on nursing research. Journal of Advanced Nursing 30(1):129–139

Hothschild AR 1983 The managed heart: the commercialisation of human feeling. University of California Press, Berkley

Huntington A 1996 Nursing research reframed by the inescapable reality of practice: a personal encounter. Nursing Inquiry 3(3):167–171

International Council of Nurses Nursing Profile 2004 Online. Available: www.icn.ch/Flash/SewDatasheet04.swf 8 Aug 2008

Jackson D 1997 Feminism: a path to clinical knowledge development. Contemporary Nurse 6(2):85–91

Janiszewski Goodin H 2003 The nursing shortage in the United States of America: an integrative review of the literature. Journal of Advanced Nursing 43(4):335–350

Jayatilaka G 2001 Rebranding feminism? Geethika Jayatilaka's talk. Online. Available: www.thefword.org.uk/features/2001/12/rebranding_feminism_geethika_jayatilakas_talk 6 Aug 2008

Jenkins E 1989 Nurses' control over nursing. In: Gray G, Pratt R (eds) Issues in Australian nursing 2. Churchill Livingstone, Melbourne

Kane D, Thomas B 2000 Nursing and the 'f' word. Nursing Forum 35(2):17–25

Kelly A 1985 The construction of masculine science. British Journal of Sociology of Education 6:33–154

Kelly NR, Shoemaker M, Steele T 1996 The experience of being a male student nurse. Journal of Nursing Education 35(4):170–174

Kitson A 2004 Drawing out leadership. Journal of Advanced Nursing 48(3):211

Lather P 1991 Feminist research in education: within/against. Deakin University Press, Geelong

Liaschenko J, Peter E 2004 Nursing ethics and conceptualizations of nursing: profession, practice and work. Journal of Advanced Nursing 46(5):488–495

Loughrey M 2008 Just how male are male nurses …? Journal of Clinical Nursing 17(10):1327–1334

Lupton D 1998 The emotional self. Sage, London

Mackintosh C 1997 A historical study of men in nursing. Journal of Advanced Nursing 26:232–236

McQueen ACH 2004 Emotional intelligence in nursing work. Journal of Advanced Nursing 47(1):101–108

McVicar A 2003 Workplace stress in nursing: a literature review. Journal of Advanced Nursing 44(6):633–642

Mann S, Cowburn J 2005 Emotional labour and stress within mental health nursing. Journal of Psychiatric and Mental Health Nursing 12:154–162

Martinez-Indigo D, Totterdell P, Alcover CM, Holman D 2007 Emotional labour and emotional exhaustion: interpersonal and intrapersonal mechanisms. Work and Stress 21(1):30–47

Mazhindu D 2003 Ideal nurses: the social construction of emotional labour. European Journal of Psychotherapy. Counselling and Health 6(3):243–262

Meadus RJ 2000 Men in nursing: barriers to recruitment. Nursing Forum 35(3):515

Morin KH 1999 Mothers: responses to care given by male nursing students during and after birth. Image: Journal of Nursing Scholarship 31(1):83–87

Myerson DE 2000 If emotions were honoured: a cultural analysis. In: Fineman S Emotion in organizations, 2nd edn. Sage, London

Neuman CE 1999 Taking charge: nursing, suffrage and feminism in America, 1973–1920 (review). Journal of Women's History 10(4):228–235

Nicolson P 1996 Gender, power and organisation: a psychological perspective. Routledge, London

Paliadelis P 2005 Rural nursing unit managers: education and support for the role. The International Electronic Journal of Rural and Remote Health Research, Education Practice and Policy 5(325). Online. Available. http://rrh.deakin.edu.au

Paliadelis P 2008 The working world of nursing unit managers: responsibility without power. Australian Health Review 32(2):256–264

Paliadelis P, Cruickshank M, Sheridan A 2007 Caring for each other: how nurse managers 'manage' their role. Journal of Nursing Management 15(8):830–837

Parker B, McFarland J 1991 Feminist theory and nursing: an empowerment model for research. Advances in Nursing Science 13(3):59–67

Peter E, Lunardi VL, Macfarlane A 2004 Nursing resistance as an ethical action: literature review. Journal of Advanced Nursing 46(4):403–416

Poliafico JK 1998 Nursing's gender gap. Registered Nurse 61(10):39–43

Rancine L 2003 Implementing a postcolonial feminist perspective in nursing research related to non-Western populations. Nursing Inquiry 10(2):91–102

Roberts SJ 2000 Development of a positive professional identity: liberating oneself from the oppressor within. Advances in Nursing Science 22(4):71–83

Rockler-Gladen N 2007 Third wave feminism: personal empowerment dominates this feminist philosophy. Online. Available: http:feminism.suite101.com/article.cfm/third_wave_feminism 6 Aug 2008

Ryan S, Porter S 1993 Men in nursing: a cautionary critique. Nursing Outlook 41(6):262–267

Sandelowski M 1997 (Ir)reconcilable differences? The debate concerning nursing and technology. Image: Journal of Nursing Scholarship 29(2):169–174

Shakespeare P 2003 Nurses' bodywork: is there a body of work? Nursing Inquiry 10(1):47–56

Sharman E 1998 The glass elevator: how men overtake women in the nursing higher education workforce in Australia. Unpublished PhD thesis, University of New South Wales, Sydney

Sharman E, Short S, Black D 1996 Why so many? The masculine mystique and men in the nursing higher education workforce in Australia. In conference proceedings of the 'Changing society for women's health conference', Australian National University, Canberra

Street A 1995 Nursing replay: researching nursing culture together. Churchill Livingstone, Melbourne

Treacy MP 1989 Gender prescription in nurse training: its effects on health provision. In: Hardy LK, Randell J (eds) Recent advances in nursing: issues in women's health. Churchill Livingstone, Edinburgh

Tronto JC 1999 Caring: gender-sensitive ethics. Hypatia 14(1):112–120

Valentine PEB 2001 A gender perspective on conflict management strategies of nurses. Journal of Nursing Scholarship 33(1):69–79

Weir H, Waddington K 2008 Continuities of caring? Emotion work in a NHS direct call centre. Nursing Inquiry 15(1):67–77

Whittemore R 1999 Natural science and nursing science: where do the horizons fuse? Journal of Advanced Nursing 30(5):1027–1033

Williams C 1992 The glass escalator: hidden advantages for men in the 'female' professions. Social Problems 39(3):253–267

Winters J, Ballou KA 2004 The idea of nursing science. Journal of Advanced Nursing 45(5):533–535

Wuest J 1997 Illuminating environmental influences on women's caring. Journal of Advanced Nursing 26(1):49–58

Wynter V 2006 Feminism is passé because it worked. Online. Available: www.onlineopinion.com.au/view.asp?article=4781 6 Aug 2008

Zebroski SA 2001 The gender lens: caring and gender. Journal of Comparative Family Studies 32(2):322–323

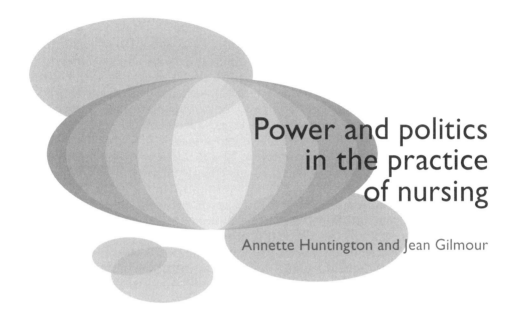

CHAPTER 13

Power and politics in the practice of nursing

Annette Huntington and Jean Gilmour

LEARNING OBJECTIVES

After completing this chapter, the reader will:

- understand the nature of power and politics
- have an awareness of different theoretical conceptions of power
- understand the way in which nurses possess power individually and collectively
- understand the advocacy role and how it relates to power, and
- appreciate the complexities of whistleblowing and its consequences.

KEY WORDS

Power, politics, agency, influence, advocacy, whistleblowing

NURSING AND POLITICS

Nursing is a political activity. Politics, in the broadest sense of the word, is part of all nurses' lives, especially in the large institutions within which many of us work. It is therefore important that we think about power and politics. At the very least, we need to understand that the health sector is a highly politicised environment at both micro and macro levels, and that the health sector is not an apolitical or neutral site. As nurses, we have considerable power in this highly political arena.

Health is fundamental to life, and nurses are intimately involved in caring for the sick and supporting the healthy, either directly or indirectly, wherever they are working. Nurses are in a privileged position in that millions of people every day put their trust in nurses and assume that nurses will always work on the public's behalf. When you become a nurse, you accept the obligations and expectations that go with being in that highly responsible and highly respected (particularly by the general public) role. When you become registered, you also accept all that registration carries with it in terms of commitment to a code of ethics, at the centre of which is the safety and wellbeing of those for whom you care. Key to this is using the power that you have wisely, and being aware of the moral and ethical obligations you have because of this position of trust.

Every nurse has a degree of power. Even as a newly registered nurse you immediately have power over patients/clients, who are nearly always in a less powerful position due to your knowledge of both health and illness, and the healthcare system. Knowledge is power, and just the ability to impart or withhold information puts you in a privileged position in relation to the people and/or communities with whom you work. Henderson's (2003) research in Western Australia exploring the power imbalance between nurses and patients clearly highlighted this, as the nurses in the study showed a reluctance to share any meaningful power with the patients. As the author says: 'This imbalance of power was most evident in information-giving and during nurse–patient interactions, where nurses used their power to maintain control' (Henderson 2003:504).

In addition to an individual nurse's power in the patient/client relationship, nurses as a collective also have considerable potential power. In many countries, nurses are the largest occupational group in the healthcare sector. In New Zealand, nurses comprise 50% of the health and disability workforce (Health Workforce Advisory Committee 2003) and, in Australia, nearly 60% (Commonwealth of Australia 2002). Many of the reforms and restructuring that have taken place in Western health systems in recent years are focused on controlling and managing this considerable workforce—often due to the perceived cost of providing nurses' services in the health sector. However, these same numbers give nurses power—power that can be used to influence the health system and improve it for both nurses and the public. As Holmes and Gastaldo (2002:563) state: 'Nurses also form a critical group that challenges the status quo and works for a more equitable society'. To be active in such a way, nurses require an understanding of power and its effects, and the way that they can use their power to enhance the health and wellbeing of people.

Power is often considered a negative and oppressive attribute. However, new definitions of the nature of power by philosophers such as Michel Foucault, who will be discussed in this chapter, incorporate the notion of power as constructive and constitutive, as well as having the potential to be destructive and oppressive. These new definitions also provide nurses with a new way of considering power, a way that means we can view nurses as being powerless in certain situations but very powerful in other circumstances. This frees us from the idea that we are inherently powerless and/or victims, simply through being nurses. This rethinking and reshaping of nurses' positioning can be particularly valuable in the current climate of global nurse shortages and shrinking health sector resources, which can result in a highly stressful environment in which nurses can feel they have little power to influence or change practices or structures.

In this chapter, we explore the concept of power and its multiple meanings and understandings. We then go on to discuss nurses' political power, followed by a discussion of power in practice, including issues of advocacy and whistleblowing.

UNDERSTANDING POWER

Power is a concept that has many meanings and definitions, and different perceptions of power will influence both people's actions and the outcomes of these actions. Simple definitions consider power to involve something one person has over another (Poggi 2001), and the potential to be influential—that is, make your ideas known to others and gain their support (Sullivan 2004).

Dye and Harrison (2005) offer a more complex definition of influence, suggesting that it is a form of power where particular effects are produced through a system of reward and punishment. They argue that power is based on access to intertwined resources such as wealth, education, political influence and economics. Resources are not evenly distributed through society, and those with 'power' control resources through rewards or the threat of deprivation of resources. An example related to nursing is when managers or clinical leaders control nurses' workload and conditions through processes such as rostering. The management role can be enacted in a range of ways, from an autocratic top-down directive with no space for personal preferences, to a participatory style of management where the nurses in a ward manage their own roster and the allocation of patient care. Ultimately, however, the manager or clinical leader has the ability to choose how they will organise work and shift allocations, and therefore has the power in this situation.

Michel Foucault (1980), a French philosopher, has another viewpoint on power. He suggests that power is exercised rather than possessed, is productive rather than mainly repressive, and furthermore emerges from below. This means that people traditionally constructed as powerless and oppressed can be seen as actually having agency—defined as the capacity to act and exert power, and therefore affecting the way it is enacted. Power circulates, rather than being localised 'never in anybody's hands, never appropriated as a commodity or piece of wealth' (Foucault 1980:98). People are simultaneously affected by power relationships and participate in those relationships.

Foucault's definition highlights the flow of power in everyday practices and relationships, and the inherent potential for the exercise of power as a productive force in social relationships. He also differentiates power relations from relations of force or violence where there is no choice and where possibilities are curtailed. The significant factor for nurses in this representation of power is that power relationships involve the possibility of resistance—the person over whom power is exercised has the capacity to react and respond in a range of ways (Foucault 1983).

Feminist writers also focus on power, as it is a central concept in any discussion of agency and/or oppression. Many feminist scholars engage with postmodern thought that considers power, in a similar way to the work of Foucault, as being a discursively constructed relationship, rather than an oppressive force requiring a victim (Peter et al 2004). As Shildrick states:

> … what becomes possible is to speak of power, not perhaps in the sense of monolithic structures, but as a field of forces held together in shifting but temporally analysable contestable configurations (Shildrick 1997:115).

While many feminist scholars consider concepts from the work of Foucault and postmodernism to be useful for feminist thinking related to power (Lupton 2003, Weedon 1997), others critique the lack of acknowledgment of the gender dimensions in such constructions of power—gender obviously being a central tenant of feminist thinking around power (Huntington & Gilmour 2001).

POLITICS AND POWER

Politics permeates all aspects of life. Mason et al (2007:4) define politics as 'the process of influencing the allocation of scarce resources'. As to who is influential, Lasswell (1958) describes them as those who get the most of what there is to get. If success in politics is judged by control over resources, nurses historically have been unsuccessful in the political arena when judged by such factors as pay parity with equivalent professional groups or satisfactory working environments. Sullivan (2004) argues that historical factors still impact on nurses' degree of influence in contemporary healthcare, with values such as personal discipline, a focus on service and obedience being seen by some as fundamental characteristics of nurses.

While many nurses have effectively engaged in politics at all levels, these values, along with the issues around the gendered culture of nursing (discussed in Ch 12), have limited the full realisation of nurses' and nursing's potential for political action, influence and advocacy. Takase et al (2001) also argue that nurses have been historically disadvantaged by their close relationship with medical colleagues. This has positioned the practice of nursing as subservient to the practice of medicine, and impacts negatively on nurses' perception of themselves. This perception can inhibit nurses from seeing the power that their increasing professionalisation confers.

Politics at state and national level is often thought of as only involving government. Governments are critical bodies for regulating behaviour in that 'government lays down the "rules of the game" in conflict and competition between individuals, organizations, and institutions within society' (Dye & Harrison 2005:198). But politics, seen as the exercise of power in the form of influence, is also part of everyday life. Engaging in political action—learning to be more influential in relation to matters that count—is therefore a possibility for all nurses. Sullivan (2004) suggests that influence exists through relationships and is more significant than authority. It is gained through position or respect for knowledge and skills. She also suggests that influence is earned through effort and that the skills of influence can be learnt, the most crucial factor being the personal decision to become influential.

Nurses tend to think that because they are good people doing a good job they should be valued and fairly rewarded and, if that does not happen, they blame themselves or the profession (Sullivan 2004). However, nurses may in fact be unrewarded due to not effectively engaging in the underlying political game—engagement, which requires adherence to a particular set of rules that they may not even know exists. Critically, we as nurses must therefore recognise the existence and reality of politics, the legitimacy and necessity of being involved in politics, and learn skills to gain greater influence if personal and professional goals are to be achieved. Sullivan (2004) identifies some possible workplace strategies for developing influence, including:

- reciprocity with other workers (i.e. exchanging favours)
- having a good understanding of the informal information that circulates within the organisation
- avoiding confrontation
- compromising when necessary to achieve a more important goal
- networking
- accepting responsibility for individual actions, both positive and negative, and
- finding a mentor.

The idea of playing workplace politics may not initially resonate with the cherished nursing ideal of teamwork, but having influence and developing assertive and satisfying interdisciplinary relationships are essential factors in nurses being active in ensuring the provision of high-quality nursing care.

NURSES' POLITICAL POWER

All people have political power as individuals, but nurses also have great potential as a collective body to exercise their power. Australian and New Zealand nurses are increasingly well educated at graduate level and have a growing evidence-based body of knowledge to support nursing practice. Nurses also work in wide-ranging roles in healthcare, spanning clinical, management, research, teaching and health policy domains that provide multiple opportunities to exert influence.

A key element of realising collective power is having formal ways to organise collectives of people for a common cause that is well articulated and appeals to broad segments of the population. In nursing, the protection, support and influence derived from the power of the collective is realised through professional organisations. This is shown clearly in situations such as collective salary bargaining or guaranteed nurse–patient ratios, such as those negotiated in Victoria, which have had a major impact on the working environment for nurses. Neither of these would be possible to negotiate at an individual level. There are many professional bodies that primarily serve to advance the interests of the nursing workforce. As nurses, you have the opportunity to be involved and shape the political activity of these organisations through contribution as a member or at governance level.

One of the most important choices you will make as a registered nurse, therefore, is the decision to join your professional body. The particular structures and focus of nursing organisations varies considerably, but their two broad areas of interest are industrial or employment concerns and what are loosely called 'professional issues'. Some organisations have two arms and encompass both these aspects, while others will focus specifically on one area. The choice of which organisation to join is up to you, but should be given careful thought, considering what each organisation's role is, the focus and achievements of each organisation, and what they can provide. An excellent overview of Australian and New Zealand organisations is provided at: www.nurses.info/organizations_australia_newzealand.htm.

While nurses are often considered an homogenous group, it is important to accept that nurses are enormously diverse. As a result, while the overall goal of nursing may be shared by everyone in the profession, individual nurses will not always share worldviews at either the macro or micro level. Therefore, using the power nurses have means being highly skilled at working not only with diverse population groups, but also with diverse nurses and nursing groups. Nurses have widely differing philosophical and political positions, and one strategy for managing this diversity is through the focus that professional organisations can bring. This means that individual difference can be accepted, but organisational power can focus on collective professional issues.

An example of nurses successfully using their collective political power to advance practice through the legislative process is the gaining of prescribing authority. Australian and New Zealand nurses have advocated for changes in legislation and governmental processes to enable nurses (usually advanced practitioners) to prescribe in their scope of practice. In New Zealand, extending prescribing rights to nurse practitioners has been contentious, with some members of the medical profession, such as general practitioners, concerned with potential competition for funding (Mackay 2003). After a drawn out and contested political process, the *Medicines (Designated Prescribers: Nurse Practitioners) Regulations* 2005 now provide a framework for nurse practitioner prescribing.

Jones' (2004) description of the approach taken by the Royal College of Nursing (RCN) in the United Kingdom notes that the implementation of nurse prescribing required 'political machination, the need to construct an effective case, and deft manoeuvring within the corridors of power' (Jones 2004:266). Initial elements of the strategy to increase political influence included focusing on a clear objective, taking advantage of an existing opportunity (which in the United Kingdom was the review of community nursing), developing alliances with the British Medical Association and pharmacists, and ensuring a unified professional position by managing internal concerns raised by groups such as practice nurses.

Table 13.1 lists some ways of developing influence through knowledge, communication skills and action.

POWER IN PRACTICE

Knowledge carries with it power and authority, but not all forms of knowledge are created equal. In the preceding section on nurses' political power, we discussed the power that nurses have as a collective. However, there is ample evidence to suggest that nurses have been conspicuously silent, or have been silenced, at times when it has been vital that patients have had vocal, assertive and knowledgeable advocates. Chiarella (2000) argues that within the legal system, nurses are seen as a separate but subordinate group to medicine, which impacts on the authority of nurses' testimony and their opportunities to speak:

> Today or tomorrow or the next day, a nurse may or may not intervene to stop a doctor from making a mistake, which might harm the patient. It will not depend on the law. It will depend on how brave they are. They operate inside (or outside) a legal framework, which insufficiently recognises their work and their presence (Chiarella 2000:198).

One instance of the devaluation of nurses' knowledge and authority by the medical profession, with lethal results, involved 12 children who died during or shortly after undergoing cardiac surgery in a Canadian hospital in 1994. Nurses involved in the cardiac surgery service had made sustained attempts to voice their concerns through the appropriate hospital channels during the preceding year, but these had not been taken seriously (Ceci 2004). Medical peers of the surgeon dismissed the validity of claims by

Knowledge	Communication skills	Action
Nursing knowledge base		
Evidence-based clinical practice knowledge Patient and family knowledge/agendas/issues Policy/legislation knowledge at government, discipline and organisational levels	Articulate and assertive verbal communication Clear and appropriate written communication meeting academic/media/political/popular conventions, depending on context	Respond in a timely and coherent manner Document using appropriate channels Take opportunities to be involved in shaping policy through submissions and committee work Use information technology competently for communication and information retrieval
Understanding power		
Relationship of knowledge with power Power as a circulating force The capacity for resistance Differentiation of power relations and force relations	Professional introductions Title parity Adhere to professional code of dress Prepare accounts demonstrating importance of nursing work	Take leadership opportunities—formal and informal Accept responsibility Use knowledge to inform patients and families Act as an advocate
The rules of the game for:		
Nursing Heathcare teams Organisations Communities	Network within and outside the profession Develop and use relationships with media and politicians	Develop respectful and communicative relationships within and outside nursing Be tenacious Enlist support from broader communities of interest in issues of concern to nursing

Table 13.1 Developing influence through knowledge, communication skills and action

several nurses that there were competency issues on the grounds that nurses did not have medical expertise. In a similar Australian example, the repeated complaints of Bundaberg Base Hospital nurses about the actions of an incompetent surgeon, who was eventually implicated in at least 13 patient deaths, were not acted upon by the Director of Medical Services (Davies 2005).

When nurses themselves feel powerless, however, they may choose not to act, and this can also have dire consequences. One example of this was revealed during New Zealand's Cartwright Inquiry into cervical cancer, which revealed unethical medical research practices and the lack of informed consent about treatment options. The approach to treatment, carried out from 1966 until the early 1980s, studied the progression of cervical cancer *in situ* in a group of women, without offering medical intervention, until progression to invasive cancer (Coney 1988). Nurses throughout this period working at this particular hospital did not openly voice their concerns or ensure the women had been provided with the information necessary to make an informed choice about participation. Judge Silvia Cartwright stated that:

> … nurses who most appropriately should be advocates for the patient, feel sufficiently intimidated by the medical staff (who do not hire or fire them) that even today they fail or refuse to confront openly the issues arising from the 1966 trial (Committee of Inquiry into Allegations Concerning the Treatment of Cervical Cancer at National Women's Hospital and into Other Related Matters 1988:172).

Although by speaking out the nurses at that time may not have been able to stop particular medical practices, their complicity through silence is something that nurses in New Zealand have to acknowledge. Constructing ourselves as powerless and lacking in agency can lead to nurses behaving unethically and not putting patients' best interests at the centre of our professional obligations.

Buresh and Gordon (2006) have offered a powerful critique of nurses' lack of visibility and voice in the public arena, and suggest many strategies for 'creating a voice of agency' (Buresh & Gordon 2006:25). Expressing agency is built upon the realisation of the importance of nurses' work and the confidence of nurses themselves. To make this agency explicit requires change at the fundamental level of day-to-day practice. Every encounter with patients, families and other staff members is an opportunity to communicate, verbally and non-verbally, messages about the competency and the knowledge base underpinning our decisions and practices.

Expressing agency begins right at the first introduction to patients and colleagues. For example, status can be reinforced through the use of both first and last names rather than just first name, along with title and role, a professional standard of dress, and non-deferential body language. Buresh and Gordon (2006) have written extensively on the necessity for nurses to take every opportunity to educate people they meet about what they do and why they do it:

> To convey the content of nursing, nurses must describe the complexity of care *they* give and the clinical judgments *they* use. They must be careful not to depict themselves as extensions of the doctor's agency in their discussions with patients and families, the broader public, the media, and political representatives (Buresh & Gordon 2006:67).

As nurses, we are highly educated practitioners with both formal education in, and considerable informal knowledge of, the culture and processes of the health system within which our clients and patients find themselves. This has important implications for power relationships between ourselves and the people for whom we care.

An example of our everyday exercise of power is the categorisation of people through the practice of assessment and the ensuing allocation of resources to them. Assessment requires recording a range of information and judging whether a person meets certain predetermined criteria for normality and/or abnormality. The distribution of a wide range of resources, including the time and expertise of nurses and other health professionals, medical equipment, pharmaceuticals, and access to the care setting is determined by nursing assessment.

From a Foucauldian perspective, the assessment process therefore needs to incorporate opportunities for patients and their families to exercise some control. This can be achieved by providing information about the purpose, scope and implications of the assessment in clear language, obtaining informed consent, and validating the documented information with the person concerned.

Power can also be used by nurses to improve practice and the experiences of the people and groups with whom we are working. We have chosen to highlight two particular situations or practices where power can be used by the individual nurse. The first of these is the advocacy role that for many nurses is an integral part of day-to-day practice, and the second is what is commonly called 'whistleblowing'.

Advocacy

Advocacy consists of taking action on behalf of a person, or supporting an individual or group to gain what they need from the system. This is now considered a fundamental element of practice at all levels and is often enshrined in nursing documents such as codes of ethics for practice (MacDonald 2006). For example, it is increasingly being included in basic texts, where it is addressed as one of the most important aspects of nurses' work (e.g. Craven & Hirnle 2003). It is also raised as a strategy or technique useful for nurse leaders (Borbasi et al 2004). The increasingly overstretched and changing world of service delivery means that, more than ever before, nurses need to understand and enact our advocacy role at the micro and macro level.

Authors such as Teasdale (1998:1) define advocacy as 'influencing those who have power on behalf of those who do not'. However, this definition could be seen as limiting the empowerment of individuals or groups—as in many instances it may be more appropriate to support a person or community to advocate for themselves (MacDonald 2006). It is important to recognise that acting as an advocate does not involve taking over the situation. This can result in a nurse acting out what he or she feels is best for the person, rather than acting to ensure that the person achieves what they want (Henderson 2003). This second form of advocacy still involves the nurse in an act of advocacy, but one that reflects a more Foucauldian approach to power, in which everyone *has* power but may need support and information to *enact* that power. If a nurse is not able to act in this way, then the appropriate action is to ensure that the person or group has access to another source of advocacy.

To be able to act effectively as an advocate, nurses need the following:

- understanding of the politics, culture and systems of health sector institutions and health service delivery
- respect for the client or community and their rights
- understanding of relevant clinical issues
- understanding of ethical issues
- commitment to the client and/or group, and
- understanding of the need for evidence and the way it can be used to support decisions.

Advocacy can be used at all levels in the health system. It can be part of day-to-day practice in relationships with patients and clients, or it can involve influencing service delivery to enhance services for a client group or community as a whole. It is important, however, that nurses understand that there are limits to their advocacy skills, and that in some areas such as mental health, people may prefer external or non-health professional advocates. External advocates can be provided by special interest sector groups, or be paid independent advocates.

Many nurses are also key players in special interest groups working with people with particular health issues. Patient and family representative groups are effective lobbyists often accorded a voice in health policy development. Joint initiatives with these groups offer productive alliances to further nurses', and health consumers', agendas focused on improving healthcare services (Davies 2004). For example, the Health and Disability Commissioner in New Zealand has established the New Zealand Code of Health and Disability Services Consumer's Rights (1996), which aims to protect consumers' rights, works in conjunction with a consumer advocate and has established a complaints system. Part of our advocacy role is to be aware of the form of advocacy that is preferred by the clients or patients concerned, and to be able to discuss this in an informed manner.

Whistleblowing

Whistleblowing, like advocacy, requires the nurse to be assertive, but also involves taking a very public stand, something that requires 'conviction, assertiveness and self-confidence' (McDonald & Ahern 1999:12). We would also add that the nurse in this situation is usually motivated by a strong sense of the moral obligation that, as noted in our introduction, comes with being a nurse.

Although authors have defined whistleblowing in a range of ways, according to Greene and Latting (2004:2) there are certain consistencies:

- it is an act of notifying powerful others of wrongful practices in an organisation
- the whistleblower is motivated by wanting to prevent unnecessary harm to others, and
- it is the action of an employee or former employee who has privileged access to information.

Or, as Dawson (2000:1) says: 'Whistleblowers are those who sound the alert on scandal, danger, malpractice, or corruption'. In situations where resources are stretched in the health sector and nurses as the biggest group are often being targeted in inevitable health cuts, events serious enough to warrant such a step may well increase (Jackson 2008).

Whistleblowing is an extremely serious action and there are major implications that must be considered by a nurse when he or she decides to take this step (Firtko & Jackson 2005). Nurses who take such action must be considered as courageous and need the support of colleagues, friends and family, rather than being subject to hostility and harassment. As McDonald and Ahern (1999) highlight in their research into the coping strategies of those considering whistleblowing, whether the nurses chose to take that final step of actually whistleblowing or not, they experienced fear, anxiety and intimidation.

Jackson and Raftos (1997) found in their research with registered nurses that whistleblowing was an extremely difficult decision, and one that left the nurses feeling exposed and unsupported. However, this study also highlights the way in which these particular nurses put their moral obligation to the residents above the possible harm they may experience themselves. The concept of 'personal resilience' is considered important in terms of being able to positively cope with adverse situations, and practice in difficult workplaces. It involves developing strategies such as productive professional networks and focusing on personal development in areas such as the maintenance of a positive attitude, work–life balance and emotional insight (Jackson et al 2007).

Greene and Latting (2004) provide guidelines for whistleblowing and stress that this is the step taken only when all other avenues have been exhausted. The box below provides a list based on their work that is applicable for nurses in this situation.

GUIDELINES FOR WHISTLEBLOWING (GREENE & LATTING 2004)

- Assess the situation and one's own preparedness to go forward. How serious is the issue? What are my motives? Can I live with myself if I stay silent? Can I cope with the results of 'going public'?
- Assume others in the organisation are concerned. Discuss the issue with colleagues, and see if there are steps that could be taken that you have overlooked.
- Obtain corroborating evidence and supporters. Collect as much evidence as possible, and discuss it with colleagues.
- Keep careful records. Keep precise and detailed documentation, as often whistleblowing can result in legal proceedings, and/or internal or government inquiries.
- Use the chain of command. Unless urgent and extremely serious, ensure you have exhausted all other avenues within the organisation for addressing the situation first.
- Obtain the advice of dispassionate, expert outsiders, such as your professional organisation, your registration body, a lawyer or employment advisers, and consult websites.
- Obtain emotional support, as this is going to be a difficult time for you. Ensure you have someone you can talk to who will encourage and support you.
- Consider going outside the organisation only as a last resort. Keep foremost in your mind that this action is for the benefit of the clients/patients/residents and that the experience of many professionals in this situation is that they do, in the end, leave the institution.

The whistleblowing actions of Toni Hoffman, the Nurse Unit Manager of the Intensive Care Unit at Bundaberg Base Hospital, Queensland, which were taken in response to concerns about the competence of a surgeon, follow the steps outlined by Greene and Latting (2004). She persistently communicated her concerns about specific cases that demonstrated issues with surgical clinical competence to the appropriate authorities, verbally and in writing. Her evidence was supported by written statements from other nurses. As a last resort she approached the local Member of Parliament and her documentation was eventually tabled in the Queensland Parliament; processes were then initiated to address major and systemic health service issues (Davies 2005).

The need and value of whistleblowing is increasingly being recognised. A number of countries, or states and territories within countries, are enacting whistleblowing protection legislation. For example, in New Zealand there exists the *Protected Disclosures Act 2000*, which has been passed with the express purpose of promoting public interest by:

> ... facilitating the disclosure and investigation of matters of serious wrongdoing in or by an organisations and by protecting employees who ... make disclosures of information about serious wrongdoing in or by an organisation (section 5(a) and (b)).

In Australia, the existence of such legislation depends on the state or territory, with examples including the South Australian *Whistleblowers Protection Act 1993*, the Queensland *Whistleblowers Protection Act 1994* and the New South Wales *Protected Disclosures Act 1994*.

Although there is considerable discussion about the extent to which employees are in fact protected by such legislation (Dawson 2000), it is essential for a nurse who has decided that this course of action must be taken to find out whether the state, territory or country has such legislation, and what this legislation provides in terms of protection. This is particularly important given that some legislation only applies to state sector employees, and does not extend to the private working environment. There are also organisations that support those who are contemplating or have already been involved in whistleblowing.

The website www.uow.edu.au/arts/sts/bmartin/dissent/ provides the names of organisations in a number of countries, which can provide information in this area.

Another extremely important issue is for nurses to understand and support those who feel that whistleblowing is their only avenue for dealing with an issue. Too often, those who choose to take a stand can feel isolated and be subject to both overt and more subtle forms of harassment. Recognising what is involved for a nurse taking such an action, even if you do not agree with it, and making this known to the person, can make a significant difference to their experience in what is an extremely stressful situation. This stress can be due to both ongoing concern for those people who have been subject to whatever practices have led to the whistleblowing, and also a very realistic concern for the fallout that the nurse will inevitably experience.

It also is important to note that not doing anything in the face of clearly inappropriate, destructive or neglectful practices can be harmful and stressful for a nurse, and a factor in that stress can be that many nurses feel, because they understand what is going on, they have a responsibility to react in some way. McDonald and Ahern (1999) note previous studies showing that those nurses who chose not to act as whistleblowers or advocates felt depressed and suffered from fatigue and moral anguish.

CONCLUSION

Nurses have traditionally been constructed as powerless by both themselves and others (Holmes & Gastaldo 2002). However, it is time that we reconsider this and acknowledge that nurses are in a very powerful position in society. More nurses than ever are both prepared at degree level and are undertaking postgraduate study that enhances their ability to provide care in the increasingly complex health services. Nursing services are pivotal in the provision of healthcare and in enacting the health goals of the international community: 'they form the backbone of health systems around the globe and provide a platform for efforts to tackle the diseases that cause poverty and ill health'

(World Health Organization 2002:vii). As nurses, we mediate between healthcare institutions, with their associated mysterious practices, language and technologies, and the person—translating and making the health system understandable for the individual or community.

Nurses are a powerful group, expert in terms of their knowledge base, their practice and their understanding of the impact of health on people and communities. This knowledge and experience places the nurse in a very powerful position in terms of being able to influence people they are working with to make particular decisions regarding their health and wellbeing. Understanding and being consciously political at both the collective and individual levels is central to using the privileged position we have to work on behalf of patients and clients, to improve their experience of healthcare and their health outcomes.

REFLECTIVE QUESTIONS

1 How can nurses as a professional group be more effective in terms of political action?

2 How can power imbalances between you and your patients be minimised in everyday practice?

3 What do patients and families need to know to be effective advocates for themselves and others?

RECOMMENDED READINGS

Buresh B, Gordon S 2006 From silence to voice: what nurses know and must communicate to the public, 2nd edn. ILR Press, Ithaca

Chiarella M 2000 Silence in court: the devaluation of the stories of nurses in the narratives of health law. Nursing Inquiry 7(3):191–199

Diers D 2004 Speaking of nursing: narratives of practice, research, policy and the profession. Jones & Bartlett, Massachusetts

Firtko A, Jackson D 2005 Do the ends justify the means? Nursing and the dilemma of whistle-blowing. Australian Journal of Advanced Nursing 23(1):51–56

Greene AD, Latting JK 2004 Whistle-blowing as a form of advocacy: guidelines for the practitioner and organization. Social Work 49(2):1–13

Jones M 2004 Case report. Nurse prescribing: a case study in policy influence. Journal of Nursing Management 12:266–272

Sullivan EJ 2004 Becoming influential: a guide for nurses. Pearson/Prentice Hall, New Jersey

Online resources

Nurses.info: www.nurses.info/organizations_australia_newzealand.htm
Suppression of dissent: www.uow.edu.au/arts/sts/bmartin/dissent/contacts
Whistleblowers Australia: www.whistleblowers.org.au

REFERENCES

Borbasi S, Jones J, Gaston C 2004 Leading, motivating and supporting colleagues in nursing practice. In: Daly J, Speedy S, Jackson D (eds) Nursing leadership. Churchill Livingstone, Sydney, pp 167–81

Buresh B, Gordon S 2006 From silence to voice: what nurses know and must communicate to the public, 2nd edn. ILR Press, Ithaca

Ceci C 2004 Nursing, knowledge and power: a case analysis. Social Science and Medicine 59:1879–1889

Chiarella M 2000 Silence in court: the devaluation of the stories of nurses in the narratives of health law. Nursing Inquiry 7(3):191–199

Committee of Inquiry into Allegations Concerning the Treatment of Cervical Cancer at National Women's Hospital and into Other Related Matters 1988 The report of the committee of inquiry into allegations concerning the treatment of cervical cancer at National Women's Hospital and into other related matters. The Committee, Auckland

Commonwealth of Australia 2002 National review of nursing education 2002: our duty of care. Commonwealth of Australia, Canberra

Coney S 1988 The unfortunate experiment. Penguin Books, Auckland

Craven RF, Hirnle CJ (eds) 2003 Fundamentals of nursing: human health and function, 4th edn. Lippincott, Philadelphia

Davies C 2004 Political leadership and the politics of nursing. Journal of Nursing Management 12:235–241

Davies G 2005 Queensland public hospitals commission of inquiry report: the state of Queensland: Online. Available: www.qphci.qld.gov.au/Final_Report.htm 30 July 2008

Dawson S 2000 Whistleblowing: a broad definition and some issues for Australia. Working Paper 3/2000. Victoria University of Technology. Online. Available: www.uow.edu.au/arts/sts/bmartin/dissent/documents/Dawson.html

Dye TR, Harrison BC 2005 Power and society: an introduction to the social sciences, 10th edn. Thomson Wadsworth, Belmont, California

Firtko A, Jackson D 2005 Do the ends justify the means? Nursing and the dilemma of whistle-blowing. Australian Journal of Advanced Nursing 23(1):51–56

Foucault M 1980 Two lectures. In: Gordon C (ed.) Power/knowledge. Pantheon Books, New York, pp 78–108

Foucault M 1983 Afterword: the subject and power. In: Dreyfus H, Rabinow P Michel Foucault: beyond structuralism and hermeneutics, 2nd edn. University of Chicago Press, Chicago, pp 208–26

Greene AD, Latting JK 2004 Whistle-blowing as a form of advocacy: guidelines for the practitioner and organization. Social Work 49(2):1–13

Health Workforce Advisory Committee (HWAC) 2003 The New Zealand health workforce future directions: recommendations to the Minister of Health. HWAC, Wellington

Henderson S 2003 Power imbalance between nurses and patients: a potential inhibitor of partnership in care. Journal of Clinical Nursing 12(4):501–508

Holmes D, Gastaldo D 2002 Nursing as means of governmentality. Journal of Advanced Nursing 38(6):557–565

Huntington AD, Gilmour JA 2001 Re-thinking representations, re-writing nursing texts: possibilities through feminist and Foucauldian thought. Journal of Advanced Nursing 35(6):902–908

Jackson D 2008 What becomes of the whistleblowers? Journal of Clinical Nursing 17(10):1261–1262

Jackson D, Firtko A, Edenborough M 2007 Personal resilience as a strategy for surviving and thriving in the face of workplace adversity: a literature review. Journal of Advanced Nursing 60(1):1–9

Jackson D, Raftos M 1997 In uncharted waters: confronting the culture of silence in a residential care institution. International Journal of Nursing Practice 3:34–39

Jones M 2004 Case report. Nurse prescribing: a case study in policy influence. Journal of Nursing Management 12:266–272

Lasswell H 1958 Politics: who gets what, when, how. World Publishing Company, New York

Lupton D 2003 Medicine as culture, 2nd edn. Sage Publications, London

MacDonald H 2006 Relational ethics and advocacy in nursing: literature review. Journal of Advanced Nursing 57(2):119–126

McDonald S, Ahern K 1999 Whistle-blowing: effective and ineffective coping responses. Nursing Forum 34(4):5–13

Mackay B 2003 General practitioners' perceptions of the nurse practitioner role: an exploratory study. The New Zealand Medical Journal 116(1170). Online. Available: www.nzma.org.nz/journal/116-1170/356/

Mason D, Leavitt J, Chaffee M 2007 Policy and politics: a framework for action. In: Mason D, Leavitt J, Chaffee M (eds) Policy and politics in nursing and health care, 5th edn. Saunders, St Louis, pp 1–16

Peter E, Lunardi AL, Macfarlane A 2004 Nursing resistance as ethical action: literature review. Journal of Advanced Nursing 46(4):403–416

Poggi G 2001 Forms of power. Polity Press, Cambridge

Shildrick M 1997 Leaky bodies and boundaries: feminism, postmoderism and (bio) ethics. Routledge, London

Sullivan EJ 2004 Becoming influential: a guide for nurses. Pearson Prentice Hall, New Jersey

Takase M, Kershaw E, Burt L 2001 Nurse–environment misfit and nursing practice. Journal of Advanced Nursing 35(6):819–826

Teasdale K 1998 Advocacy in health care. Blackwell Science, Oxford

Weedon C 1997 Feminist practice and poststructuralist theory. Blackwell Publishers, Oxford

World Health Organization (WHO) 2002 Strategic directions for strengthening nursing and midwifery services. WHO, Geneva

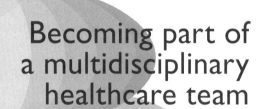

CHAPTER 14

Becoming part of a multidisciplinary healthcare team

Patrick Crookes, Rhondha Griffiths and Angela Brown

LEARNING OBJECTIVES

Having read and understood this chapter, the reader will be able to:

- describe the characteristics of multidisciplinary healthcare teams
- discuss the advantages of multidisciplinary teams as a model of providing healthcare
- discuss the attributes that contribute to high levels of satisfaction and effectiveness among members of multidisciplinary teams
- outline ways in which conflict may come about in multidisciplinary teams, and
- describe strategies for managing conflict in multidisciplinary teams.

KEY WORDS

Models of healthcare, multidisciplinary teams and teamwork, communication, roles, socialisation, oppressed group behaviour, values, leadership, shared governance, magnet hospitals, managed care, transformational leadership

---

INTRODUCTION

In contemporary healthcare much greater attention is being paid to the importance of good teamwork in healthcare for a range of reasons (Baker et al 2006). Perhaps most importantly this is because evidence has emerged which shows that a significant number of adverse events in healthcare can be attributed to poor communication and poor teamwork among health professional teams (Manjolovich et al 2008). Quality and safety can be compromised where these issues exist with negative consequences for those on the receiving end of healthcare.

Research has also demonstrated that members of a multidisciplinary team may not be well informed about the nature and scope of practice of their colleagues (While & Barriball 1999). This has led to work designed to improve ways of better preparing health professionals in their undergraduate education for optimum healthcare teamwork on graduation. This includes, in particular, ensuring that graduates are aware of the role and function of the multidisciplinary healthcare team. Graduates (regardless of their specific health profession) need to understand the roles of all team members and the characteristics of effective teamwork, and have a strong appreciation of the importance of good communication in healthcare teams and implications for health outcomes of poor teamwork and communication. They need to be able to function effectively and optimally in a team context in healthcare (Baker et al 2006).

In Australia, work is underway to improve interprofessional learning (also referred to as multiprofessional learning) in healthcare to improve interprofessional teamwork and consequently patient care. For examples, see the Clinical Excellence Commission, New South Wales (www.cec.health.nsw.gov.au), and the National Health Workforce Taskforce (www.nhwt.gov.au). This has application to both students in the health professions and also currently practising health professionals.

The multidisciplinary team brings cross-discipline expertise to healthcare consumers in a collaborative and coordinated way. The aims of this model are to enhance the quality of care received, support a planned and holistic approach to care, and to optimise resources. Some authors who discuss this concept use the title 'interprofessional teams' in place of 'multidisciplinary teams'. We have chosen to use 'multidisciplinary team' in this chapter. Our discussion of teamwork and team dynamics applies to a range of healthcare settings. These can include hospitals, and a range of other health agencies, including community care.

As a student of nursing who is being prepared to work in a contemporary healthcare system, whether it be in a hospital or within a community setting, it is imperative that you recognise the significance and responsibilities of being an active participant in multidisciplinary healthcare teams. To do this requires not only an awareness of the role of nurses, but also that of others within such teams. It is also useful to be aware of factors that impact upon the nature of teams, and how they form and function. Additionally, it is helpful to be aware of what affects their success.

WHAT IS A MULTIDISCIPLINARY TEAM?

In its simplest form, a team is a group of people. However, Gallagher (1995:276) draws an interesting distinction between 'groups' and 'teams'. She asserts that while both are composed of a number of individuals with some unifying relationship, the two can be differentiated by virtue of the members of a team being 'associated together in specific work or activity'. The key point to be made, then, is that while people participate in all sorts of groups, a team is characterised by common goals, interdependence, cooperation, coordination of activities, division of effort and shared language (Pfeffer & Schnack 1995).

A dictionary definition of a multidisciplinary (healthcare) team is a 'team of professionals including representatives of different disciplines who coordinate the contributions of each profession, which are not considered to overlap, in order to improve care' (O'Toole 2005:1737).

The ideals encompassed by a multidisciplinary approach to care require a culture conducive to collaborative working, as well as professional ideals that are complementary to the aim of improving client/customer experiences and outcomes. Effective communication and the ability to work in groups are important characteristics of team members, if the team is to function effectively.

Lenkman and Gribbins (1994) describe the values healthcare organisations must demonstrate for multidisciplinary care to become reality. These include being patient-focused and service-oriented, with attention to organisational, technical and professional issues. Staff who feel empowered to 'make a difference', who are also expert in systems thinking, who feel involved, and who are dedicated to the achievement of the goals of the organisation, form the basis of effective multidisciplinary teams.

To achieve such a culture, healthcare facilities need to move from individualistic or parochial group activity to multidisciplinary activity. This point is raised again later in this chapter, when factors impacting upon the effectiveness of multidisciplinary healthcare teams are discussed. The literature provides a number of examples of multidisciplinary healthcare teams working in a range of settings and populations, including: acute care (Scheuren et al 2006); aged care (Scherer et al 2002); the community (Inglis et al 2006); adolescents with diabetes (Strawhacker 2001); and inpatient rehabilitation (Ellis et al 2008). The reader is encouraged to explore these and other readings to build knowledge and understanding of multidisciplinary teams across contexts of healthcare.

WHY DO MULTIDISCIPLINARY TEAMS EXIST IN HEALTHCARE?

Extending from the definition provided by O'Toole (2005) above, it could be said that the purpose of a multidisciplinary healthcare team is to involve professionals from various health-related disciplines, whose contributions do not overlap, in the planning and provision of ever-improving standards of healthcare.

This definition is simplistic and not truly reflective of clinical environments because it gives the impression that health professionals perform functions that are prescribed and confined by their discipline base. However, it does reinforce the fact that this multidisciplinary healthcare team has (or should have) as its focus, high-quality care. In practice, the demarcations that previously defined the functions and roles of each discipline are becoming blurred and increasingly complementary as collaborative models of care emerge. For example, shared care (Moser et al 2007) and managed care (Hillegass et al 2002) support collaborations between public and private healthcare providers.

Healthcare needs to be a team effort because no one person or any single discipline can provide the care and services required by the range of clients wishing to access health services, particularly in Western societies. This is indeed the case if one accepts the view that healthcare is wider than the services provided by hospitals and health centres (Hill & Becker 1995). The whole is (or should be) greater than the sum of the parts.

MEMBERSHIP OF MULTIDISCIPLINARY HEALTHCARE TEAMS

A comprehensive overview of the role of disciplines common to multidisciplinary healthcare teams is beyond the scope of this chapter. You are encouraged to extend your knowledge and understanding of the special roles of the wide range of professionals who can comprise a multidisciplinary healthcare team. Team members may include medical practitioners (e.g. physicians, surgeons, psychiatrists), registered nurses, enrolled nurses, social workers, nutritionists, occupational therapists, physiotherapists, podiatrists, exercise physiologists, welfare workers, radiographers, psychologists, pharmacists, ministers of religion, or others who may provide spiritual guidance. The role and function of the professional nurse is described throughout this text. It is important to note that at times the coordination and leadership of the multidisciplinary healthcare team rests with the professional registered nurse. In many cases, the contribution of nurses to multidisciplinary teams is fundamental, given their close relationship to patients; they can be pivotal to the success of this process.

DYNAMICS OF MULTIDISCIPLINARY HEALTHCARE TEAMS

Yukl (2006:319) identifies that organisations usually comprise of 'small subunits' with defined tasks and that the types of teams that can be found in organisations can sometimes be very different. He identifies different types of teams and these can be readily identified in healthcare: functional operating teams (nursing); cross-functional teams (multidisciplinary); self-management operating teams (ancillary services); and top executive teams (healthcare executive teams).

Interestingly, Yukl (2006) also identifies another type of team—the virtual team. This type of team is emerging and it is suggested will be more commonplace in the future—a possibility enhanced by technological advances such as mobile telephones, email and teleconferencing. Whatever the description of the team, however, the success of a multidisciplinary team is identified not only by improved effectiveness, but also by the client's experience of that team.

Borrill et al (2002) highlighted that the quality of team working is powerfully related to the effectiveness of healthcare teams, while according to Arthur et al (2003) teams are critical to person-centred care. The importance of this is very topical. Kitson and colleagues are currently exploring the impact of multidisciplinary teams and outcomes of care for the older person (Jordon 2008). The ideals of effective teams are identified by the Royal College of Nursing's work (2007) on developing and sustaining effective teams. They summarise Borrill and West (2002) who:

> … show us that effective teams are ones that:
> • have clarity of, and commitment to, team objectives
> • fully involve all team members in the processes and activities of the team
> • focus on quality through regular review and feedback on performance, in relationship to team functioning and the achievement of team objectives
> • support creativity and innovation (Royal College of Nursing 2007:4).

In practice, few multidisciplinary healthcare teams fully meet these ideals, especially relating to clearly defined tasks (a point discussed later in this chapter). Nurses (and indeed other professionals within their own discipline) may therefore feel themselves to be more clearly a member of a unidisciplinary team (e.g. the nurses on a ward or unit, or in community settings) than a multidisciplinary one, though there are of course many specialties within the profession of nursing.

THE IMPACT OF TRADITION

Multidisciplinary healthcare teams are like all teams, in that each member has expected roles and functions that are influenced partly by members of the team and partly by external factors. Health services have traditionally been organised around functional areas of professional expertise (e.g. nursing, medicine, nutrition) with a strong hierarchical structure. Individuals bring with them expectations associated with their discipline, which coalesce with the established social roles and rules (written and unwritten) associated with healthcare facilities. As a result, multidisciplinary healthcare teams tend to develop along traditional hierarchical lines, partly because of the varying skill levels of members, but also 'because that's the way it's always been' (reflecting organisational norms). The result is that relationships within multidisciplinary healthcare teams perpetuate the hierarchical approach to decision making (Cott 1997) and, as such, are dominated by those with legitimated power (e.g. managers) or historical/authority-based power (e.g. medical doctors).

From the discussion presented thus far, it would seem obvious that this situation is at odds with the concept of multidisciplinary teams, which implies seamless care, equal recognition of skills of members, and equal recognition of members' contribution (Warelow 1996).

HEALTHCARE CULTURE

One association that has attracted attention in the literature is the nurse–doctor relationship. This association is not generally discussed within the context of multidisciplinary teams, but over the years this has been rather more commonly situated within the literature on power and how it is exercised over others (Farmer 1993, Gjerberg & Kjolsrod 2000, Matheson & Bobay 2007, Porter 1992, Roberts 1983, Warelow 1996). The origins of 'traditional' nurse–doctor interactions and the nature of their association are both relevant to a discussion about multidisciplinary teams. It has been argued that, regardless of the expected roles of team members, the most powerful team members direct the contribution of others. In that scenario, the medical profession invariably dominates, and nurses (and to a lesser extent other allied health professionals) are generally submissive. This situation is maintained through an effective socialisation (societal and professional) based on gender and role differences.

Roberts (1983) in a now classic paper, presents a range of suggestions for nurses and nursing to free itself from domination by (particularly) the medical profession, within an excellent discussion of oppressed group behaviour and its implications for nursing. Included in her recommendations is that nurses and nursing should seek to have a public voice, clearly stating what is valuable about nursing's contribution to healthcare teams and healthcare more generally. How this might be best achieved is discussed in the excellent text, *From Silence to Voice: What Nurses Know and Must Communicate to the Public* (Buresh & Gordon 2006). It is unfortunate that multidisciplinary teams in healthcare still tend to function in ways that perpetuate the power differences. At some time in the future, we may see increasing numbers of multidisciplinary teams in which the contribution of each member, regardless of professional background, will be recognised and the ideal of equality among members will be achieved. One way that this will be more readily achieved will be when nurses accept that they do play a vital role in healthcare, and are confident to assert that fact when working with colleagues from other health disciplines.

Senior managers in the organisation also need to recognise that, intentionally or unintentionally, they are instrumental in establishing the values and norms that set the tone of the organisation. The organisational culture is based on, and reflects the policies, procedures and practices that are supported and reinforced at all levels. Individuals and groups then internalise the values and act out their roles accordingly. Therefore, any organisation that claims to be committed to an integrated and multidisciplinary approach to healthcare needs to identify clear goals for its teams, as well as putting into place the communication and organisational structures discussed earlier. If this is not the case, then the subcultures based on departments, disciplines and charismatic individuals will continue to direct the team, the consequence of which will be that the advantages of the multidisciplinary approach will be lost to the organisation, team members and, of course, recipients of healthcare.

EFFECTIVENESS OF MULTIDISCIPLINARY HEALTHCARE TEAMS

A multidisciplinary team brings together individuals from diverse disciplinary and functional backgrounds. The experience and skill that members bring to the team can be a significant asset when used in problem solving, decision making, conflict resolution and other activities that enable the team to achieve its goals. The outcomes will depend largely on how effectively the group of individuals is transformed into a team with common goals (Liberman et al 2001). To ensure these teams do function effectively, complex communication procedures must be established and maintained.

The literature on multidisciplinary teams indicates clearly that functional groups have elements in common (Hein 1998, Ivancevich et al 2008, Kelly-Thomas 1998). The most frequently identified attribute is the presence of effective communication. Other factors include clear roles (including leadership) and conflict resolution strategies. Inherent in these attributes is the importance of a sense of common purpose for the team, demonstrated by a mission statement and agreed goals (Kouzes & Posner 2007, Marriner-Tomey 2008, Wright 2003, Yukl 2006).

Effective communications

Organisations require elaborate channels of communication, both formal and informal, to ensure that everyone in the team shares a sense of common purpose—in this case, the provision of high-quality healthcare. This may seem relatively straightforward, but in reality the various members of multidisciplinary healthcare teams may have very different views.

Fargason and Haddock (1992) present an interesting illustration of how poor communication can impact on the outcomes of a multidisciplinary team. In their example, a delivery-room patient record form, intended for use by obstetric and paediatric staff, was developed and approved by senior obstetric physician staff without input from other user groups. It was not surprising that the form did not fulfil its intended purpose. Fargason and Haddock conclude that in order for teams to make high-quality decisions, attention needs to be paid to group processes, including selection of team members and group decision making.

An example of a clinical specialty where one could expect to find a shared sense of purpose across the team is the hospice environment. Since the early 1970s, the hospice movement, under the influence of visionaries such as Cicely Saunders, has developed to the point where there is clear agreement between the various disciplines working in this area. They concur that the focus of hospice care should be patient/family centred and holistic (not merely the relief of physical symptoms) so as to facilitate as peaceful a death as possible (Fisher 1988, Stedeford 1984). They also agree that hospice care should be provided in an environment in which staff do not see death as a failure, where staff are experts in their field yet accepting, even welcoming, the skills of others when focused towards the goal of patient comfort and wellbeing, all within a supportive, humanistic environment (Fisher 1988, Stedeford 1984). One outstanding feature of these teams is the sense of common purpose that is almost palpable when one comes into contact with such organisations.

Other subsets of 'effective communication' and their importance to the functioning of multidisciplinary healthcare can be identified within the literature. It is important, for example, that team members have a clear idea of what colleagues in other disciplines do (Crowell 2000), and the professional language they use (Jenkins et al 2001), to avoid the problems of care being fragmented through lack of a coordinated plan (Joy et al 2003). Communication between team members from different disciplines offers the opportunity to observe and acknowledge the unique contributions being made by colleagues (Benierakis 1995). Such clarity of purpose and awareness of the roles and expertise of colleagues should then enable team members to work together to achieve the (preferably) clearly stated goals of the team (Jenkins et al 2001). This synergy is only achieved when all members of the team are willing to cooperate (Yoder Wise 2006).

Potter and Palmer (2003) discuss the importance of peers within teams supporting and valuing each other, rather than being critically destructive of each other. If mutual appreciation occurs, then trust will also tend to build up between team members, leading eventually to everyone feeling that they can put forward ideas and suggestions for improvement. Brown et al (2003) reinforce the significance of peer support, and add the view that managers should regard innovation and encourage personal accountability, perhaps through the use of a participative management style—in effect, encouraging collaboration in decision making about care, as well as actually providing that care.

Members of multidisciplinary healthcare teams potentially benefit greatly from the sharing of expertise and insight, not least because decisions reached and actions agreed tend to be well planned, informed by relevant experience, and 'owned' by the parties concerned, thus enhancing the chances of effecting successful change (Brown et al 2003, Dion 2004).

Clear roles

In effective teams, the role each member of the team is expected to assume is generally well established and understood, albeit tacitly at times. When people fulfil these roles (norms of behaviour), the team is likely to be functional. However, conflict can arise when team members assume a role that is different from that expected of their position in the team, or when the notion of 'equal recognition' is overlooked. As previously mentioned, it is crucial that all members of the multidisciplinary team have a clear understanding of their role, its responsibilities, boundaries and capabilities.

The roles of nurses (who are numerically dominant in health) and doctors (who are undisputedly the dominant power group in health) have been described and analysed within the context of multidisciplinary teams (Braithwaite & Westbrook 2004, Warelow 1996, West et al 2002). In the main, the assumed roles maintain the status quo, with the nursing literature tending to nominate the doctor as team leader. This situation could change, albeit slowly, as new roles emerge; nurse consultant posts are increasing in number and the nurse practitioner role is now established in a wider range of clinical settings.

Pfeffer and Schnack (1995) describe the 'shared governance' approach to leadership of a multidisciplinary team providing care to people with HIV/AIDS. Shared governance is a dynamic process that requires team members at every level to play key roles in the decision making that affects the team and the people it serves. As is the case in other healthcare environments, the nurses in that team were the only full-time primary care providers, and as a result had responsibility for clinical decisions, including triaging patients, quality assurance, crisis management and conducting team meetings. As it gains momentum, shared governance will lead to changes in the structure and functioning of multidisciplinary healthcare teams of the future.

Leadership

The style of the leader influences significantly the performance and morale of a team (Kelly-Thomas 1998:344), although, as Barnum (1998) notes, the best leader may not always be the manager. Traditionally, the leader does have responsibility for the day-to-day activities of the team. However, contemporary leadership models focus on the need for a leader to have, and to be able to articulate, a vision of what is intended and expected of the team, and to create the 'social environment' in which this can happen (Kouzes & Posner 2007). According to Barnum, this shift in emphasis from manager as supervisor to that of visionary is reflective of changing professional and community expectations. Leaders with vision are vital in healthcare situations where the system is changing at such a rate that health professionals require an environment that enables them to interpret, create and grow with change. The reader who is new to nursing would benefit from further reading in the area of the management of change (see, for example, Crookes & Davies 2004, Wright 2003).

For a variety of reasons, doctors are often cast in the role of leaders of healthcare teams. One reason for this is that when medical care is sought, the initial contact is usually with a medical practitioner (particularly GPs) and, in cases where onward referral is required, it is often to other specialist doctors. Given that many people only seek to access health services when they are sick or injured, it is not unreasonable for doctors to be considered necessary and important. However, there are issues related to the conventions of this assumption of power that nurses and those in professions allied to medicine may find problematic. It is also the case that medical practitioners may not always be the best people to take the lead in multidisciplinary healthcare, particularly when outcomes are not 'curative' (e.g. in rehabilitation and developmental disability services). It must, however, be acknowledged that doctors occupy a key role in the care of people requiring health services, not only because the public see doctors in this light (convention again), but also because modern Western health services continue to be orientated towards being essentially 'sick services' (Crookes 1992:228).

Globally, there is a call for leadership in healthcare (Leeder et al 2007). Locally, *Health: Working as a Team* (New South Wales Health 2000) and *A Framework for Building Capacity* (New South Wales Health 2001) identified a need for leadership development within the workforce. As a result, much attention is being given to developing clinical leadership skills within all members of the multidisciplinary team, with the emphasis on the development of transformational leadership qualities (a concept introduced by

Burns 1978). There has been a proliferation of clinical leadership development globally, as it is seen as being central to achieving healthcare reform. For example, in New South Wales, the Clinical Excellence Commission clinical leadership program identifies that 'strategies for sustainable patient safety and system improvement are dependent on strong clinical leadership capabilities' (Clinical Excellence Commission 2008). This notion is also supported by the magnet hospital principles, where there is evidence of measurable differences to patients and staff where strong, collaborative, clinical leadership exists (Joyce & Crookes 2007, Kramer & Schamlenberg 1988a 1988b).

The preceding discussion of roles and leadership and their impact upon the effectiveness of the multidisciplinary team leads us to the final issue related to effective teams: conflict.

THE NATURE OF CONFLICT

Organisations are, in fact, a collaboration of people; when they come together as a group, there will be differences in attitudes and behaviours (Axelsson & Axelsson 2006). This can result in conflict, despite the need for collaborative activity. Conflict in teams may originate from the tasks to be performed or relationships between team members (De Dreu & Vianen 2001). While the adoption of multidisciplinary teams is one strategy to increase the performance of individuals (Fay et al 2006), the traditional hierarchical nature of the work environment (Brown et al 2000) and the multidisciplinary nature of healthcare teams (Katz 2007) contribute to the development of conflict in healthcare environments.

This section will focus on potential conflict arising from relationships between people because that is a more common cause of conflict in healthcare teams. While conflict between colleagues is associated with reduced job satisfaction and increased stress and sick leave (Montoro-Rodriguez & Small 2006), it is not necessarily destructive. Functional conflict can actually enhance and benefit the organisation's performance. For example, two community health teams may agree that community-based aged care is a priority; however, there may be a conflict regarding how that can best be achieved. Each team applies a different model, both of which result in improved access to services for the elderly. There is not always only one 'answer'. However, the potential for dysfunctional conflict to interfere with the harmony and outcomes of the group is considerable, and must be addressed effectively.

Umiker (1988) identifies six common causes of conflict: unclear expectations; poor communication; lack of clear jurisdiction; incompatibilities or disagreements based on difference; conflict of interest; and operational or staffing changes. Increased demand for specialists has also been identified as contributing to conflict (Ivancevic et al 2008), as has the potential for conflict in stressful, volatile clinical areas where outcomes are subject to high scrutiny (Katz 2007). As would be expected, teams that work well together demonstrate the opposite characteristics: agreed goals; an agreed plan; effective communication styles; clear team roles; and competent leadership (Burke et al 2000).

Team members may be unclear about their role in the team, policies and procedures, or how outcomes will be measured. As we have discussed previously, effective communication between members of teams, and between the team and organisation, is arguably the most significant contributing factor to the team's success. Jurisdiction refers to accountability, authority and responsibility within the team. Conflict can arise when members do not comply with established expectations, either via a failure to assume expected roles, or a failure to recognise positions with legitimate authority. Conflict arising from incompatibilities, or differences of opinion, are complex situations that can spring from factors as diverse as politics, ethics, values or gender. Conflicts of interest may arise between departments, shifts and individuals, and may be precipitated by operational or staff changes (Burke et al 2000).

Conflict resolution

Resolving conflict requires clear procedures for communication (discussed earlier in this chapter), decision making and commitment to team building. Other factors such as the number of team members and their personalities also need to be taken into account in conflict resolution activities. The association between the size of a team and job satisfaction is significant in the discussion about health teams.

Fargason and Haddock (1992) proposed that the optimum number of members in a team is five, and that a greater number predisposes to conflict manifested by increased absenteeism and reduced job satisfaction. However, multidisciplinary teams working in clinical areas usually have more than five members, some significantly more. Team size is therefore potentially a major cause of conflict within multidisciplinary healthcare teams.

The model described by Tuckman and Jensen (1977) for group formation (forming, storming, norming, performing and adjourning) can be used as a framework for conflict resolution. Groups engaged in this process agree on aims, structure, leadership (forming), and then go through a stage of discussion and debate, which may include conflict (storming) to achieve cooperation, collaboration and establishment of team norms (norming). The group is then functional (performing). Depending on the purpose of the group, it may then adjourn. A common theme in all techniques is the requirement for constructive negotiation via effective communication between the parties.

Behfar et al (2008) identified three criteria for team viability: the needs of members are satisfied by the team experience; individual needs of members are satisfied; and the processes used to resolve conflict when it develops enhance the team's ability to work together. Problem solving requires meetings between the groups to debate differences and negotiate agreement (Behfar et al 2008). Resolving the conflict also requires groups to display a willingness to work together. This requires all members to contribute to the solution, and, in most cases, there will be compromise and trade-offs. Compromise can be used effectively when the goals can be divided equitably, and therefore is most useful when the conflicting parties have relatively equal power and are strongly committed to mutually exclusive goals (Behfar et al 2008). Nevertheless, conflict between individual members of the team may be difficult to resolve (De Dreu & Vianen 2001).

Good communication is necessary to resolve conflict, and a variety of approaches have been developed (Montoro-Rodriguez & Small 2006). These authors tested the effect of three approaches to conflict resolution with nurses working with long-term residents in aged care facilities: aggressive and uncooperative behaviour that requires members to conform; working together and cooperating to identify a solution; and avoidance, which used indirect strategies of non-confrontation to address conflict. Their data supported the hypothesis that the psychological morale, occupational stress and job satisfaction of nurses are influenced by the style of conflict resolution.

Confrontational and avoidance styles have been shown to contribute to reduced levels of psychological morale, while collaborative styles have been shown to have the opposite effect (Montoro-Rodriguez & Small 2006).

The traditional, department-based, hierarchical decision-making model is not new to those who have worked in health services. In that environment, failure to attend to the 'health' of the team and/or absence of organisational commitment impose considerable risks to outcomes. Lenkman and Gribbins (1994) refer to the 'human resource perspective', which seeks to achieve a balance between organisational and team needs. Failure to achieve that balance results in job dissatisfaction manifested in the inability to retain valued employees and attract new team members.

These authors have identified six general areas, which, if addressed effectively, will significantly enhance the success of multidisciplinary teams and reduce conflict:

1. Allow for flexibility within the team and be alert to opportunities and strategies for effective change.
2. Identify potential barriers to success.
3. Agree on and implement the framework to be adopted (e.g. shared care, case management) by the multidisciplinary team.
4. Identify opportunities and strategies to assist and promote change within the organisation.
5. Take advantage of educational opportunities and team-building exercises provided by the organisation.
6. Managers within the organisation must recognise that some health professionals find working in teams more difficult than others, and support must be provided to those individuals.

CONCLUSION

Multidisciplinary teams are formed to achieve objectives; the most obvious (but certainly not the only) reason is to achieve measurable outcomes that are beyond the capacity of individuals or groups from the same discipline. The complexity of new therapies, increasing specialisation (and the emergence of new specialties), and the increasing diversity of services consumers expect, point to the team approach as an efficient and effective model of care. The professions represented in a multidisciplinary team will reflect local needs, priorities and resources.

Health services have traditionally been structured around functional areas of professional expertise; therefore, multidisciplinary teams are unlikely to be successful until the organisation is committed to change, and group processes are in place to support communication within the group, and between the group and the organisation. The culture within the organisation will largely determine the productivity of teams and the degree of satisfaction experienced by the members.

There are potential barriers to the success of multidisciplinary teams, and these must be dealt with at both the group and organisational level. We have discussed precipitating factors for group conflict and, very briefly, presented strategies to prevent, or at least minimise, the effect of conflict on the team. Opportunities for professional development of members, which includes team-building activities, must be provided and supported by the organisation, and evidence of successful problem solving, negotiation and compromise rewarded.

REFLECTIVE QUESTIONS

1 What do you believe to be the strengths and weaknesses of multidisciplinary teams?

2 How could multidisciplinary teams benefit nurses and the nursing profession?

3 Reflect on ways in which nurses in general, and you personally, could positively impact on the efficacy of the multidisciplinary team you may work within.

RECOMMENDED READINGS

Baker D, Day R, Salas E 2006 Teamwork as an essential component of high reliability organizations. Health Services Research 41:1576–1598

Buresh B, Gordon S 2006 From silence to voice: what nurses know and must communicate to the public, 2nd edn. Cornell University Press, New York

Daly J, Speedy S, Jackson D 2004 Nursing leadership. Churchill Livingstone, Sydney

Manjolovich M, Barnsteiner J, Bolton LB, Disch J, Saint S 2008 Nursing practice and work environment issues in the 21st century: a leadership challenge. Nursing Research 57(1):S11–S14

Royal College of Nursing (RCN) 2007 Developing and sustaining effective teams. RCN, London. Online. Available: www.rcn.org.uk/data/assets/pdffile/0003/78735/003115.pdf

REFERENCES

Arthur H, Wall D, Halligan A 2003 Team resource management: a programme for troubled teams. Clinical Governance 8(1):86–91

Axelsson R, Axelsson B 2006 Integration and collaboration in public health: a conceptual framework. International Journal of Health Planning and Management 21:5–88

Baker D, Day R, Salas E 2006 Teamwork as an essential component of high reliability organizations. Health Services Research 41:1576–1598

Barnum BS 1998 Leadership: can it be holistic? In: Hein EC (ed.) Contemporary leadership behaviour: selected readings, 5th edn. Lippincott, New York

Behfar KJ, Paterson RS, Mannix EA, Trochin WM 2008 The critical role of conflict resolution in teams: a close look at the links between conflict type, conflict management, and team outcomes. Journal of Applied Psychology 93(1):170–188

Benierakis CE 1995 The function of the multidisciplinary team in child psychiatry: clinical and educational aspects. Canadian Journal of Psychiatry 40:348–353

Borrill C, Carletta J, Carter AJ, Dawson JF, Garrod S, Rees A, Richards A, Shapiro D, West MA 2002 The effectiveness of healthcare teams in the National Health Service report. Aston University, Aston

Borrill C, West M 2002 Team working and effectiveness in healthcare: findings from the healthcare team effectiveness project. Ashton Centre for Health Service Organisation Research, Birmingham

Braithwaite J, Westbrook M 2004 A survey of staff attitudes and comparative managerial and non-managerial views in a clinical directorate. Health Services Management Research 17:141–166

Brown B, Crawford P, Darongkamas J 2000 Blurred roles and permeable boundaries: the experience of multidisciplinary working in community mental health. Health and Social Care in the Community 8(8):425–435

Brown MS, Ohlinger J, Rusk C, Delmore P, Ittmann P, Group C 2003 Implementing potentially better practices for multidisciplinary team building: creating a neonatal intensive care unit culture of collaboration. Pediatrics 111(4, Pt 2):482–488

Buresh B, Gordon S 2006 From silence to voice. what nurses know and must communicate to the public, 2nd edn. Cornell University Press, New York

Burke D, Herrman H, Evans M, Cockram A, Trauer T 2000 Educational aims and objectives for working in multidisciplinary teams. Australasian Psychiatry 8(4):336–339

Burns JM 1978 Leadership. Harper & Row, New York

Clinical Excellence Commission 2008 The clinical leadership program. Online. Available: www.cec.health.nsw.gov.au/moreinfo/CLP.html#background 1 Sept 2008

Cott C 1997 'We decide, you carry it out': a social network analysis of multidisciplinary long-term care teams. Social Science Medical 45(9):1411–1421

Crookes PA 1992 The politics of healthcare. In: Boddy J, Rice V (eds) Health: perspectives and practices, 2nd edn. Dunmore Press, Palmerston North, pp 216–32

Crookes PA, Davies S (eds) 2004 Essential skills for reading and applying research in nursing and healthcare: research into practice, 2nd edn. Baillière Tindall, Edinburgh

Crowell DM 2000 Building spirited multidisciplinary teams. Journal of Perianesthesia Nursing 15(2):108–114

De Dreu D, Vianen A 2001 Managing relationship conflict and the effectiveness of organisational teams. Journal of Organisational Behaviour 22:309–328

Dion X 2004 A multidisciplinary team approach to public health working. British Journal of Community Nursing 9(4):149–154

Ellis T, Katz DI, White DK, DePiero TJ, Hohler AD, Saint-Hilair M 2008 Effectiveness of an inpatient multidisciplinary rehabilitation program for people with Parkinson's disease. Physical Therapy 88(7):812–819

Fargason CA, Haddock CC 1992 Cross-functional, integrative team decision-making: essential for effective QI in healthcare. Quality Review Bulletin May:157–163

Farmer B 1993 The use and abuse of power in nursing. Nursing Standard 7(23):33–36

Fay D, Borrill C, Amir Z, Haward R, West M 2006 Getting the most out of multidisciplinary teams: a multi-sample study of team innovation in healthcare. Journal of Occupational and Organisational Psychology 79:553–567

Fisher M 1988 Death and loss: hospice nursing. Nursing 3(32):8–10

Gallagher R (ed.) 1995 Team building. In: Yoder Wise PS (ed.) Leading and managing in nursing. Mosby, St Louis, pp 275–99

Gjerberg E, Kjolsrod L 2000 The doctor–nurse relationship: how easy is it to be a female doctor co-operating with a female nurse? Social Science and Medicine 52:189–202

Hein EC (ed.) 1998 Contemporary leadership behaviour: selected readings, 5th edn. Lippincott, Philadelphia

Hill MN, Becker DM 1995 Roles of nurses and health workers in cardiovascular health promotion. The American Journal of the Medical Sciences 310(Suppl):S123–S126

Hillegass BE, Smith DM, Phillips SL 2002 Changing managed care to care management: innovations in nursing practice. On the Scene 8(13):33–46

Inglis SC, Pearson S, Treen S, Gallasch T, Horowitz JD, Stewart S 2006 Extending the horizon in chronic heart failure: effects of multidisciplinary, home-based intervention relative to usual care. Circulation 114:2466–2473

Ivancevich JM, Konopaske R, Matteson MT 2008 Organizational behavior and management, 8th edn. Irwin, Boston

Jenkins V, Fallowfield L, Poole K 2001 Are members of multidisciplinary teams in breast cancer aware of each other's informational roles? Quality in Healthcare 10(2):70–75

Jordon Z 2008 A kaleidoscope of possibilities: the joy and frustration of nursing practice. Joanna Briggs Institute. PACEsetter S5(2)

Joy EA, Wilson C, Varechok S 2003 The multidisciplinary team approach to the outpatient treatment of disordered eating. Current Sports Medicine Reports 2(6):331–336

Joyce J, Crookes P 2007 Developing a tool to measure 'magnetism' in Australian nursing environments. Australian Journal of Advanced Nursing 25(1):17–23

Katz J 2007 Conflict and its resolution in the operating room. Journal of Clinical Anaesthesia 19:152–158

Kelly-Thomas KJ 1998 Clinical and nursing staff development, current competence, future focus, 2nd edn. Lippincott, New York

Kouzes JM, Posner BZ 2007 The leadership challenge, 4th edn. John Wiley, San Francisco

Kramer M, Schamlenberg C 1988a Magnet hospitals: part 1 institutions of excellence. Journal of Nursing Administration 18(1):13–23

Kramer M, Schamlenberg C 1988b Magnet hospitals: part 2 institutions of excellence. Journal of Nursing Administration 18(2):1–19

Leeder S, Raymond S, Greenberg H 2007 The need for leadership in global health. Medical Journal of Australia 187(9):532–535

Lenkman S, Gribbins R 1994 Multidisciplinary teams in the acute care setting. Holistic Nursing Practice April:81–87

Liberman RP, Hilty DM, Drake RE, Tsang HWH 2001 Requirements for multidisciplinary teamwork in psychiatric rehabilitation. Psychiatric Services 52(10):1331–1342

Manjolovich M, Barnsteiner J, Bolton LB, Disch J, Saint S 2008 Nursing practice and work environment issues in the 21st century: a leadership challenge. Nursing Research 57(1):S11–S14

Matheson LK, Bobay K 2007 Validation of oppressed group behaviors in nursing. Journal of Professional Nursing 23(4):226–234

Marriner-Tomey A 2008 Guide to nursing management and leadership, 8th edn. Mosby, St Louis

Montoro-Rodriguez J, Small F 2006 The role of conflict resolution styles on nursing staff morale, burnout, and job satisfaction in long-term care. Journal of Ageing and Health 18:385–406

Moser A, Houtepen R, Widdershoven G 2007 Patient autonomy in nurse-led shared care: a review of theoretical and empirical literature. JAN: Review Paper. Blackwell Publishing, pp 357–65

New South Wales Health 2000 Health: working as a team: the way forward. New South Wales Health Department, Sydney

New South Wales Health 2001 A framework for building capacity: capacity to promote health. New South Wales Health Department, Sydney

O'Toole M (ed.) 2005 Miller-Keane encyclopedia and dictionary of medicine, nursing and allied health. WB Saunders, Philadelphia

Pfeffer GN, Schnack JA 1995 Nurse practitioners as leaders in a quality healthcare delivery system. Advance Practice Nurses Quarterly 1(2):30–39

Porter S 1992 A participant observation study of power relations between nurses and doctors in a general hospital. Journal of Advanced Nursing 16:728–735

Potter TB, Palmer RG 2003 360-degree assessment in a multidisciplinary team setting. Rheumatology 42(11):1404–1407

Roberts SJ 1983 Oppressed group behaviour: implications for nursing. Advances in Nursing Science 5(4):21–30

Royal College of Nursing (RCN) 2007 Developing and sustaining effective teams. RCN, London. Online. Available: www.rcn.org.uk/data/assets/pdffile/0003/78735/003115.pdf

Scherer S, Jennings C, Smeaton M, Thompson P, Stein M 2002 Innovations in aged care: a multidisciplinary practice guideline for hip fracture prevention in residential aged care. Australasian Journal of Ageing 21(4):203–209

Scheuren L, Baetz B, Cawley MJ, Fitzpatrick R, Cachecho R 2006 Pharmacist designed and nursing-driven insulin infusion protocol to achieve and maintain glycemic control in critical care patients. Journal of Trauma Nursing 13(3):140–145

Stedeford A 1984 Facing death: patients, families and professionals. Heinemann, London

Strawhacker M 2001 Multidisciplinary teaming to promote effective management of type 1 diabetes for adolescents. Journal of School Health 71(6):213–217

Tuckman BW, Jensen M (eds) 1977 Stages of small group development revisited, 3rd edn. Irwin, Boston

Umiker W 1998 Collaborative conflict resolution. In: Hein EC (ed.) Contemporary leadership behaviour: selected readings, 5th edn. Lippincott, New York

Warelow PJ 1996 Nurse–doctor relationships in multidisciplinary teams: ideal or real? International Journal of Nursing Practice 2(1):33–39

West MA, Borril CS, Dawson JF, Brodbeck F, Shapiro DA, Haward B 2002 Leadership clarity and team innovation in healthcare. Online. Available: www.modern.nhs.uk/115/23713/25415/Leadership%20Clarity.pdf

While A, Barriball KL 1999 Qualified and unqualified nurses' views of the multidisciplinary team: findings of a large interview study. Journal of Interprofessional Care 13(1):77–89

Wright S 2003 Changing nursing practice, 3rd edn. Arnold, London

Yoder Wise PS 2006 Leading and managing in nursing, 4th edn. Mosby, St Louis

Yukl G 2006 Leadership in organizations, 6th edn. Pearson Prentice Hall, New Jersey

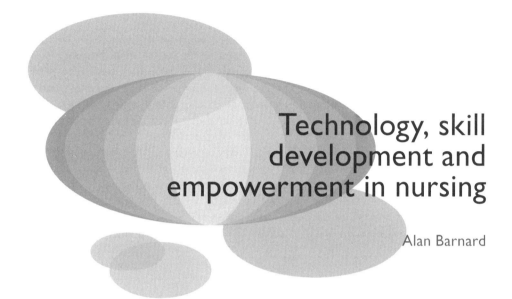

CHAPTER 15

Technology, skill development and empowerment in nursing

Alan Barnard

LEARNING OBJECTIVES

When you have read this chapter, you should be able to:

- explain the importance of technology for nursing practice and skills development
- describe characteristics associated with technology that are important for healthcare
- outline implications of technology for nursing care with specific reference to empowerment, and
- describe key principles and values important for fostering excellence in nursing practice.

KEY WORDS

Technology, empowerment, skill, nursing, technique, clinical, healthcare, knowledge

NURSING AND TECHNOLOGY

This chapter considers the role and importance of technology for nursing practice, with specific reference to skill development and empowerment. Principles important to understanding technology are outlined and the implications of technology for nursing and healthcare are discussed, along with guiding principles and values important to appropriate integration of technology into clinical practice. It is argued that technology is a phenomenon that must be understood adequately to address the many challenges it presents for current and future nurses.

Technology influences the practice of nursing both from the perspective of what we do and how we understand ourselves as practitioners. Nurses talk about technology, develop skills and knowledge to apply technology, interpret technology, praise the qualities of the latest computer applications, worry about loss of human contact and work in a changing workplace. Technology is used, for example, to deliver accurate treatment, to hold water, to cover patients and to observe the internal workings of the human body. Technology advancement is linked to a range of experiences, including shorter length of admission to hospital, greater efficiency, changing skills and knowledge, alteration to employment patterns, specialisation and standardisation of care (Locsin 2001, Rinard 1996, Sandelowski 2000). These outcomes of technological development combined with the interests of dominant social groups, increasing legal liability and the maintenance of technology have produced healthcare practices that are focused sometimes on functionality, sameness, conformity, automation, safety, predictability and logical order.

Technology is significant to the history, contemporary practice and future of nursing. It has always been a part of nursing and in order to understand nursing as a discipline we need insight into the social, theoretical and practical implications that emerge as a result of our links with technology. Prior to the twentieth century, technical knowledge and skills developed by trial and error, and were passed down through generations via a practical and oral culture. Nurses relied on experience and faith. Technical skills included magical and aesthetic components that equated with moral and psychic life. Nursing practice relied less on scientific knowledge and explanation than on a personal and intuitive understanding developed and refined through practice (Barnard & Cushing 2001).

The rapid growth of scientific and technological knowledge has bought about enormous changes for nursing and healthcare over the past hundred years, and technology has figured prominently as both a protagonist for development and an influential partner in our practice. Technology remains integral to healthcare and has significantly influenced our workplace, not only in terms of the artefacts and resources we use, but also how we do things, how we organise ourselves as nurses and what we value. In fact, over 15 years ago Cooper (1993) warned that the process of technological change had advanced to such an extent that many areas of nursing practice had come to be defined by technology. For example, the haemodialysis machine is associated with renal nursing and the ventilator is associated with intensive care practice. The warning would appear to be confirmed as a result of an increasing emphasis on competency-based education and practice, which is linked directly to the use of technology(ies). But regardless of whether the warning of Cooper is proving to be entirely accurate, it is acknowledged widely that nurses in all specialties are required to manipulate a significant amount of technology and accept increasingly complex roles and responsibilities associated with its ongoing importance in healthcare (Barnard & Locsin 2007, Sandelowski 1997).

INTERPRETING TECHNOLOGY

The word technology (tech.nol.ogy) refers to the practical arts, specific implements and the knowledge and/or activity of a group (i.e. technologist). The phenomenon is subject to varied and sometimes inadequate explanation in nursing and is influenced by social status, culture, gender and politics (Barnard 2002, Pelletier 1989, Rinard 1996). Technology is more than the sum of things we use in healthcare. It has characteristic features that include the development of skills, knowledge and the incorporation of social arrangements and values (Feenberg 1999, Pacey 1999, Winner 2003).

One way to interpret and portray technology is as three concentric circles (see Fig 15.1). Concentric circles highlight the characteristics of technology, and together they therefore emphasise a character-ological interpretation of the phenomenon. The interpretation is useful because it focuses our attention on not only the 'things we use in nursing and society' (at the centre), but also their relations with other characteristics that are integral to meaning.

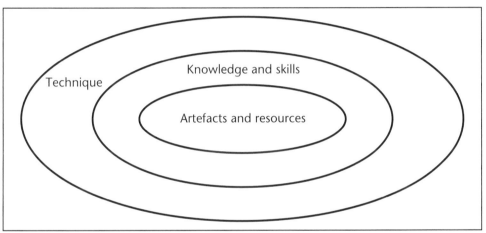

Figure 15.1   A character-ology of technology

Artefacts and resources

The smallest and central concentric circle depicted in Figure 15.1, *artefacts and resources*, is technology at its most obvious and refers to the integration, use and application of the 'things' of nursing. Rinard (1996) noted that in modern nursing there have been three key periods of change that have been significantly influenced by technology. The first period was 1950–65 and was characterised by new medical techniques and a significant introduction of pharmaceuticals to care. The second period was 1965–80 and was associated with increasing machinery and specialisation. The third period was from 1980–90 and was associated with increasing technical control, streamlining and prediction of care. A more recent period has not been identified by Rinard, but it could be argued that current nursing is within a period of informational retrieval and computerisation.

We are required to use and maintain increasing amounts of technology in daily practice, and it is useful to clarify the various types of technology that are often found in our practice. We use simple, sophisticated, old, new, unique and commonplace technologies that continue to evolve in design and application. It can be observed that there are at least 12 different types of technologies that are artefacts and resources of nursing. These include *clothes* (e.g. shroud, pyjamas), utensils (e.g. bedpan, kidney dish), structures (e.g. hospital ward, isolation room), apparatus (e.g. Jordan frame, wheelchair, trolley), utilities (e.g. electricity, gas), tools (e.g. urinary catheter, syringe), resources (e.g. pharmaceuticals, sterile dressing), machines (e.g. intravenous infusion pump), automata (e.g. computer, refrigerator), tools of doing used to enact clinical practice (e.g. nurse's watch, stethoscope), objects of art or religion (e.g. nurse's uniform), and toys/games used for diversion (e.g. chessboard).

Although some machinery, apparatus, tools and so on are new, increasingly accurate and powered by utilities such as electricity, it is worth noting that there is also a lot of *simple* technology that remains fundamental to daily care (e.g. a shower chair, a stethoscope and a bedpan). Artefacts and resources assist to enact complex assessment and treatment, while supporting us to meet the daily needs of each patient. They can manifest as things to be held in our hand, pharmaceuticals we dispense to patients, volumetric pumps we use to assist enteral feeding, and occasionally as various noises and visual stimuli that we observe, such as colour screens and digital displays.

While an extended debate could be undertaken to examine what constitutes technology that is specific to nursing, for the purposes of this chapter nursing technologies include any technology that we use and/or claim to be fundamental to our daily practice. However, in stating this, it must be recognised that a lot of commonplace and simple nursing technology is not acknowledged as significant (e.g. bedpan) (Barnard & Locsin 2007). That is, it lacks recognition as technology by nurses both in clinical practice and in nursing literature. The reasons for the lack of acknowledgment are speculative, but include our emphasis on the application of sophisticated technology, our inclination to uncritically embrace new technologies, a de-emphasis on technology associated with the 'dirty work' of nurses, limited investigation into the historical development of nursing technologies and a lack of substantive scholarship examining the phenomenon (Sandelowski 2000).

Knowledge and skills

The second or middle concentric circle in Figure 15.1 portrays technology as *knowledge and skills*. Artefacts and resources have associated meaning(s) and these are in many ways determined by the knowledge and skills associated with the way we use, repair, design and interpret them. Knowledge and skills contribute to the successful use of artefacts and resources, and are as much technology as the objects themselves. Without required knowledge and skills for the use and application of technology, it has limited ability to meet the needs of nursing practice and care. For example, without the skills necessary to use a computer, it is not much more than plastic, metal and electricity, and will not assist daily practice.

Nursing is a practical occupation and our knowledge is expressed most often through the way we perform our work. We focus often on what we do as practitioners and explain technology from perspectives that emphasise daily roles and responsibilities. For example, there has been debate concerning the increasing role of nurses in the use and maintenance of machinery and equipment. It has been argued that nurses have to fulfil the role of technician, and this is significantly distracting us from focusing on the experience of each patient (Boykin & Schoenhofer 2001).

Nurses rely on experience, continuing education, personal development and peer mentors to maintain and develop knowledge and skills that are associated with technology. Failure to establish and develop knowledge and skills is inadequate for practice and unhelpful to patient care, colleagues and the requirements of the healthcare sector. Knowledge takes many forms and relates to not only competencies related to nursing intervention, but also organisational policy, current research and changing evidence. These all form part of the development of technological competence, which is central to technology–nurse–patient relations and is vitally important for care.

The outcome of technological competence is not only the development of skills for technology use, but also to know 'the other' (i.e. the person whom you nurse) in terms related to who they are as individuals. Thus in integrating technology in care we must seek to know their preferences, culture and beliefs. This significant part of caring for another is achieved as an outcome of purposefully seeking to know the other and through making appropriate use of technological data and resources for their benefit (Locsin 2001). One of the most important behaviours that patients look for from nurses is our competence when using technology. Demonstrating competence reduces anxiety and fear and increases the likelihood of successful care outcomes. Advances in organ transplantation, genetics, pharmaceuticals, microsurgery, virtual reality, e-health, telehealth, and so on, demand the ability to update and adapt knowledge, while maintaining technological competence as an essential element of quality care.

Knowledge and skills alter regularly, and thus an active interest in maintaining and advancing competence is a sign of a caring and responsible practitioner who is accountable for the quality of their practice. Attitudes that reflect an offhand and neglectful interest in updating knowledge and skills are inadequate, and reflect a failure to value the importance of the person. It is a denial of the many possible contrary indicated outcomes that might arise from inadequate technology integration and is unprofessional.

Technology introduces options for care and can make clinical practice more efficient, quicker and more accurate. Skills alter as a result of technology, and this fact should encourage personal reflection on the nature, relevance and impact of change on individual and collective practice (Locsin 2001). For example, an automatic blood pressure monitor de-emphasises manual skills related to assessing a person's blood pressure, but demands new skills in terms of integrating electronic data. Many skills that were required previously for nursing are no longer necessary for contemporary practice and new skills emerge regularly to become part of daily care. For example, the practice many years ago of boiling urine in a test tube to analyse urine was replaced by the use of a coloured test strip, and the electronic blood pressure monitor often replaces the use of a hand-operated sphygmomanometer. We are engaged in an ongoing and regular process of deskilling and reskilling in practice.

The outcomes of technological change are associated with changing technical complexity that should be integrated into the organisation of work. Technological sophistication is always about achieving greater efficiency and logical order, and technological change should be associated with better use of your time and resources and better patient care. For example, the intravenous infusion pump permits nurses to undertake 'other duties' while intravenous therapy is being delivered to their patient at a determined rate. However, the intravenous infusion pump de-emphasises skills associated with manually determining flow rate. An infusion pump is often a good thing for time saving and control in daily practice, but at a higher level we are reminded that an often unasked question in relation to technology and nursing is 'what skills need to be retained' and 'what skills can fall away' as a result of specific technological change(s).

These are important questions and are fundamentally necessary for current and future professional development. For example, although we have been proactive in acquiring new skills and knowledge for care, we are required sometimes to revisit older, less common ways of undertaking certain assessment(s) and treatment(s), especially in less resourced clinical areas.

But amidst all this change, some nurses interpret the process as skills loss, especially when skills associated with caring and human relationships are devalued or ignored. Rinard (1996) postulated that the evolution of technology and nursing is a story of deskilling in which nurses have purposefully gendered nursing knowledge in line with vocational and societal expectations of what is (was) valued culturally as 'feminine', at the cost of serious analysis of skills.

Deskilling and reskilling are issues worthy of analysis, but little has been undertaken within the profession. In fact, over the past 60 years nursing has seemingly been reluctant to critically analyse technological change within the contexts of skills alteration, societal trends and the changing nature of nursing work (Barnard 2002, Barnard & Cushing 2001, Fairman 1998, Rinard 1996, Sandelowski 1999b, 2000). Although new clinical activities have been added to the professional role of the nurse, these additions have been regarded as secondary to a more generalised growth in the sophistication of nursing work.

Most technological development in nursing has arisen as a result of technology replacing older procedures with newer more efficient and reliable technology, and among this there are significant changes occurring to nursing labour. We do things more quickly, more efficiently, with more automation and at times with more accuracy, yet there is a clear disjunction between the social–scientific nature of nursing work, analysis of changing healthcare, theoretical interpretation of nursing and the realities of nursing work. The effects of technological change on the skill of each nurse have been analysed poorly by nurses, but at a practical level changes are linked to increasing technical complexity and alteration to practitioner discretion/autonomy.

Technique

The influence of technology on practitioner discretion/autonomy is most obviously illustrated in the third and most inclusive concentric circle in Figure 15.1, which highlights the concept of *technique*. The third circle extends our character-ology of technology to include the way systems, policy, politics, economics, ethics, organisational management and human behaviour are organised for the benefit of technology. The way nursing practice is organised for, as well as by, artefacts and resources is as much technology as the first and second levels of meaning. Technique is not an entity or a specific thing. It is a way of thinking, and is an attitude that has an enormous influence upon us and society.

A transformation is occurring in which many aspects of our practice that were once instinctive, reflexive, natural and particular to individuals and cultures are being transformed into rational method and instruction. In craft-based technology the worker is able to express themselves with a sense of creativity, pride in personal agency and autonomy in determining action and expression. In automated technology environments these values and experiences have a tendency to be replaced by a sense of dependency on predetermined actions and protocols, a partial exercise of personal ability and preference, and knowledge that personal input can be replaced by another (Ferre 1995).

Technique is a mentality, a discourse and an objectification of naturally occurring phenomena such as reflective thinking, communication and human behaviour. An example to illustrate technique might be the difference between a caring moment with a patient motivated by nothing more than a nurse's compassion for another, versus the preplanned use of efficient communication strategies for the fulfilment of predefined goals and outcomes. The latter has all the hallmarks of technique because there is emphasis, for example, on a 'one best way' to efficiently undertake the activity. According to Lovekin (1991), technique is the consciousness that gives machines force, that sees everything else as machine-like or as needing to serve the machine-like, the ideal towards which technique strives.

Technique reduces the means of production, whether they be machines or nurses, to that which is most technological (i.e. efficient and rational), in order to create a unified activity. Examples of technique in the management of healthcare services are economic rationalism, protocols, risk assessment, action planning, communication strategies, benchmarking, patient dependency models, systems theory, clinical pathways management and standardised care plans.

Technique is a complex phenomenon that is constituted by three subtle yet important characteristics. First, technique adheres to a *primacy of reason* to govern practice. It is a way of thinking, acting and living by which people attempt to control the internal, passionate and emotional world of everyday life via protocols, rules, evidence and general observance to a logical order. Second, it requires a *desire for efficiency* in order to assist its goal and to justify its activity. The desire for efficiency is akin to the inventor or factory owner who seeks to streamline methods and actions in order to obtain certain outcomes. Efficiency seeks practical utility and a guaranteeing of results. There is a striving to reduce waste and the construction of systems that simplify and systematise previously uncontrolled or random activity. We nurses are free to engage in clinical practice, but this freedom is limited much like that of a clock. There is freedom for the hands to move around the clock face as long as nothing 'gets in the way'. The gears and springs move freely within the mechanism, yet there is a clear expectation that behaviour is determined and replicable.

It must be stressed that there is nothing wrong or dangerous per se with a desire for reasoned activity or efficiency. In fact, there is nothing new about rationality or efficiency as reasonable and worthwhile goals. They have both guided invention and activity throughout human history and, after all, who wants to be exposed to ineffective care?

However, the third characteristic of technique brings about new and different activity because it stresses primacy of efficiency in *every realm of human activity and thinking*. Technique has become so prevalent in society, organisations and nursing that people are increasingly incapable of thinking outside its boundaries in their search for meaning. A world has been created that has a tendency to override or minimise the importance of subjectivity and human experience. There is emphasis on control, efficiency and order within a climate of litigation (Harvey 1997, Neuhaus et al 2002, Sinclair & Gardner 2001, Wagner 1992, 1994).

Technique reduces thinking and human-centred activities such as nursing to measurable and predictable outcomes. It has potential to change previously natural worlds of human experience to *other*. That is, technique brings about qualitative transformation(s) in care. Under these conditions nursing practice risks becoming a robotic-like activity that does not require its practitioners to be particularly caring, compassionate or necessarily understanding of the experiences of people (except if it is preplanned as an efficient activity). As a result of technique, a new struggle has emerged for nursing and we need to find ways to authentically respond to individual need(s), cultural difference(s) and personal choice.

TECHNOLOGY, NURSING AND PROFESSIONAL EMPOWERMENT

Empowerment can be measured at an individual, organisational and community level, and is associated with the ability to make independent decisions and maintain individual autonomy at a personal level (Masi et al 2003). It is characterised by a sense of control, goal attainment and competence. Professional empowerment is linked to ownership of knowledge, especially knowledge that is attributed to a specialist group or professional elite. Unfortunately, power for nursing has arisen less often in association with our ownership of knowledge because nursing knowledge is associated often with gendered skills of caring that are valued less by society and healthcare (Henderson 2003, Rinard 1996). Notwithstanding we continue to seek recognition as a discipline and seek to produce competent practitioners for clinical environments where technical performance is prized highly (Barnard & Locsin 2007).

We have accepted new roles and responsibilities that have originated from the introduction of technology and the reassignment of duties from medicine (e.g. diagnostics and assessment). As a result, there is consistent reliance within healthcare sectors on our knowledge and skills, and this fact has been interpreted as a demonstration of our success (Almerud et al 2008, Sandelowski 2000). Nurses are often the only healthcare workers who possess the knowledge and skills required to operate particular machinery and tools in clinical environments. Technology cultivates for nurses enhanced respect, importance and uniqueness and, when it is used well, these qualities transfer to nursing as a profession (Fairman 1992, Sandelowski 1997).

However, it must be noted that despite the growth of knowledge and skills in nursing and the expansion of roles and responsibilities, the legal, clinical and political responsibility for technology continues to remain predominantly in the control of medicine. It is noted by Patel (2002) that even though physicians make up less than 10% of the workforce in the United States, they determine why, how, when, and the frequency with which biomedical technologies will be used, not only in the diagnosis of patients, but also in their treatment. Nurses and other healthcare workers provide well-defined and restricted services that are reflective of the physician's orders. Doctors admit patients to hospital, order most diagnostic procedures and, by and large, have been the decision makers and gatekeepers who determine treatment(s) that patients will receive.

With this continuing reality and the growth of technique in many realms of human activity, empowerment is a significant challenge, both because we lack clear avenues for franchisement and our autonomy is limited by the continual search for efficiency in care delivery to which we nurses must best fit.

From where then might empowerment arise?

It is commonplace for nurses to judge the effects of technology from perspectives that award it either a positive or negative influence upon clinical practice (known commonly as the optimism versus pessimism debate) (Sandelowski 1997). Debates between nurses have been reliant upon whether, for example, technology is believed to reduce menial work, increase comfort, emphasise a harmony between technology and caring, and expand knowledge (optimism), or undermine patient care, cause fragmentation of health services, foster a lack of caring behaviour and deskill nurses (pessimism).

Either perspective (optimism or pessimism) is to some degree an expression of specialist and class interests and value judgments concerning technological development. In reality, both perspectives contain elements of truth. For example, problems related to enhancing a person-focused approach in high-technology areas reflect individual nursing experience(s), assumptions about the role of technology in clinical practice and the organisation of healthcare, rather than any essential or fundamental conflict between technology and nurses (Barnard 2000, McGrath 2008, Sandelowski 1999a, Rudge 1999). In a critical essay on the semiotics of the nursing–technology relationship, Sandelowski (1999a, 2000) highlighted the way(s) that language/depiction/sign within nursing has served to create a presumed problem between nurses and technology. It was argued that there is growing evidence that current representation of the relationship between nursing and technology does not support the development of practice informed by critical reflection, nor the development of strategies that best enable clinical decisions to be made about the appropriate use of technology.

Future professional advancement will demand deeper insight into technology, and this growth will empower nurses because it will equip us to better engage in debate and decision making (Barnard & Sinclair 2006, Fairman 1998, Fairman & D'Antonio 1999). Expertise in clinical practice will be enhanced through our ability to: assess the suitability of technology for healthcare provision; advance person-focused care; sustain effective healthcare initiatives; and reinvigorate cultural, spiritual, moral and social values important to healthcare professions. Thus, it was encouraging to note that the United States Institute of Medicine 2001 report, entitled 'Crossing the quality chasm: a new health system for the twenty first century', emphasised the need for patient-centred and performance-based care that is devised around healing relationships and the provision of healthcare founded on needs and values.

The following guiding principles and values related to technology and nursing are important for empowerment in practice, will equip us to engage in healthcare debate(s) and should foster a desire to reinvigorate social and public service.

Good healthcare matters because people matter

Healthcare and nursing practice must be guided fundamentally by principles that promote, establish and protect human dignity. Protection of dignity is central to all that nurses engage in, and is central to the utilisation and integration of technology in care. Each person and their family have intrinsic value. Their uniqueness and importance must be acknowledged in even the most sophisticated technological environments. Episodes of objectification and loss of human dignity have been linked with technology (Almerud et al 2008, Locsin 2001, Rinard 1996, Sandelowski 2000), yet so often an emphasis on the experience and uniqueness of the person is possible with foresight and courage. For example, Barnard and Sandelowski (2001) highlight that even during high-intervention experiences such as emergency resuscitation, clinical measures can be adopted in order to place human experience and dignity central to care. Good healthcare matters because people matter, and this moral value must be continually emphasised, especially within healthcare systems dominated increasingly by technique.

Technology is political

The practice environment of a specialist unit, community facility or an institution impacts on the usefulness of technology. For example, a hospital unit that is designed poorly or resourced inappropriately is unsuitable to accommodate modern machinery and automata. Nurses can spend excess time and effort attending to technology and compensating for the inadequacies of poor resources. When resources do not foster adequately the use of technology, when they are defective or deficient, and support is not provided to foster skills and knowledge, the practice of nursing becomes difficult and stressful. Technology under these conditions becomes a burden to our practice. Funding, ward design, appropriate equipment and resources such as power and gas supply are crucial. When the practice environment is inadequate, the experience of integrating technology into care can be one of frustration, compromised health and safety for patients and staff, inadequate patient care and decreased efficiency and effectiveness (Barnard 2000, Lumley 1987, McConnell 1990, McGrath 2008).

Central to nursing practice is the need to create order in busy, demanding and complex clinical environments because practice alters regularly, policies and procedures are governed by external authorities, and patients are very often acutely sick. Nurses can experience a lack of certainty in clinical practice (unpredictability, varying demands on time, numerous roles and responsibilities) due to the demands of busy and complex clinical practice environments, and we rely upon appropriate technology. In the following quotation a nurse explains her experience of technology and states that:

> [T]echnology has so many advantages that if you are without it and you are busy, you do notice the difference. You tend to be more rushed and you don't have as much time to stop and chat … to your patients (Barnard 1998:169).

When technology operates effectively and is appropriately resourced, it provides substantial assistance to establishing safe and predictable patient care and coordinates various elements of clinical practice. Therefore, we need to be involved in determining the direction(s) of technological change and influencing decision making (Fairman 1996, Harding 1980, Hiraki 1992, McGrath 2008, Sandelowski 1997, 2000, Walters 1995). Decisions regarding access to particular technology, or the acquisition and use of machinery and equipment, are always political. Decisions related to technology will impact directly on the practice of each nurse, the organisation, and the patients for whom we care.

The right to quality care

Each person has a right to healthcare resources and quality nursing. Even though access to technology is sometimes restricted as a result of factors such as physical location and managed-care initiatives that place limitations on available resources (e.g. types of pharmaceuticals available in Australia), the dignity and worth of each life supports the view that we are responsible to effectively utilise and integrate appropriate technology.

Technology reveals only part of each person's experience and condition

Sophisticated electronic and computerised technology emphasises a reliance on quantitative evidence that is made available for us as digital displays, computer screens and printouts. Although technology offers real and worthwhile indicators as to the physical condition of a patient, an excessive reliance on technology can result in a tendency to accept quantitative evidence in preference to, and in spite of, the thoughts, experiences and feelings of the person. The following quotation from a nurse explains a typical scenario:

> [Y]ou've got this patient who is really grey, sinking in the bed, more and more you've got to be saying, what's happening? Is it just because of his oxygen saturation levels? Is there nothing else going wrong? Should I be checking other things? We've got to have faith in ourselves to go and check through and say, what is happening with this patient? (Barnard 1998:189).

It is unprofessional to replace patient assessment skills with a singular reliance on information from machinery and equipment. Excessive focus on information from technology without adequate consideration of a patient's total physical and emotional condition can result in treatment and intervention that is inappropriate and insensitive.

Technology is not a neutral object and nurses are not its master

Technology assists to achieve care outcomes that are complex and significant. However, technology is *not* neutral to care and sometimes overrides consideration of cultural, spiritual, emotional, physical and psychological needs along its path to bring about efficient outcomes (Almerud et al 2008, Barnard 1997, McGrath 2008, Sandelowski 2000). That is, it always has seen and unseen impact(s) upon activity, goals and outcomes. It does *not* lead always to outcomes acceptable for patients and nurses, but it is *not* a demonic force leading always to uncaring nurses in inhospitable wards. The use of technology will lead to care which ranges across all possibilities from positive to negative, and expertise in practice needs to be based upon a holistic framework that informs awareness and planning. Holism emphasises the centrality of the person and by extension the values, choices and individual lives that come into our care and management. The increasing emphasis within healthcare upon, for example, standardisation, protocols and integrated systems to manage healthcare delivery have to be balanced against the values and expectations of the person for whom we profess to care.

Technology to a greater or lesser extent alters our capacity to determine and accomplish individual goals, professional approaches to care and principles of nursing practice. It influences what Walters (1994) described as the ability of each nurse to *focus* his or her energies on the person and their ability to *balance* technology with the qualities of caring. Technology can positively and negatively shape a nurse's available time to establish a nurse–patient relationship and be involved in personal care. For example, technology in a clinical environment that malfunctions often will not save time nor allow each nurse to concentrate on practice principles that place the person at the point of primary concern. Poorly integrated technology can make the daily practice of nursing more demanding, time consuming and distracted. In addition, when clinical practice is dominated by excessive policies, protocols and limited resources, as well as constant demands to check equipment, administer drugs and respond excessively to inappropriate alarms, technology becomes a compelling and sometimes annoying influence upon a nurse's time, physical commitment and intellectual attention.

The demands of technology can sometimes intervene independent of strategies used to ensure the smooth operation of a clinical area. Choice of technology affects people's lives and requires users to formulate different ways to do things. It is not surprising that when problems arise from technology it can affect available time to, for example, care for a person's body (e.g. mouth care, hygiene, bathing). We are required to manage the effective integration of technology sometimes at the cost of other roles and responsibilities. The demands of telephones, buzzers and equipment checking can draw us away from the other things we need to do. In the following quote from a nurse, the experience is explained:

> All those alarms and monitors, they're geared to catch your attention aren't they? I mean, that's why they have alarms. So the first thing you do when you have alarms is go to it. It's like telephones at home. The first thing that you do when the telephone rings, it doesn't matter how busy you are, you drop everything to go and answer the phone, instead of saying, it's just a phone, leave it ring. I mean you put telephone answering machines on telephones these days, because the phone has to be answered doesn't it? We're geared these days to attend to noises and equipment before we attend to people (Barnard 1998:193).

You cannot use technology without also, to some extent, being influenced by its use. Our ability to display many of the caring behaviours associated commonly with nursing (i.e. a focus on personal experience, empathy, compassion) can be challenged, not often by a lack of compassion, empathy or desire to be involved more with people, but by the influence of technology on roles and responsibilities. The amount of technology in nursing practice does not alter our ability to feel compassion for the experience of others. It is simply not true to claim that the majority of nurses do not desire to engage in patient-focused practice founded on compassion and concern. It is true, however, to claim that sometimes technology and the way(s) we use it gets in the way of our ability to express the desire.

CONCLUSION

When technology is used appropriately in clinical practice it improves the effectiveness and efficiency of nursing, empowers carers and establishes predictable measures, assessment and behaviour. It assists greatly in our ability to understand the physical condition of the patient, and saves time by making patient assessment increasingly accurate and potentially reliable. These advantages are extended further when we properly integrate technology into personalised care and our practice is one of expertise and competence. Technology–nurse relations are more than just being able to manage equipment. Nursing practice continues to change in association with technology. It influences the practice of nursing, both from the perspective of what we do, how we think and how we understand ourselves as practitioners. There is nothing secondary about the experience of technology as it has continued to have an ongoing role in changing healthcare (Barger-Lux & Heaney1986, Barnard 2002, DeVries & Barroso 2000, Sandelowski 2000).

Nurses are increasingly responsible for technology in healthcare systems within administrative and bureaucratic structures. Knowledge and skills associated with nursing practice have altered over time, the ends to which we find ourselves working have changed, and clinical practice continues to broaden despite a paucity of understanding and explanation as to ongoing changes to arise from technology. For example, Gordon (2006) highlights how there is emerging in literature and practice an apparent disjunction between the technical aspects of care and the embodied experience of people. Nursing discourses highlight an emphasis on mechanistic and reductionist explanations of technical aspects of care without an equal emphasis on the experience and personal nature of the healthcare experience that each patient (person) embarks upon when they are cared for by each nurse. Gordon describes the situation as a new cartesianism: a new dualism in which the technical is separated from the embodied and experiencing person.

More scholarship and research is needed that addresses technology and nursing from perspectives that examine how we use artifacts and resources in practice, the relationship of clinical practice to theoretical models of nursing and caring, competency development, and a range of philosophical and sociological issues associated with power, gender, human experience and discipline development. Technology is a complex phenomenon that places before us an abundance of puzzles and questions. It is influential in every realm of social and professional life. Our profession continues to seek recognition, and technology has implications for nursing practice, education, theory and research.

Finally, the question remains, what do we do about technique in our clinical practice in order that we might begin to empower ourselves and the people for whom we care? The answer to the question lies probably in political action, individual activism, making informed choices in care and being willing to create a certain detachment from the imperatives that technique engenders. Being willing to question the use of technology when it does not meet the needs of people or promote quality care is paramount, and we should not underestimate the challenge that is before us.

Technique is integrated within the sociocultural context of society and nursing, and person-focused practice(s) is a freedom to be won. Being determined by specific technology(ies) is not the issue. In fact, the idea is nonsense because the act of freedom lies in victory over necessity, rather than over individual machines and automata. That is, empowerment is most likely to arise through individual and collective acts of resistance to the use of every possible means available in care and the technological order that is increasingly part of us. Healthcare practice that is not wholly determined by technique is a prize to be won in the first instance by our awakening to what is before each of us. Our duty is to occupy ourselves with the dangers, errors, advantages, difficulties and temptations of technology for the benefit of people. In undertaking this duty, we empower ourselves as significant contributors to healthcare.

REFLECTIVE QUESTIONS

1 What does this chapter tell us about the relations between nursing, technology and empowerment?

2 What important issues need to be addressed in order to further our skills in the appropriate use of technology in clinical practice?

3 Based on this chapter, what future research and practice development could be initiated in a clinical practice environment that you have experienced?

RECOMMENDED READINGS

Barnard A, Locsin R (eds) 2007 Technology and nursing practice. Palgrave-Macmillan, London

Barnard A, Sandelowski M 2001 Technology and humane nursing care: (ir)reconcilable or invented difference? Journal of Advanced Nursing 34:367–375
Locsin R 2001 Advancing technology, nursing and caring. Auburn House, Westport
Nelson S, Gordon S (eds) 2006 The complexities of care: nursing reconsidered. Cornell University Press, London
Sandelowski M 2000 Devices and desires: gender, technology and American nursing. University of North Carolina, Chapel Hill

REFERENCES

Almerud S, Alapack R, Fridlund B, Ekebergh M 2008 Caught in an artificial split: a phenomenological study of being a caregiver in the technologically intense environment. Intensive and Critical Care Nursing 24(12):130–136
Barger-Lux MJH, Heaney RP 1986 For better or worse: the technological imperative in health care. Social Science Medicine 22(12):1313–1320
Barnard A 1997 A critical review of the belief that technology is a neutral object and nurses are its master. Journal of Advanced Nursing 26:126–131
Barnard A 1998 Understanding technology in contemporary surgical nursing: a phenomenographic examination. Unpublished PhD thesis, University of New England, Armidale
Barnard A 2000 Technology and the Australian nursing experience. In: Daly J, Speedy S, Jackson D (eds) Contexts of nursing: an introduction. MacLennan & Petty, Sydney, pp 163–76
Barnard A 2002 Philosophy of technology and nursing. Nursing Philosophy 3:15–26
Barnard A, Cushing A 2001 Technology and historical inquiry in nursing. In: Locsin (R) (ed.) Advancing technology, caring and nursing. Auburn House, Westport, pp 12–21
Barnard A, Locsin R (eds) 2007 Technology and nursing practice. Palgrave-Macmillan, London
Barnard A, Sandelowski M 2001 Technology and humane nursing care: (ir)reconcilable or invented difference? Journal of Advanced Nursing 34:367–375
Barnard A, Sinclair M 2006 Spectators and spectacles: nurses, midwives and visuality. Journal of Advanced Nursing 55(5):578–586
Boykin A, Schoenhofer SO 2001 Nursing as caring: a model for transforming practice. National League for Nursing, Massachusetts
Cooper MC 1993 The intersection of technology and care in the ICU. Advances in Nursing Science 15(3):23–32
DeVries R, Barroso R 2000 Midwives among the machines: recreating midwifery in the late 20th century. Online. Available: www.stolaf.edu/people/devries/docs/midwifery.html
Fairman J 1992 Watchful vigilance: nursing care, technology, and the development of intensive care units. Nursing Research 41:56–60
Fairman J 1996 Response to tools of the trade: analysing technology as object in nursing. Scholarly Inquiry for Nursing Practice: An International Journal 10:17–21
Fairman J 1998 The nurse–technology relationship in the context of the history of technology. Nursing History Review 6:129–146
Fairman J, D'Antonio P 1999 Virtual power: gendering the nurse–technology relationship. Nursing Inquiry 6:178–186
Feenberg A 1999 Questioning technology. Routledge, New York

Ferre F 1995 Philosophy of technology. University of Georgia Press, London

Gordon S 2006 The new cartesianism. In: Nelson S, Gordon S (eds) The complexities of care: nursing reconsidered. Cornell University Press, London, pp 104–21

Harding S 1980 Value laden technologies and the politics of nursing. In Spicker SF, Gadow S (eds) Nursing: images and ideals, New York, Springer, pp 49–75

Harvey J 1997 The technological regulation of death: with reference to the technological regulation of birth. Sociology 31(4):719–736

Henderson S 2003 Power imbalance between nurses and patients: a potential inhibitor of partnership in care. Journal of Clinical Nursing 12:501–508

Hiraki A 1992 Tradition, rationality, and power in introductory nursing textbooks: a critical hermeneutics study. Advanced Nursing Science 14(3):1–12

Locsin R (ed.) 2001 Advancing technology, nursing and caring. Auburn House, Westport

Lovekin D 1991 Technique, discourse and consciousness: an introduction to the philosophy of Jacques Ellul. Associated University Press, New Jersey

Lumley J 1987 Assessing technology in a teaching hospital: three case studies. Paper presented at the 'Technologies in health care: policies and politics conference', Canberra

McConnell EA 1990 The impact of machines on the work of critical care nurses. Critical Care Nursing Quarterly 12(4):45–52

McGrath M 2008 The challenges of caring in a technological environment: critical care nurses' experiences. Journal of Clinical Nursing 17(8):1096–1104

Masi C, Suarez-Balcazar Y, Cassey M, Kinney L, Piotrowski H 2003 Internet access and empowerment. Journal of General Internal Medicine 18:525–530

Neuhaus W, Piroth C, Kiencke P, Gohring UJ, Mallman P 2002 A psychosocial analysis of women planning birth outside hospital. Journal of Obstetrics and Gynaecology 22(2):143–149

Pacey A 1999 Meaning in technology. MIT Press, Cambridge

Patel KRM 2002 Health care policy in an age of new technologies. ME Sharpe, New York

Pelletier D 1989 Health care technology: sharpening the definition and establishing aspects of the social context. Australian Health Review 12(3):56–64

Rinard R 1996 Technology, deskilling, and nurses: the impact of the technologically changing environment. Advances in Nursing Science 18(4):60–70

Rudge T 1999 Situating wound management: technoscience, dressings and 'other' skins. Nursing Inquiry 6:167–177

Sandelowski M 1997 (Ir)reconcilable differences? The debate concerning nursing and technology. Image: Journal of Nursing Scholarship 29:169–174

Sandelowski M 1999a Culture, conceptive technology, and nursing. International Journal of Nursing Studies 36:13–20

Sandelowski M 1999b Venous envy: the post-World War II debate over IV nursing. Advances in Nursing Science 22(1):52–62

Sandelowski M 2000 Devices and desires: gender, technology and American nursing. University of North Carolina, Chapel Hill

Sinclair M, Gardner J 2001 Midwives' perceptions of the use of technology in assisting childbirth in Northern Ireland. Journal of Advanced Nursing 36(2):229–236

Wagner M 1992 Appropriate birth care in industrialised countries. Paper presented at the 'Future birth conference', Sydney

Wagner M 1994 Pursuing the birth machine. Ace Graphics, Sydney

Walters AJ 1994 An interpretative study of the clinical practice of critical care nurses. Contemporary Nurse 3:21–25

Walters AJ 1995 Technology and the lifeworld of critical care nursing. Journal of Advanced Nursing 22:338–346

Winner L 2003 Social constructivism: opening the black box and finding it is empty. In: Scharff RC, Dusek V (eds) Philosophy of technology: the technological condition. Blackwell, Oxford, pp 233–44

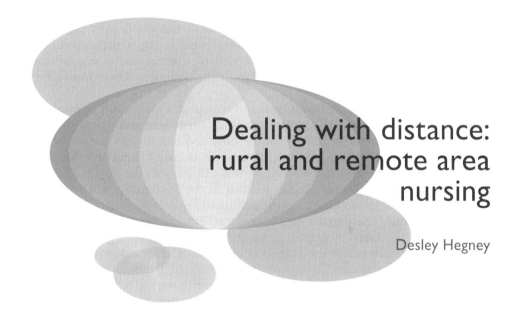

CHAPTER 16

Dealing with distance: rural and remote area nursing

Desley Hegney

LEARNING OBJECTIVES

On completion of this chapter, the reader will be able to:

- demonstrate an understanding of the impact of rural life on the health of rural Australians
- explain how the Australian rural and remote environment impacts upon the scope of practice of the nurse
- demonstrate an understanding of the differences between rural, remote area and metropolitan nursing
- describe the role and function of the rural and remote area nurse in Australia, and
- explain the issues currently impacting upon the practice role of the rural and remote area nurse.

KEY WORDS

Rural, remote nursing, diversity, health status, service delivery, recruitment and retention, professional development

RURAL AND REMOTE NURSING

This chapter provides an overview of the nature and different health status of rural and remote communities. In this chapter, the words 'regional', 'rural' and 'remote' refer to the 32% of Australians who live outside a major city (population equal to or greater than 250,000). There is no 'one' rural or remote community; rather, each community in Australia has a different economic base and different demographics that impact upon the health and health needs of rural and remote residents. Many rural researchers have argued that despite images of rural Australia as being a healthy place to live, rural Australians have poorer health than those living in larger population centres. While this health disadvantage is still acknowledged, current studies suggest that the effect is more from socioeconomic factors and risky occupations than from the rural environment itself.

A description of the role of both rural and remote area nurses will be provided, as well as an examination of the similarities and differences in their scope of practice. It will be demonstrated that the role of the rural and remote area nurse is different from that of the nurse employed in health facilities in major cities, and that the core difference is the generalist practice role, which can be from the novice to advanced practice level. This generalist role has resulted in the devaluing of the role of these nurses by other nurses working in more specialised fields.

Identified issues that impact on the scope of practice of rural and remote area nurses will be discussed—issues such as inadequate preparation for the role, lack of access to education and training, personal and professional isolation, and the lack of anonymity associated with working in small rural and remote towns. While some aspects of the role are highly valued by these nurses (e.g. the higher level of professional autonomy), the isolation and lack of preparation for the role often results in low retention rates, especially in the more remote communities (Dowd & Johnson 1995).

For those who stay in rural and remote practice, the work is both professionally and personally rewarding. To quote Western Australian nurse Andrew Cameron: 'So the work is varied and on the whole, I find it tremendously rewarding' (Cameron 2004).

RURAL COMMUNITIES

Rural Australia is seen by most Australians as 'the bush'. When visualising 'the bush', most Australians have images of wide-open spaces, clean air, a healthy lifestyle and primary production (agriculture, mining, forestry, fishing). They do not have images of poverty and of Indigenous populations with Third World health status. Despite this reality, the myths of 'mateship', 'hardiness', and people surviving through hard times caused by environmental factors (such as drought and flood) and/or economic factors (such as the value of the Australian dollar), still dominate the descriptions of rural Australia. To understand rural life today, however, requires the inclusion of images such as poverty, economic problems and underserviced healthcare needs.

The dominant image of rural Australia is one of being reliant on agriculture. Yet the 768 million hectares, which is the land area of Australia, have a great diversity of resources, opportunities and alternatives for future development (Lovett 1993). The key consideration in modern rural Australia is diversity. That is, no two rural areas are alike and some areas are more advantaged than others. For example, settlements that are in close proximity to capital cities, those on the coastal fringe, those with tourist potential, mining communities and the regional centres, are more likely to sustain growth and survive. In contrast, the more remote areas face a more tenuous and difficult future (Lovett 1993).

RURAL POPULATIONS

Approximately 32% of Australians live in rural or remote areas. Using the Australian Standard Geographical Classification, which classifies Australia's population into five areas (major cites, inner regional, outer regional, remote and very remote), 29% of the 32% live in regional areas and only 3% live in remote areas (Australian Institute of Health and Welfare 2008a). When interpreting rural and remote health data, it should be remembered that in remote areas, a large proportion of the population is Indigenous (24% of the population in remote areas and 45% of the population in very remote areas) (Australian Institute of Health and Welfare 2008a). The Australian Institute of Health and Welfare (2008a:81) note: 'this means that information about the health of Australians living in remote areas is often influenced by the generally poorer health status of the Indigenous population living in those areas'.

Rural and remote settlements do not have an homogenous economic base. Rather, their economic base ranges from mining, Indigenous settlements, coastal resorts, retirement communities, regional service centres and towns which could be considered to be commuter suburbs (as they are located on the periphery of a major city), to those dependent on agriculture, forestry and fishing (Frager et al 1997).

The composition of the population residing in rural areas of Australia has changed enormously over time. For example, since 1976, there has been a 60% decline in the number of farmers in their 20s. Instead of young people, those entering farming were more likely to choose farming as a mid-career option and therefore be aged 40 years or older. Additionally, younger people's disinterest in farming has meant that many farmers stay longer into their later years. All of these changes have meant that the median age of a farmer has increased from 44 in 1981 to 50 in 2001 (Land and Water Australia 2004).

Farms have been subject to severe cost/price pressures, resulting in many farmers being asset rich and income poor (Rolley & Humphreys 1993). In the early twenty-first century, farm incomes have become diverse, with on-farm income comprising only a small proportion of earnings. The economic pressure on farmers has meant that farms have become larger. Thus, as smaller farms are merged to make larger economic units, the farming population has declined (Land and Water Australia 2004). Additionally, many family-owned farms have been replaced by corporate farming. In the late twentieth century, the rural landscape had changed considerably with only one in ten people in the non-metropolitan workforce employed in agriculture, and with many people living in retirement in rural coastal areas (Australian Institute of Health and Welfare 2004a).

Rural and remote Australians have some characteristics that are quite different from Australians living in major cities. For example, they:

- have larger families
- are less likely to be aged between 15 and 34 years
- are less likely to be one-parent families
- are more likely to live in a house (rather than an apartment) and less likely to pay rent

- are more likely to own a car
- are more likely to have both partners of the marriage in employment, and
- are more likely to be employers rather than employees (Australian Institute of Health and Welfare 2004a).

It must be remembered that rural Australia is composed of much more activity than agricultural pursuits and that the income generated by rural women is a vital part of the rural landscape. In a 2004 report on *Women in business in rural and remote Australia*, it was found that the income derived by regional businesswomen around Australia was diverse and generated income in the order of $1.2 billion per annum (Houghton & Strong 2004). The authors noted that regional women ran businesses which ranged from 'bed and breakfasts and traditional "country craft" business to business in professional and health services, education, manufacturing, and personal and business services' (Houghton & Strong 2004:2). In some cases, the income provided much-needed off-farm income, while in other cases, the women lived in town and had no link with agriculture (Houghton & Strong 2004).

While much is made about the isolation of rural communities (and isolation from services will be the focus later in this chapter), some argue that communities are far less isolated than they were in the past. Epps and Sorensen (1993) stated that in the 1970s a typical rural life was one where incomes were largely dependent on seasonal conditions and fluctuations of commodity prices, housing was cheap and functional, and food prices were high. In addition, less emphasis was placed on educational attainment than today, services were fewer and of poorer quality than those of larger cities because of low population density and insufficient demand to make delivery of services worthwhile, and many rural communities experienced outmigration of the young and energetic. People were concerned about the weather, isolation and road conditions, had a strong work ethic and viewed impersonal city life with suspicion (Bessant 1980).

It is argued that rural Australia has been transformed since the 1970s in that technology has reduced the sense of isolation, deregulation of transport has facilitated overnight parcel deliveries to many rural areas, people can travel further by road to obtain goods and services, and larger regional centres often have cultural visits by national and international artists (Epps & Sorensen 1993, Rolley & Humphreys 1993).

Recognising that the face of rural Australia is constantly changing, and that there is no one standard rural town or area, it is time now to examine the claims that rural and remote Australia is a healthy place to live.

RURAL AUSTRALIA: A HEALTHY PLACE TO LIVE?

The myth of rural Australia as a healthy place to live seems to have dated from the nineteenth century and it appears that, in comparison to industrialised and urbanised Europe, it may have been so (Walmsley & Sorensen 1988). Rural people have been reported to have a more self-reliant attitude to health (Lovett 1993). They are renowned for their independence, resourcefulness, capacity for hard work, stoicism in the face of adversity, generosity and community-mindedness (Rolley & Humphreys 1993).

In the late 1990s and early 2000s, there have been several publications focusing on the health of rural and remote Australians (e.g. Strong et al 1998, Australian Institute of Health and Welfare 2004a). The major findings of these reports suggested that rural and remote Australians have considerable differences in morbidity and mortality rates to those Australians living in major cities. These studies have been confirmed by recent publications (Australian Institute of Health and Welfare 2008a), which suggest that:

- life expectancy decreases with increasing remoteness
- people living in rural and remote areas are more likely to have certain chronic diseases (e.g. cancer, depression, diabetes, arthritis) than people living in major cities
- children tend to have more decayed, missing or filled teeth
- mortality rates are higher, the main contributions being coronary heart disease, 'other' circulatory disease and motor vehicle accidents; additionally, for people less than 65 years of age, injury (e.g. motor vehicle accidents and suicide) are notable contributors to deaths, particularly among males
- perinatal death rates increase with remoteness
- rural and remote people are more likely to smoke
- the intake of other drugs and alcohol is higher with consumption of alcohol increasing with remoteness, and
- these populations are more likely to be overweight or obese and report sedentary behaviour.

The causes of this health disparity are linked strongly to the socioeconomic and environment factors impacting on rural and remote Australians (Australian Institute of Health and Welfare 2008a, Smith et al 2008). An important factor within the environment is the distance that rural people are forced to travel to access equivalent health services taken for granted by people living in larger population centres (Smith et al 2008).

Socioeconomics

Socioeconomic disadvantage is now higher in rural districts than in major cities and is a significant variable in terms of rural health. The factors that influence this disadvantage include: high unemployment rates in rural and remote areas; decreased education opportunities; a higher proportion of unskilled labour in the workforce; and, with the exception of some remote mining communities, a lower family income (Australian Institute of Health and Welfare 2008a, Frager et al 1997). A number of studies have found links between low socioeconomic status and the health of the individual in rural areas (Australian Institute of Health and Welfare 2008a, Frager et al 1997, Smith et al 2008, Strong et al 1998). Smith et al (2008:59) note that 'much of the variation between rural and urban health status can be explained by socioeconomic factors affecting the use of health services'.

Use of health services: problems posed by distance

Rural Australia is characterised by low population densities and varying distances between towns (Strong et al 1998). These low population densities are of 'critical importance in understanding problems of service provision' (Humphreys & Rolley 1991:23). Rural people 'in need' are more dispersed and isolated in their distribution than city residents in major cities, and this makes the provision of even basic services extremely expensive (Rolley & Humphreys 1993).

It is well documented that accessibility is the main issue for rural residents (Australian Institute of Health and Welfare 2004a, Humphreys & Rolley 1991, Macklin

1991, Smith et al 2008). This lack of accessibility is caused by remoteness. Remoteness has been defined as:

> ... access to a range of services, some of which are available in smaller and others in larger centres: the remoteness of a location can thus be measured in terms of how far one has to travel to centres of various sizes (Department of Health and Aged Care and Geographical Information Systems Classification of Australia 2001, cited in Australian Institute of Health and Welfare 2004a:2).

Populations in Australia (and thus the health status of these populations) are now reported on according to one of three 'remoteness classifications'. However, all of these classifications have limitations, and the readers of this chapter are referred to the discussion about these strengths and weaknesses as outlined in 'Rural, regional and remote health: a guide to remoteness classifications' (Australian Institute of Health and Welfare 2004a).

Accepting that rural and remote Australians are affected by remoteness, and despite Macklin's (1991) statement that universal coverage and equity of access 'to the healthcare system are two important principles which are widely accepted' (Macklin 1991:5), in rural and remote areas of Australia, the reality is that the majority of residents do not have access to the range of services available in major cities. The barriers of access to health services by the rural and remote population have been identified as: lack of healthcare professionals; cost and limited access to specific services; and lack of culturally acceptable services.

Lack of healthcare professionals

There is wide agreement that rural and remote Australian communities are underserved by appropriately trained health professionals. Additionally, there is evidence that urban-background medical practitioners are less likely to remain in rural practice for more than 3–5 years. This contrasts with medical practitioners with a rural background, who are more likely to choose a rural career and remain in practice for longer (Hays et al 1997). Further, in many of the more remote areas of Australia, communities are unable to attract a medical practitioner and are dependent upon rural and remote area nurses to provide their healthcare (Macklin 1992). The shortage of rural registered nurses is also now impacting on healthcare delivery in rural and remote areas (Australian Institute of Health and Welfare 2004a).

The problem of recruitment and retention of medical practitioners to rural areas has been the subject of several discussion papers (e.g. 'The future of general practice', Macklin 1992). Schemes focusing primarily on medical practitioner recruitment and retention such as the Rural Incentive Program (Hays et al 1997), the Rural Clinical Schools (Australian Government 2004b) and the University Departments of Rural Health (Humphreys et al 2000) have been introduced to address this problem.

The same level of attention has not, to date, been given to the issues of the recruitment and retention of other health professionals such as nurses and allied health, mainly because medical practitioners are seen as 'employees' of the Australian Government (through Medicare reimbursement), whereas nurses and allied health professionals are normally employees of state or territory governments (Hegney 1996). However, as the shortage of nurses has increased, the state/territory governments, the Australian Government and private enterprise have begun to offer incentive programs for nurses. For example, the Australian Government now offers the aged care nursing scholarship scheme, as well as the rural and remote nurse scholarship program, which provides support for undergraduate, reentry, upskilling, postgraduate and conference scholarships (Australian Government 2004a, 2004b). Examples of state and territory government scholarships include:

- the New South Wales Nursing and Midwifery Innovation Scholarships: www.health.nsw.gov.au/nursing/scholar.html
- the Australian Rotary Health Research Fund: Parnell Rural and Remote Nursing Scholarship: www.arhrf.org.au/main.asp?pageName=Rural%20 Medical%and%20Nursing
- the Queensland Health Rural Scholarship Scheme: www.health.qld.gov.au/orh/ qhrss/default.asp

Since 1991, when the first national rural health conference was held in Toowoomba, Queensland, there has been a plethora of rural health organisations. For example, the National Rural Health Alliance (NRHA), which is an organisation comprised of key professional and consumer rural organisations, is now responsible for most of the lobbying to governments for adequate rural health policies. Professional organisations, such as the Rural Doctors' Association of Australia (RDAA), the Services for Australian Rural and Remote Allied Health (SARRAH), the Council of Remote Area Nurses of Australia (CRANA), the Isolated Children's Parents Association (ICPA), and the Country Women's Association of Australia (CWA), are all member bodies of the NRHA. Despite the work of these organisations, in 2008 there was still a shortage of Australian-born medical practitioners, nurses and allied health professionals in rural and remote Australia. This lack of a 'stable, efficient and well-educated workforce' directly impacts upon the viability of rural health services (Kenny & Duckett 2003).

Cost and limited access to specific services

Several authors, in their examination of the health resources available to rural and remote residents, have noted that:

- nurses provide a higher proportion of healthcare in rural and remote Australia than in metropolitan Australia (Strong et al 1998)
- nursing home beds are less likely to be available as remoteness increases (Australian Institute of Health and Welfare 2008a, Strong et al 1998)
- Medicare data indicate that people living in rural and remote zones use less services than those living in major cities (Australian Institute of Health and Welfare 2008a, Strong et al 1998), and
- the number of doctors (including medical specialists) and pharmacists declines as an area becomes more remote (Australian Institute of Health and Welfare 2008a, Strong et al 1998).

People in rural areas therefore, while experiencing increasing levels of poverty, have to face increased costs of travel and accommodation should they require anything other than basic primary care services. While schemes such as the Isolated Patients' Travel Assistance Scheme have been available for some time, patients usually have to pay the costs up-front and seek reimbursement later. This can be problematic if the rural person was unaware of their entitlement or wishes to claim after they have sought treatment (McGrath et al 1999). The financial and personal cost of travel for treatment in a major centre does mean that some rural people will either choose more radical initial surgery options (e.g. women will choose to have a mastectomy for breast cancer rather than radiotherapy and chemotherapy) or they will delay treatment until it can no longer be avoided (Hegney et al 2005a, Humphreys & Rolley 1993, McGrath et al 1999). A Senate Inquiry into patient travel schemes in 2007 (Parliament of Australia, Senate 2007) made 16 recommendations, including the establishment of a taskforce to drive the development of national standards to ensure equity of access to medical services.

One way to overcome the need to travel to services is to bring the service to the population. One such method is the use of telehealth services. These services were initiated in the 1990s by leaders such as Professor Peter Yellowlea who provided psychiatric clinics using telehealth services. Australian telehealth service provision appeared to stall in the late 1990s and early 2000s. However, there are some excellent examples of telehealth services currently under trial. For example, Professor Len Gray, a geriatrician located at the Princess Alexander Hospital in Brisbane, provides a telehealth service to the rehabilitation unit at the Toowoomba Health Service (approximately 130 kilometres west of Brisbane, Queensland). The service provision overcomes the lack of availability of a geriatrician in Toowoomba, and provides support to both patients and staff of the service in Toowoomba.

Lack of culturally acceptable services

This has been one of the reasons for the 'Fourth World' health status of the Aboriginal and Torres Strait Islander people (Peach et al 1998, Strong et al 1998). As there is a chapter on Indigenous health for this book (see Ch 20), I will not replicate the information but refer you to that chapter. There are also substantial culturally and linguistically diverse populations living in rural and remote areas of Australia. It is evident that there are few culturally appropriate services delivered for these populations.

RURAL AND REMOTE AREA NURSING

A remote area nurse is:

> ... a registered nurse whose day-to-day practice encompasses all or most aspects of primary healthcare. This practice most often occurs in an isolated or geographically remote location. The nurse is responsible, either solely or as a member of a small team, for the continuous, coordinated and comprehensive healthcare in that location (CRANA 1993, cited in Dowd & Johnson 1995:36).

In contrast, 'rural nursing' has no one agreed definition. The most cited definition defines rural nursing as the practice of nurses in the rural environment and where no medical practitioners are employed full time in a hospital, but are 'located within the town' (Hegney 1997a). This definition has its limitations, as it defines rural nursing 'by default'. That is, it does not define rural nursing by what rural nurses do; rather, it states that rural nursing practice is defined by the absence of other health professionals. However, the definition does recognise that it is the rural environment that determines the context of rural nursing practice and, therefore, the generalist/specialist practice nature of the rural nurse's role.

Both definitions highlight the similarities and differences between rural and remote area nursing. Remote area nurses are isolated from medical and allied health support staff, and therefore their practice is more autonomous than that of the rural nurse, who often has medical and allied health staff located within the town. For remote area nurses, medical support is usually provided by a medical practitioner located in a distant location (e.g. the Royal Flying Doctor Service). Remote area nurses are often the only health professionals providing healthcare to the community—with or without the support of Indigenous health workers. In contrast, rural nurses are more likely to work in an interprofessional team, with at least one medical practitioner practising in the town and experiencing varying levels of support from allied health professionals, depending on the size of the town and its surrounding area.

Another difference between rural and remote area nurses is the model of healthcare delivery on which their practice is based. Remote area nurses provide, on the whole, a primary healthcare service, whereas rural nurses predominantly work from a medical model health service (Cramer 1994, Hegney 1996, Wakerman & Field 1998). The similarities and differences of the practice of rural and remote area nurses are also reflected in their workforce profile.

Demographic characteristics of the rural and remote area nursing workforce

In 2005, of the 244,360 registered and enrolled nurses employed in Australia, 91,471 (or about 37.5%) were employed in rural or remote areas (Australian Institute of Health and Welfare 2008b). This was an increase in nurses employed in rural and remote areas, with the largest rise occurring in outer regional areas and very remote areas (Australian Institute of Health and Welfare 2008b).

Nurses employed in inner regional areas were older, with an average age of 46.1 years, than any other region, particularly compared with nurses in major cities (average age 44.6 years). Compared to the national figure of 7.9%, the portion of male nurses was lower in outer regional areas (6.1%) and remote areas (4.9%) (Australian Institute of Health and Welfare 2008b).

Nurses in remote areas (average 34.7 hours per week) and very remote areas (average of 38.2 hours per week) were more likely to work longer hours (compared to the national average of 33 hours per week) (Australian Institute of Health and Welfare 2008b). The Australian Institute of Health and Welfare (2008b) noted that for nurses in both remote and very remote areas, hours of work were increasing at a greater rate than the national figure of 2.3 hours per week.

The scope of practice of the rural and remote area nurse

Nursing roles in rural and remote Australia are different not only from the role of nurses employed in major cities, but also from each other. The role differences are caused by many factors, including:

- geographical location (e.g. a nurse working closer to a regional or major city will usually have easier access to medical and allied health services and be more likely to work in an interprofessional team)
- the population density of the area (as the population increases the more cost-effective are generalist and specialist medical and allied health services; this means that either on-site or visiting services are available)
- the type of employing institution (e.g. community compared with hospital facility)

- the type of community, its economic base and health needs (e.g. remote area nurses working in Indigenous communities have a different role from remote area nurses working in mining communities), and
- the number and type of services available within the community, which also impact on health (e.g. generalist and specialist healthcare services, access to transport, educational facilities, levels of public sanitation).

It is the context of practice, it has been argued, that determines the role and function of the nurse (Hegney 1996). The increased level of responsibility and autonomy within the practice role accepted by rural and remote area nurses is described as high compared with nurses employed in major cities (Dowd & Johnson 1995). The level of responsibility has been linked to the high job satisfaction level of rural and remote area nurses (Cramer 1994, Hegney et al 1997).

Research in Australia on the role and function of rural and remote area nurses has revealed that the majority of the community believe these nurses are competent in a vast array of nursing skills, acquired by education and experience, and possess skills that are highly valued by the community in which they work (Burley & Harvey 1993, Kreger 1991).

This advanced practice role, which has been described as 'Jack-of-all-trades', or 'extended', 'expanded' and 'multiskilled', is not new to these nurses; rather, it has been the norm for rural and remote area nursing practice since white settlement (Hegney et al 1997). In small rural and remote health facilities, the broad scope of the role means that nurses are providing care, as well as dealing with situations external to the health environment, including the wellbeing, development and safety of the local community in which they work (New South Wales Health 1998). Rural and remote area nurses, therefore, must have skills and knowledge:

> ... beyond that acquired in basic nursing education, as well as the advanced knowledge and skills to meet the needs of the population unserved, or underserved by the medical services normally available in urban communities (McMurray et al 1998:9–10).

Until relatively recently, with the introduction of the nurse practitioner program in Australia, the advanced practice role of rural and remote area nurses was not recognised or legitimised in law (Dowd & Johnson 1995, Hegney et al 1997). In 2008, there were advances in the numbers of practising nurse practitioners (approximately 130), many of whom are now employed in metropolitan settings. However, the first nurse practitioner in Australia was employed in New South Wales in the remote setting of Lightning Ridge. Nurse practitioners in rural and remote areas mostly deliver primary healthcare. Similar to all nurse practitioners in Australia, the nurses' scope of practice is limited by their inability to access the Australian Pharmaceutical Benefits Scheme (PBS) and the Medical Benefits Scheme (MBS). At the time of writing this chapter, with a change of government, it appears action may take place to overcome these barriers and thus allow nurse practitioners to work within their wide scope of practice.

In Queensland, and increasingly in other states such as Victoria, legislation is being or has been changed to widen the scope of practice of rural and remote area registered nurses. In Queensland, changes were made to the *Health (Drugs and Poisons) Regulations* to allow registered nurses (who were not nurse practitioners) in rural and remote areas who were endorsed for an advanced role to administer and supply restricted and controlled drugs (as listed on a Drug Formulary). These drugs are linked to protocols (called a Health Management Protocol). The changes to Queensland's *Health (Drugs and Poison) Regulations* have ensured that registered rural and remote area nurses endorsed for rural and isolated practice now have legislation which legitimises their medication practice (Hegney et al 2005b).

Factors impacting upon rural and remote area nursing practice

To ensure a stable rural and remote nursing workforce, several factors need to be addressed. These include educational preparation, access to continuing professional education, recruitment and retention issues, dealing with personal and professional isolation, lack of anonymity, promoting rural and remote area nursing as a desirable career, and strengthening communication between rural and urban health authorities, and professional groups. This chapter will now discuss some of these issues.

Anonymity

In small towns people know each other and are often related. For the rural and remote area nurse, this knowing and being known by the community has advantages and disadvantages (New South Wales Health 1998). Several authors have described the lack of anonymity of remote area nurses and the need for those in small communities to have 'time out' because of their high visibility within the small community (Cramer 1992, Kreger 1991, Siegloff & Hegney 1996). Additionally, remote area nurses who are employed in Indigenous communities experience a level of visibility within the community for which they often have not been prepared (Cramer 1992).

The rural nurse employed in a small rural community, and the remote area nurse, are often well known by the rural community, as the majority of nurses remain in one health service for long periods of time (Hegney et al 1997). In contrast to remote area nurses, it is not uncommon for rural nurses to have grown up in the area in which they are employed, and to have kinship ties with other members of the community (Hegney et al 1997). This means that the nurse often has to provide care to relatives and friends. Thus, in adverse advents, the nurse has to cope with personal feelings of loss, as well as those of the patient and/or family (Siegloff & Hegney 1996).

As well as being a member of a small community, rural and remote area nurses can provide healthcare to several generations of the same family. This aspect of their role has been described as 'womb to tomb care' (Hegney 1996). Studies have suggested that rural nurses have a 'unique insight' into their community and its needs because of the length of time that most rural nurses work in rural communities (Burley & Harvey 1993). In contrast, the majority of remote area nurses do not have the same work history within one community as do rural nurses.

Rural communities have the expectation that the nurse will be an integral member of the community. Thus it is suggested that nurses lose their anonymity by virtue of their rural and remote area practice—they are never off-duty (Hegney 1996). Leaving the community or 'getting out' is, for some nurses, an important coping mechanism. To do this, however, nurses must have access to relief staff locums (New South Wales Health 1998). The lack of locum relief is a barrier that has been identified as impacting not only on the nurse's ability to leave the community for 'time out', but also for continuing professional education.

Education and training

Education and training levels have a significant impact upon rural and remote area nursing practice.

Lack of preparation for the role

A feature of the literature with regard to the role of the nurse employed in remote area and small rural communities is the lack of preparation for their role (Cramer 1992, 1994, Dowd & Johnson 1995, Hegney et al 1997, Kenny & Duckett 2003, Kenny et al 2004). A study of 57 remote area nurses (Cramer 1992) found that the majority believed they were totally unprepared for their role. A major contributing factor to their lack of preparation for the role is the lack of orientation to practice (Cramer 1992, Hanna 2001, Hegney et al 1997). For remote area nurses the lack of preparation for working in Indigenous communities has resulted in 'reality shock' (Cramer 1994, Hanna 2001). Additionally, the lack of preparation for remote area practice has been linked to the higher turnover rate (as much as 300% per annum in some locations), as well as burn-out (Cramer 1992, Dowd & Johnson 1995).

Attempts have been made to address this lack of preparation, with orientation courses for remote area nurses now conducted in some states (e.g. Queensland and Western Australia). As the majority of the remote area nursing workforce is employed in Indigenous communities, cultural awareness programs are considered an essential part of this orientation (Dowd & Johnson 1995). Several studies, however, indicate that there remain inadequacies in access to education (and career-enhancing opportunities) between nurses who are employed in major cities and nurses who work in rural and remote areas (Courtney et al 2002b, Hegney et al 2003a).

Undergraduate, postgraduate and continuing education and training

Since 1991, there has been recognition that rural and remote area nurses require adequate preparation for their role in the form of formal higher education programs and orientation courses (Wakerman & Field 1998). In response to these criticisms, several universities have introduced either an undergraduate double degree (e.g. Monash University) or a 4-year undergraduate degree, which focuses on rural nursing practice (La Trobe University). Kenny et al (2004) believe that their 4-year undergraduate degree particularly addresses the underpreparation of new graduates to practice in rural and remote areas. Other universities, particularly those in regional areas, have specifically focused their clinical preparation to prepare nurses for rural and remote areas (Lea et al 2008).

The shortage of clinical practice placements for students in rural areas, as well as a lack of preceptor/mentors who can supervise students during the program, is another barrier to access (Hegney 1996, Lea & Cruickshank 2007). While some states provide some funding for clinical placements, the majority of undergraduate students are required to self-fund clinical placements in the rural or remote area health facility. This is an added cost, which often means that a rural clinical placement is limited for many nurses (Neill & Taylor 2002).

In addition to these undergraduate degrees, several universities have introduced postgraduate programs which either prepare nurses for rural and remote practice or specifically prepare the nurse as a nurse practitioner to practise in a rural or remote area (e.g. the University of South Australia, the University of Queensland, Flinders University). Because of changes to Australian Government funding, the majority of university postgraduate courses are now fee-paying. The cost varies between universities, but it affects the ability of rural and remote area nurses to enrol in a course. There have been some attempts to address this barrier. For example, in 1998 the Australian Government provided funding in the form of rural and remote scholarships (through the Royal College of Nursing Australia) for rural and remote area nurses to attend formal and informal education and training courses (Australian Government 2004a). Since this time, several states have also introduced scholarship schemes to assist with undergraduate and postgraduate education and training. Several industrial organisations (such as the Queensland Nurses Union and the New South Wales Nurses Association) have also ensured funding is enshrined in nursing awards, with funds and/or study days now part of the enterprise agreement for employed registered and enrolled nurses.

Mentoring nurses employed in rural and remote areas has been a focus of a federally funded project which had a twofold aim: to develop the capacity of rural nurses to mentor effectively; and to provide support to them during the mentoring experience (Mills et al 2006). The successful project made several recommendations, including the need for planned mentoring to support both experienced rural nurses and new graduates (Mills et al 2006).

To meet the ongoing professional education and training needs of rural and remote area nurses, there are now many offerings available through organisations such as university departments of rural health, regional and metropolitan universities and hospitals, and other employers. However, studies of rural and remote area nurses suggest that remote area nurses in particular still have problems accessing education and training programs (Hegney et al 2003a). The Australian literature contains a wealth of information on the lack of access to education and training of rural and remote area nurses. It particularly focuses on the need for appropriate, accessible and flexible programs delivered within the rural clinical environment (Dowd & Johnson 1995, Lampshire & Rolfe 1993, McMurray et al 1998). Barriers to education and training that have been identified include family commitments, inability to afford unpaid leave, lack of locum relief staff, lack of finance, lack of information on what courses are available, lack of employer support, and the unsuitability of many courses for rural nursing practice (Hanna 2001, Hegney et al 1997, Hegney et al 2003a, McMurray et al 1998).

The extensive literature on education and training for rural and remote area nurses recommends that they be educationally prepared for their role prior to employment, have access to suitable education and training after their employment, and be able to enrol in programs which give articulation between higher education providers (Hegney et al 1997, Kenny & Duckett 2003). It was also recommended that the clinical environment be an equal partner in the preparation and continuing education of rural nurses (Hegney et al 1997, Lea & Cruickshank 2007).

Professional isolation

Related to the need for an adequately prepared nurse is the ability of the nurse to provide a health service in relative isolation from the nursing profession and other healthcare providers. Distance does not necessarily mean isolation. Nurses can feel isolated in metropolitan settings, especially if they are working as a sole practitioner (such as midwife or occupational health nurse). The literature suggests that rural and remote area nurses do feel isolated in their practice, and the major cause of this isolation is the distance between health services and, therefore, nursing, medical and allied health support (Dowd & Johnson 1995, Hegney et al 1997, Neill & Taylor 2002). Distance, in these cases, limits the ability of nurses to form peer networks with other nurses and healthcare professionals (New South Wales Health 1998).

To address the isolation of remote area nurses, the Council of Remote Area Nurses in Australia (CRANA) received federal government funding for the provision of a 'Bush Crisis Line'. This crisis line, which has a toll-free number, can be used by rural and remote area nurses 24 hours a day.

Relationships with other healthcare professionals

A factor that often influences the level of responsibility of rural and remote area nurses is the number of medical and allied health professionals employed by or appointed to the health service. This varies between health facilities, ranging from remote area nurses often working alone and relying on off-site medical services (such as the Royal Flying Doctor Service) to rural nurses who have resident medical officers, medical specialists and a wide range of allied health professionals working in the town.

In small rural hospitals and remote communities where there are no resident medical officers, the first patient contact in an emergency is the nurse. General practitioner contact can be unavailable for periods ranging from 30 minutes to 4 hours, depending on locale and travelling time for the doctor. Additionally, in many of these facilities there may be no allied health staff, such as pharmacist, radiographer, physiotherapist or occupational therapist. In these facilities, nurses dispense medications on a telephone order from an off-site practitioner (or an endorsed rural and isolated practice nurse or nurse practitioner may work from a protocol), take X-rays and provide allied health services. For those nurses who rely on the orders of part-time or distant medical and allied health professionals, role relationships are vitally important, not only to the nurse but also to the quality of healthcare which is delivered to rural and remote residents (Blue & Fitzgerald 2002).

Despite the rhetoric of interdisciplinary teams in rural areas, there is often role conflict between the nurse and the medical officer (Blue & Fitzgerald 2002, Hegney 1998). A major cause of the conflict between rural nurses and medical officers occurs when the off-site medical officer is required to attend a patient in the hospital. During the day, it may be that the medical officer is conducting a consulting session with private patients. During the evening and night it is often the case that the nurse, having assessed the patient, must discuss the patient with the off-site medical officer. These telephone conversations are reported to be a source of stress for many rural nurses, as often the medical practitioner does not wish to attend the patient in the hospital (unless it is an emergency) (Hegney 1998, Hegney et al 2003b, Kenny et al 2004).

Additionally, many medical practitioners undervalue the skills of rural nurses by not recognising their experience and expertise. This may lead to a situation where medical practitioners limit the nurse's ability to deliver holistic care and only allow them to deliver fragmented care (e.g. requesting that a community nurse check on a client's blood pressure without giving a concise picture of the client's condition or any prescribed medication, or a referral to the nurse for care) (Lampshire & Rolfe 1993). The pressure that medical practitioners place on rural and remote area nurses to work outside their role is associated with a higher rate of medication violations (McKeon et al 2003).

Recruitment and retention

While much has been written about the shortage of medical practitioners in rural and remote areas, until recently very little attention has been paid to the increasing shortage of rural and remote area nurses and midwives in Australia (New South Wales Health 1998, Senate Community Affairs References Committee 2002). A report by New South Wales Health (1998:4) stated that the top specialties for which positions were being actively recruited for the rural nursing workforce were 'generalist, mental health, intensive care, midwifery, operating theatre, emergency department, orthopaedic, community health and paediatrics'. Similarly, the shortage of experienced remote area nurses has been well documented (Dowd & Johnson 1995).

Factors that have been linked to poor retention include lack of understanding of the role, poor accommodation, the lack of a career pathway, little to no child-minding facilities, the lack of access to affordable and relevant education and training, lack of employer support, the level of work-related stress, legal aspects of the role (particularly with regard to the administration and supply of medications), relationships with medical officers, inadequate locum relief, mentoring, and the violence often experienced by remote area nurses (Cramer 1992, Dowd & Johnson 1995, Hegney et al 1997, 2003a, 2003b, 2003c, Mills et al 2006).

A major outcome of shortages of registered and enrolled nurses is the increased workload placed on those who remain. McKeon et al (2006) have noted that this increase in workload results in the inability of nurses to work safely. Work pressures, they note, not only decrease the safety of the environment, but often encourage nurses to work outside their legitimised scope of practice. The shortage of both nurses and doctors in rural and remote areas therefore, 'often lead[s] to informal crossing of boundaries, that is, nurses making decisions about treatment without consulting a doctor' (McKeon et al 2006:121).

As with the shortages of remote area nurses, the recruitment of rural nurses is becoming problematic in Australia. The factors that have a negative impact on the decision of nurses to work in rural areas include the lack of promotion of rural nursing as a desirable career option, the low number of clinical placements that are available for pre-registration undergraduate nursing students, and the lack of graduate year placements in rural health facilities (Courtney et al 2002a, Hegney et al 1997, Lea & Cruickshank 2007, McMurray et al 1998, New South Wales Health 1998).

CONCLUDING REMARKS

The majority of nurses who practise in rural and remote areas find their practice rewarding, despite the demands of autonomous practice and the hardships associated with isolation. The provision of healthcare to rural and remote communities would not occur without this nursing workforce. The introduction of a legitimised advanced nurse practitioner role is, therefore, a positive step and will lead to improvements in the quality of healthcare provision in rural and remote areas. This is particularly important in remote areas of Australia where population densities make the employment of a medical officer uneconomical. This is not to say that the rural or remote advanced practice nurse is a medical officer replacement—rather, with their focus on the delivery of primary healthcare, these nurses provide a different health service. In the twenty-first century, as in the nineteenth and twentieth centuries, it is nurses who provide the majority of healthcare services to rural and remote Australians.

REFLECTIVE QUESTIONS

1 Working in relative isolation from other healthcare professionals, how can the rural and remote area nurse implement primary healthcare with a focus on prevention in the community in which they are employed?

2 What programs could be introduced to attract and retain rural and remote area nurses?

3 What is the level of educational preparation that would best suit the beginning rural and/or remote area nurse? Note that this may involve several different programs—before commencement of employment and during employment.

RECOMMENDED READINGS

Australian Institute of Health and Welfare (AIHW) 2004 Rural, regional and remote health: a guide to remoteness classifications. AIHW, Canberra

Australian Institute of Health and Welfare (AIHW) 2008 Australia's health 2008. AIHW, Canberra

Bushy A 1998 Rural nursing in the US: where do we stand as we enter a new millenium? Australian Journal of Rural Health 6:65–71

Smith KB, Humphreys JS, Wilson MGA 2008 Addressing the health disadvantage of rural populations: how does epidemiological evidence inform rural health policies and research? Australian Journal of Rural Health 16:56–66

Strong K, Trickett P, Titulaer I, Bhatia K 1998 Health in rural and remote Australia: the first report of the Australian Institute of Health and Welfare on rural health. AIHW, Canberra

Online resources

Australian Government, Department of Health and Ageing: www.health.gov.au. This site gives you access to various information on rural health policy.

Australian Institute of Health and Welfare: www.aihw.gov.au. This site contains the statistical reports on rural health and the labour force.

National Rural Health Alliance: www.ruralhealth.org.au. This site gives you access to all the member bodies of the alliance. It is the most useful site for rural health.

REFERENCES

Australian Government 2004a Online. Available: www.health.gov.au/internet/wcms/publishing.nsf/Content/ruralhealth-studying-in 1 Dec 2004

Australian Government 2004b Online. Available: www.health.gov.au/internet/wcms/publishing.nsf/Content/ruralhealth-scholarship 1 Dec 2004

Australian Institute of Health and Welfare (AIHW) 2004a Rural, regional and remote health: a guide to remoteness classifications. AIHW, Canberra

Australian Institute of Health and Welfare (AIHW) 2004b Rural, regional and remote health: a study on mortality. AIHW, Canberra

Australian Institute of Health and Welfare (AIHW) 2008a Australia's health 2008. AIHW, Canberra

Australian Institute of Health and Welfare (AIHW) 2008b Nursing and midwifery labour force 2005. AIHW, Canberra

Bessant G 1980 Rural schooling and the rural myth in Australia. Comparative Education 14:121–132

Blue I, Fitzgerald M 2002 Interprofessional relations: case studies of working relationships between registered nurses and general practitioners in rural Australia. Journal of Clinical Studies 11:314–321

Burley M, Harvey D 1993 Nurses and their small rural communities. In conference proceedings of the 'Nursing the country conference of the Association for Australian Rural Nurses Inc'. Warrnambool, Victoria, pp 149–58

Cameron A 2004 Rural nursing brings rewards. Australian Nursing Journal 12:27

Courtney M, Edwards H, Smith S, Finlayson K 2002a The impact of rural clinical placement on student nurses' employment intentions. Collegian 9:12–18

Courtney M, Yacopetti J, James C, Walsh A, Finlayson K 2002b Comparison of roles and professional development needs of nurse executives working in metropolitan, provincial, rural or remote settings in Queensland. Australian Journal of Rural Health 10:202–208

Cramer J 1992 Remote area community health services. In: Braum F, Fry D, Lennie I (eds) Community health: policy and practice in Australia. Pluto Press, Sydney, pp 235–48

Cramer J 1994 Finding solutions to support remote area nurses. Australian Nursing Journal 2:21–25

Dowd T, Johnson S 1995 Remote area nurses—on the cutting edge. Collegian 2:36–40

Epps R, Sorensen T 1993 Introduction. In: Sorensen T, Epps R (eds) Prospects and policies for rural Australia. Longman, Melbourne, pp 1–6

Frager L, Gray EJ, Franklin RJ, Petrauskas V 1997 A picture of health? A preliminary report of the health of country Australians. Australian Agricultural Health Unit, Moree

Hanna L 2001 Continued neglect of rural and remote nursing in Australia: the link with poor health outcomes. Australian Journal of Advanced Nursing 9:36–45

Hays RB, Veitch PC, Cheers B, Crossland L 1997 Why doctors leave rural practice. Australian Journal of Rural Health 5:198–203

Hegney D 1996 The windmill of rural health: a Foucauldian analysis of the discourses of rural nursing in Australia, 1991–1994. Unpublished PhD thesis. Southern Cross University, Lismore

Hegney D 1997a Defining rural and rural nursing. In: Siegloff L (ed.) Rural nursing in the Australian context. Royal College of Nursing Australia, Canberra, pp 25–44

Hegney D 1997b Rural nursing practice. In: Siegloff L (ed.) Rural nursing in the Australian context. Royal College of Nursing Australia, Canberra, pp 25–44

Hegney D 1998 The advanced practice role of the rural nurse: challenging the culture of nursing, pharmacy and medicine. In conference proceedings of 'The cultures in caring, 4th biennial Australian rural and remote health scientific conference', pp 1.200–1.228. Toowoomba Hospital Foundation, Toowoomba

Hegney D, McCarthy A, Rogers-Clark C, Gorman D 2003a Why nurses are resigning from rural and remote Queensland health facilities. Collegian 9:33–39

Hegney D, Pearce S, Rogers-Clark C, Martin-McDonald K 2005a Close, but still too far. The experiences of people with cancer commuting from a provincial town to a major city for radiotherapy treatment. European Journal of Cancer Care 14:75–82

Hegney D, Pearson A, McCarthy A 1997 The role and function of the rural nurse in Australia. Royal College of Nursing, Canberra

Hegney D, Plank A, Parker V 2003b Nursing workloads: the results of a study of Queensland nurses. Journal of Nursing Management 11:307–314

Hegney D, Plank A, Parker V 2003c Workplace violence in nursing in Queensland. International Journal of Nursing 9:261–268

Hegney D, Plank A, Watson J, Raith L, McKeon C 2005b Provision of patient education and consumer medicine information: a study of Queensland rural and remote area registered nurses. Journal of Clinical Nursing 14: 855–862

Houghton K, Strong P 2004 Women in business in rural and remote Australia: growing regional economies. Rural Industries Research and Development Corporation. Australian Government, Canberra

Humphreys JS, Lyle D, Wakerman J, Chalmers E, Wilkinson D, Walker J, Simmons D, Larson A 2000 Roles and activities of the Commonwealth Government university departments of rural health. Australian Journal of Rural Health 8:120–133

Humphreys J, Rolley F 1991 Health and health care in rural Australia. University of New England, Armidale

Humphreys JS, Rolley F 1993 Neglected factors in planning rural health services. In: Malko K (ed.) A fair go for rural health: forward together. University of New England, Armidale, pp 47–54

Kenny A, Carter L, Martin S, Williams S 2004 Why 4 years when 3 will do? Enhanced knowledge for rural nursing practice. Nursing Inquiry 11:108–116

Kenny A, Duckett S 2003 Educating for rural nursing practice. Journal of Advanced Nursing 44:613–622

Kreger A 1991 Report on the national nursing consultative committee project: enhancing the role of rural and remote area nurses. Unpublished.

Lampshire Rolfe 1993 The realities of rural district nursing: a study of practice issues and education needs—Loddon–Mallee Region. Victorian In-service Nurse Education and Department of Health and Community Services, Victoria

Land and Water Australia 2004 Australia's farmers: past, present and future. Australian Government, Canberra

Lea J, Cruickshank M, Paliadelis P, Parmenter G, Sanderson H, Thornberry P 2008 The lure of the bush: do rural placements influence student nurses to seek employment in rural settings? Collegian 15:77–82

Lea J, Cruickshank MT 2007 The experience of new graduate nurses in rural practice in New South Wales. Rural and Remote Health 7:814. Online. Available: www.rrh.org.au

Lovett J 1993 Foreword. In: Sorensen T, Epps R (eds) Prospects and policies for rural Australia. Longman, Melbourne, pp vii–ix

McGrath P, Patterson C, Yates P, Treloar S, Oldenbury B, Loos C 1999 A study of postdiagnosis breast cancer concerns for women living in rural and remote Queensland. Part II: support issues. Australian Journal of Rural Health 7:43–52

McKeon CM, Fogarty GJ, Hegney DG 2003 Organisational factors contributing to violations by rural and remote nurses during medication administration. In: Katsikitis M (ed.) Proceedings of the 38th APS Annual Conference, 2–5 October 2003, Perth, pp 128–32

McKeon CM, Fogarty GJ, Hegney DG 2006 Organisational factors: impact on administration violations in rural nursing. Journal of Advanced Nursing 55:115–123

McMurray A, St John W, Lucas N, Donovan A, Curry A, Hohnke R 1998 Advanced nursing practice for rural and remote Australia: report to the National Rural Health Alliance. Griffith University, Gold Coast

Macklin J 1991 The Australian health jigsaw: integration of health care delivery. Background Paper No. 1, Department of Health, Housing and Community Services, Canberra

Macklin J 1992 The future of general practice. Issues Paper No. 3, Department of Health and Housing, Canberra

Mills J, Lennon D, Francis K 2006 Mentoring matters: developing rural nurses knowledge and skills. Collegian 13:32–36

Neill J, Taylor K 2002 Undergraduate nursing students' clinical experiences in rural and remote areas: recruitment implications. Australian Journal of Rural Health 10:239–243

New South Wales Health 1998 Rural and remote nursing summit report. New South Wales Health, Sydney

Parliament of Australia: Senate 2007 Highway to health: better access for rural, regional and remote populations. Commonwealth of Australia, Canberra

Peach HG, Pearce DC, Farish SJ 1998 Age-standardised mortality and proportional mortality analysis of Aboriginal and non-Aboriginal deaths in metropolitan, rural and remote areas. Australian Journal of Rural Health 16:36–41

Rolley F, Humphreys JS 1993 Rural welfare: the human face of Australia's countryside. In: Sorensen T, Epps R (eds) Prospects and policies for rural Australia. Longman Cheshire, Melbourne, pp 241–57

Senate Community Affairs References Committee 2002 The patient profession: time for action. Australian Government, Canberra

Siegloff L, Hegney D 1996 Recognition for their role: the nurse practitioner project, Wilcannia, New South Wales. In conference proceedings of 'The windmills, wisdom and wonderment' conference. Association for Australian Rural Nurses, Roseworthy

Smith KB, Humphreys JS, Wilson MGA 2008 Addressing the health disadvantage of rural populations: how does epidemiological evidence inform rural health policies and research? Australian Journal of Rural Health 16:56–66

Strong K, Trickett P, Titulaer I, Bhatia K 1998 Health in rural and remote Australia: the first report of the Australian Institute of Health and Welfare on rural health. AIHW, Canberra

Wakerman J, Field P 1998 Remote area health service delivery in central Australia: primary health care and participatory management. Australian Journal of Rural Health 6:27–31

Walmsley D, Sorensen AD 1988 Contemporary Australia. Longman Cheshire, Melbourne

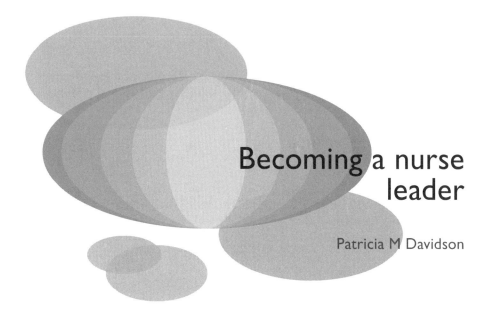

CHAPTER 17

Becoming a nurse leader

Patricia M Davidson

LEARNING OBJECTIVES

At the completion of this chapter, the reader will be able to:

- describe the social, economic and political trends influencing contemporary nursing practice
- identify the differences between the terms leadership and management
- recognise strategies for undergraduate nurses to develop to become nurse leaders
- appreciate the importance of evidence-based practice in facilitating optimal patient outcomes, and
- identify professional and organisational factors that facilitate effective leadership and strategic management.

KEY WORDS

Clinical leadership, clinical management, nurse practitioner, transformational leadership, evidence-based practice

INTRODUCTION

Nursing leadership facilitates evidence-based, ethical practice that promotes optimal clinical outcomes and excellence in nursing care. This chapter describes contemporary trends influencing clinical practice and models of nursing care delivery. The characteristics and attributes of leaders in the clinical workplace are identified and the importance of expert clinical practice in forging a professional identity for nursing is justified. The chapter also provides insights into the way expert practitioners, functioning as leaders in the clinical setting, can face challenges, and successfully implement strategies to improve patient care and advance nursing practice.

As you read through this chapter, it is important as a beginning nurse to consider the attributes that you need to develop to become a nurse leader. It is never too early to start this process as effective leaders cultivate a reflective and iterative process, involving appraisal of their personal strengths and weaknesses and developing strategies for personal empowerment. It is also important for you to consider that leadership is evident and crucial at all levels of nursing practice—from novice to expert. As you observe the behaviours of your colleagues, you can see the characteristics of future nursing leaders. Perhaps, most importantly, even in your early days of practice you can shape the future of patient care and the nursing profession through engaging in critical discussion, reflective practice and developing your leadership skills (Allan et al 2008, Daly et al 2006, Morgan 2000).

Internationally, contemporary clinical, administrative and policy environments of healthcare provide challenges to both professionals and consumers. Increased demands for clinical services, rising healthcare costs and health workforce shortages are just some of the issues you will face as you begin your nursing career. In spite of these obstacles, the healthcare setting has never been so welcoming for dynamic nurse leaders and managers. This is because contemporary healthcare systems are no longer based upon hierarchical medical leadership but are more inclusive and interdisciplinary (Aiken et al 2000). At many levels of organisations you will see nurse leaders functioning in general as well as nursing-specific leadership positions (Davidson et al 2006a). Further, the growth of nursing research and scholarship has been able to demonstrate the unique and valuable contributions of nurses to health-related outcomes, particularly related to promoting care continuity and coordination of care.

In order for nurses to function effectively in dynamic clinical environments and, importantly, exert their influence to optimise patient care, they need to appreciate the multiple factors that impact upon nursing practice and healthcare delivery. These factors are as diverse as the nature of nursing practice itself. It is also important to consider that regardless of the healthcare system in which you will work, healthcare delivery is provided in a political context that is strongly influenced by economic factors and prevailing cultural and social values (Aldrich et al 2003, Beaglehole et al 2007b). The crucial role of leadership has been recognised in the introduction of a clinical nurse leader role by the American Association of Colleges of Nursing (AACN) (Poulin-Tabor et al 2008, Stanley et al 2008). In this chapter, we explore clinical leadership within the current healthcare environment.

HEALTHCARE IN CONTEXT

Contemporary healthcare systems are often portrayed as a system in crisis as they battle increasing demands and diminishing resources (Harris 2000). Population ageing and the increasing burden of chronic conditions challenges a healthcare system largely designed for acute procedural care. Currently, the worldwide nurse staffing shortage continues to attract government and public comment (Cooper 2008, Siela et al 2008). Nurses, along with many other professional groups, are experiencing workforce shortages (Cummings et al 2008). In healthcare systems commonly portrayed as being in a crisis state, pointing the finger at nurses and nursing models of education are an all too easy scapegoat (Jackson & Daly 2008). Yet the challenges facing health are global and strongly mediated by factors such as epidemiological transitions, increased migration and globalisation of economic factors (Davidson et al 2003). Taking the time to consider these forces is critical in assessing current clinical situations and planning for the future.

As you begin your nursing journey and struggle with acquiring skills and terminology, terms such as leadership and mentorship can appear distant and remote. However, it is important to consider that you and your colleagues are the nurse leaders of the future. Further, leadership is rarely an historical accident; rather, it is a set of knowledge, skills and attributes that is developed over time (Morgan 2000). Therefore, as you read over this chapter, consider the factors that you will need to develop to prepare yourself for a leadership role. As the skill mix of nursing diversifies in the clinical setting with growing numbers of enrolled nurses and assistant roles, the registered nurse role will increasingly take on a role of leadership and coordination. No matter how small or large your clinical team is, you will need to inspire and motivate and lead your team to achieve negotiated goals and deliver effective clinical care. Skills such as reflection, listening and critical thinking are crucial in developing these roles. Take the time to develop these skills and to seek feedback from your peers.

OPPORTUNITIES FOR CLINICAL NURSING LEADERS

A commitment to equity and access are driving healthcare reforms in many countries, such as Australia, New Zealand and the United Kingdom (Australian Commission on Safety and Quality in Health Care 2008). Nurses undertake a crucial role in these reforms from the primary to tertiary care sectors. Technological innovation has improved clinical outcomes. Rates of deaths from infectious diseases continue to fall globally and we face an international burden of chronic conditions, such as heart disease and stroke (Beaglehole et al 2007a).

Healthcare professionals are increasingly challenged to deliver healthcare in an equitable and accessible manner, while dealing with issues of quality and safety (Ramanujam et al 2008, Rogers et al 2008). Further, the increasing trend towards globalisation means that we have to consider issues beyond our local environment in healthcare policy and delivery (Ben-Shlomo & Kuh 2002, Davidson et al 2003). The threats of avian influenza and increasing rates of tuberculosis are just some recent examples of living in a globalised world. Frequent travel, migration and other social and political factors can impact on the health and wellbeing of individuals and community through the spread of disease.

Within a climate of healthcare reform, nurses now also have increasing opportunities to influence healthcare policy and practice. This new position of power is evidenced by nurses holding influential positions and driving practice changes following credible scientific research. For example, in the United States, the National Institute for Nursing Research is the lead institute within the National Institute for Health (NIH) for end-of-life research, as recognition of nursing's substantial contribution to palliative and supportive care.

Significant barriers continue to exist, such as opposition from powerful groups, including medical organisations, which challenge advanced practice nursing roles. However, these challenges are not insurmountable. There are examples across a range of nursing and midwifery practice where innovative models of care have improved patient outcomes by challenging traditional views and perspectives. Innovative models of midwifery care, such as early discharge care, have improved the experiences of mothers and their babies. Recognising that the greatest power base for nurses exists within the practice domain, with demonstration of clinical excellence and innovation, is an important factor in overcoming scepticism surrounding the role of nurses (Sorensen et al 2008). For example, nurses in the management of chronic heart failure have demonstrated their ability to influence patient outcomes and policies through nurse-coordinated programs and advanced practice nursing roles (Grady et al 2000, McAlister et al 2004).

As a consequence, clinical leadership in the practice domain is an important tool, and strategies to achieve this are discussed below. A clinical leader is a nurse who demonstrates the ability to influence and direct clinical practice (Lett 2002). This clinical leader also has a vision for the direction of nursing practice. This vision is informed by expert knowledge and analysis of the social, political and economic trends influencing healthcare. Fedoruk and Pincombe (2000) suggest that current and future nurse leaders need to let go of traditional managerial practices and behaviours to focus on achieving change management and process reengineering. To achieve this goal, contemporary nursing leaders have to adopt flexible, innovative and collaborative practice models. Pressures on the healthcare system—for example, financial pressures and increasing chronic disease burden—represent significant challenges for nurses. However, innovative models of care, increasing emphasis on independent nursing practice, and institution of clinical governance structures will likely serve nurses in addressing these challenges (Davidson et al 2006b).

POLICY FRAMEWORKS FOR NURSING PRACTICE

In order to engage an organisational system, direct change and assert leadership, it is important to appreciate what 'drives' this process. This observation is relevant at both a macro and a micro level of operation. Politics can be just as intriguing and complex within a hospital ward or community health centre as at the bureaucratic or parliamentary levels. However, at all levels it is important to be aware of social, political and economic factors that influence healthcare delivery (Davidson et al 2006a, 2006b). Politics in nursing is discussed in more detail in Chapter 13 of this text.

The working environment of nurses is influenced by the social, economic and political systems of the healthcare system. Table 17.1 compares the policy environments and roles of nurses in Australia, New Zealand, the United Kingdom, Taiwan and the United States. In some instances, policy can be either a barrier or facilitator to clinical leadership. The emerging role of the nurse practitioner in Australia is an example where significant policy and legislative reform has created a context to promote advanced nursing practice in spite of opposition and scepticism from some medical professional groups (Driscoll et al 2005, Gardner & Gardner 2005). Internationally, healthcare professionals strive to ensure the delivery of safe and effective evidence-based care. Frameworks such as clinical and shared governance serve as a structure to achieve this goal.

	Australia	New Zealand	United Kingdom	Taiwan	United States
Healthcare system	Universal coverage	Universal coverage	Universal coverage	National health insurance program	Fragmented user-pays system
Role of nurses within the healthcare system	Collaborative Interdisciplinary practice	Collaborative Interdisciplinary practice	Collaborative Interdisciplinary practice	Collaborative Interdisciplinary practice	Independent nursing practice Collaborative interdisciplinary practice
Nurse practitioner role	Newly established	Newly established	Established	Established	Well established
Key health issues	Increasing burden of chronic illness Population ageing Diversity health where the needs of culturally and linguistically diverse groups is considered Adverse outcomes for Indigenous Australians Access and equity for rural and remote Australians Mental health Control of escalating health costs	Increasing burden of chronic illness Population ageing Improving health outcomes for Maori population Control of escalating health costs	Increasing burden of chronic illness Population ageing Control of escalating health costs Mental health	Increasing burden of chronic illness Population ageing High rates of hepatitis Mental health Control of escalating health costs Integrating traditional Chinese and Western medicine	Increasing burden of chronic illness Population ageing Inequity of access Control of escalating health costs Mental health
Impact on clinical leadership	Striving to nurture a clinical progression strand Retention and recruitment issues	Striving to nurture a clinical progression strand Retention and recruitment issues Midwifery-specific programs	Striving to nurture a clinical progression strand Retention and recruitment issues Shared governance	Promoting nurses' welfare Providing continuing education Development of nurse specialist programs establishing clinical career ladders	Striving to nurture a clinical progression strand Retention and recruitment issues Shared governance

	Australia	New Zealand	United Kingdom	Taiwan	United States
Nursing workforce	National nursing shortages Ageing workforce Pressure to deregulate healthcare workers	National nursing shortages Ageing workforce	National nursing shortages Ageing workforce	Low nursing wages Professional issues Integrating traditional and Western medicine	National nursing shortages Ageing workforce
Nursing education	Technical and further education programs (enrolled nurse) University undergraduate degree (registered nurse) programs Postgraduate programs	University undergraduate degree programs Postgraduate programs	Vocational entry Diploma programs University undergraduate degree programs Postgraduate programs	Vocational schools Junior college Undergraduate university, masters and doctoral programs	Undergraduate diploma, associate and baccalaureate programs Postgraduate programs
Levels of nursing care provision	Nursing assistant Enrolled nurse Registered nurse Nurse practitioner Physician assistant	Enrolled nurse Registered nurse	Nursing assistant Practice nurse Registered nurse Level 1 and Level 2 nurses (Parts 1–15)	Nursing aide Physician assistant	Practical nurse Registered nurse Nurse practitioner Clinical nurse specialist Clinical leader Physician assistant

Table 17.1 Policy environments and nurses' roles in Australia, New Zealand, the United Kingdom, Taiwan and the United States

Sources: Australian Institute of Health and Welfare 2007, Cicatiello 2000, Driscoll et al 2005, Hinshaw 2000, Jackson & Daly 2008, Needleman et al 2002, Poulin-Tabor et al 2008, Sheer & Wong 2008, Tzeng 2004.

Clinical governance is a mechanism through which healthcare organisations are held accountable for adhering to evidence-based practice standards, continuously improving the quality of their services and ensuring high standards of care (Marshall 2008). As you engage in your clinical placements and nursing studies, consider the factors in which nursing care can shape the outcomes of patients. Falls prevention, mouth care and pressure care are examples of essential nursing care that influence patient outcomes (Berry & Davidson 2006).

CHANGING MODELS OF CARE DELIVERY

A variety of care delivery models are used in healthcare—some relate to nursing only and are historic, while others are interdisciplinary and responsive to emerging practice trends (see Table 17.2) (Davidson et al 2006b). The changing healthcare environment— characterised by increasing short-stay surgery, decreasing lengths of stay and numbers of acute beds, combined with increasing patient acuity related to co-morbidities— requires vastly different models of care delivery from even a decade ago. Novel models of care are commonly developed in response to actual or perceived deficits in existing care delivery (Davidson et al 2006b).

Care delivery model	Characteristics
Functional nursing	Ward-based care with allocation of specific clinical tasks, such as medication administration, to nursing staff
Team nursing	Ward-based care where a small team of nurses (perhaps with different educational preparation, skills and competencies) provides care to a designated number of patients
Patient allocation/total patient care	Ward-based care provided by a registered nurse on a shift-by-shift basis to a defined number of patients
Primary nursing	Ward-based care with a registered nurse assigned to patients for their entire admission period. Within this model a plan of care is developed, implemented and evaluated by the 'primary' nurse, with 'associate' nurses continuing the plan in the absence of the 'primary' nurse
Care management/clinical pathways	Ward or hospital-based multidisciplinary coordinated patient care for a specific case type (e.g. patients with total hip replacement). This model frequently incorporates a 'critical' or 'clinical path' tool to 'map' and document care, including the sequence and timing of interventions and variances from expected outcomes
Case management	Hospital, outreach and/or community-based multidisciplinary care that provides continuity of care for a specific case-type of patients (e.g. patients with heart failure and chronic obstructive pulmonary disease) across the entire episode of care from hospital to community

Table 17.2 Common care delivery models
Source: Davidson PM, Hickman L 2009 Managing client care. In Crisp J, Taylor C (eds) Fundamentals of nursing, 3rd edn. Elsevier, Sydney, pp 230–330.

Patients are admitted to acute care hospitals primarily for collaborative or independent nursing care, as many medical diagnostic and therapeutic procedures can now be conducted in ambulatory care settings, except in critical or emergent circumstances. However, efficient and effective care also requires continuity of patient management beyond the traditional hospital admission period to encompass the entire episode of care, particularly for those with continuing chronic disease. Programs that promote nurse coordination of care are emerging across many diagnostic conditions, including diabetes, heart disease, arthritis and chronic obstructive pulmonary disease. Similarly, there are programs in early childhood and midwifery care. As you consider your options for nursing in the future, it is important to remember that in the future, a large proportion of nursing care will be provided in the community-based setting (Pascoe et al 2005). In addition, increasing adoption of technology will see nursing interventions delivered by telehealth and web-based media (Clark et al 2007). This will likely require the development of a suite of skills and resources to work in this setting effectively.

WHAT IS LEADERSHIP?

Leadership is an attribute of an individual to work with, inspire and motivate others to work towards a defined goal or mission (Weber 2007). The dynamic and changing healthcare systems place change as a focus in contemporary health environments. Unless nurses choose to be swept along by change, they need to actively engage the process on both a personal and political level. An important attribute of a leader is to formulate an action plan and support their team in achieving negotiated goals (Porter-O'Grady et al 2006). There is an increasing discourse and discussion of leadership within the nursing profession. The concepts that make nursing leadership unique are the requisites for evidence-based healthcare: responsibility for the care and safety of patients; and the need for evaluation of clinical practice (Porter-O'Grady & Malloch 2008).

Leadership has long been an important part of the function of any organisational structure. Leadership styles vary along a continuum from authoritative to participatory, although common characteristics for leaders include being a visionary and having a plan to take individuals and services to the future. O'Rourke (2001) defines a visionary leader as one who can simultaneously have a vigilant focus on promoting health, with the capacity to build teams, articulate and demonstrate what others cannot see and address immediate challenges, as well as leading their team into a future of often unchartered waters. Leadership is influenced by the values of individuals and organisations, as well as society. Values are a set of beliefs and concepts derived from knowledge, experience and aspiration (Heller 1999). Values can be: personal, such as the importance placed on honesty and integrity; professional, such as the emphasis placed on reflective practice and continuing professional development; and organisational, such as the emphasis placed on patient outcomes. In order to function effectively and avoid role conflict, there needs to be a congruency between the values and beliefs of the individual and the organisation in which they work (Stanley 2008). As you choose your work setting, it is important that you take the time to understand the mission and values of the organisation and ensure that these are congruent with your own belief system.

Figure 17.1 describes the relationship between personal, professional and organisational values, and leadership styles. It is generally considered that for leaders to be effective they need to demonstrate honesty, integrity and inspiration (Heller 1999).

Figure 17.2 demonstrates the influence of vision and direction on clinical leaders. This leadership is linked to the cultural values of the systems, resources and support available. Policy and practice environments, as described in Tables 17.1 and 17.2, also have significant influence on leadership direction.

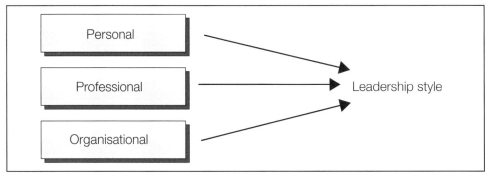

Figure 17.1 Value systems contributing to leadership style

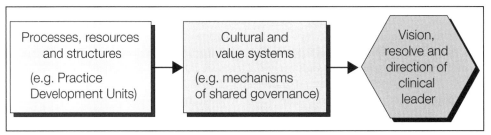

Figure 17.2 Relationship between organisational resources, values and culture, and the vision, resolve and direction of the clinical leader

A distinction of leadership characteristics is made between transactional and transformational leaders. Transactional leadership focuses on transactions or exchanges between leaders and others, with self-interest the key motivator. In contrast, transformational leaders create a culture of leadership for all stakeholders, generating empowerment, open dialogue and inclusive decision making (Davidson et al 2006a). An additional concept, 'breakthrough leadership', incorporates role modelling, clarification of own values, and respect for others' views (Lett 2002). Role modelling, mentoring and succession planning are vital aspects in preparing current and future nursing leaders. Jackson describes servant leadership as an important and emerging trend where the servant-leader does not work in isolation, but rather actively searches for opportunities to build connections to promote creativity and enabling and mutually beneficial relationships (Jackson 2008).

WHAT MAKES A CLINICAL LEADER?

In organisations, such as hospitals and community health settings, there are different nursing leaders functioning at all levels. The individuals who readily come to mind are often those who are very visible in organisations, such as directors of nursing. However, it is important to differentiate between management and leadership (Fedoruk

& Pincombe 2000). Management refers to the planning and organisation of services. The term leadership infers that an individual is visionary and pivotal in directing and shaping clinical practice (Allan et al 2008). Implicit in functioning as a clinical leader is a significant mentoring role. Table 17.3 describes the attributes of a clinical leader (Lett 2002). These attributes show that the clinical leader is not only an expert clinician but uses his or her skills to address the needs of patients and colleagues. Cook (2001) states that we must question the assumption that the leader making the difference to care is at the hierarchical apex of the organisation. He believes that the most influential individuals, in terms of improving direct care provision, are those who directly deliver nursing care. Therefore, clinical leaders are involved in the provision of patient care and are implicitly clinical experts in their field.

• expert clinician	• dynamism
• patient focused	• confidence
• vision	• selflessness
• stamina	• assertiveness
• innovation	• collaboration

Table 17.3 Attributes of a clinical leader

Further, Cook (2001) compared nursing practice in two clinical practice settings, and noted that the factor differentiating a vibrant research-based, evidence-based practice culture and one based upon routine and ritual was the nursing leader. Organisations that stimulate nursing leadership through their involvement in organisational decision making and promoting nursing research and innovative practice frequently have better outcomes (Aiken et al 2000).

It is clear that patients with complex disorders, particularly in the context of psychosocial considerations, require the professional services of different occupational groups. Nurses have demonstrated their ability to work as part of a team and be collaborative and participatory in their actions and decision making (for more on teamwork, see Ch 14). Hall and Weaver (2001) identify two emerging issues in healthcare as clinicians face the complexities of current patient care: the need for specialised clinical experts; and the need for these professionals to collaborate. Interdisciplinary healthcare teams with members from many disciplines increasingly work together to optimise patient care. Examples of these teams are found in trauma, neonatal retrieval, geriatric assessment, and drug and alcohol areas of clinical practice.

PROMOTING LEADERSHIP IN THE PRACTICE SETTING

Given the challenges facing contemporary health systems, focusing on clinical leadership development strategies is of crucial importance. In order to address these factors, a number of strategies have been implemented. These include: clinical professoriate positions (Dunn & Yates 2000); clinical development units (Atsalos et al 2007); practice development strategies (Wilson & McCormack 2006); clinical leadership programs (Cunningham & Kitson 2000); and initiatives focusing on promoting evidence-based practice (Rycroft-Malone 2008). The outcomes of these strategies are variable and commonly influenced more by local contextual and management factors rather than the value and the ethos of these programs.

An example of successful leadership models is embedded in the 'magnet' programs, which have been widely implemented in the United States and in two Australian sites (Aiken et al 2000). Magnet status is an award status administered by the American Nurses' Credentialing Center (ANCC), an affiliate of the American Nurses Association, to hospitals that satisfy a set of criteria designed to measure the strength and quality of their nursing. Many of these organisations have demonstrated optimal nursing outcomes in respect of nurse-sensitive patient outcome indicators, such as pressure areas and falls. These programs have a strong influence across all levels of the organisation from human resources to customer relations. Programs that employ such an approach are likely to have a greater chance of sustainable integration, of strategies to promote clinical leadership. Further strategies that foster clinical leaders within interdisciplinary care models espouse and profile the important role of nurses in improving health outcomes. As you move through practice areas during your clinical placements, observe and critically evaluate strategies that you consider enabling for clinical leaders. Strategies that support a culture of collaborative clinical decision making, as well as an emphasis on education and reflective practice, are just some examples.

Professional societies and organisations to promote clinical leadership

Professional societies play an important role in terms of not only providing an environment of collegiality, but also leadership, mentorship and promotion of clinical excellence (Astley et al 2007). These aims are achieved through development of policy documents, publication of professional journals, conduct of scientific meetings, and sponsorship of research and attendance at professional meetings. Some organisations serve the nursing profession broadly, focusing on an array of nursing issues, while others maintain a specialty focus. Examples of this in Australia are specialty groups such as the Australian College of Critical Care Nurses (ACCCN) and the Australasian College of Cardiovascular Nurses (ACCN), and more generic organisations such as the College of Nursing (incorporating the New South Wales College of Nursing), the Royal College of Nursing Australia and, internationally, Sigma Theta Tau International and the International Council of Nursing.

Sigma Theta Tau International is an international organisation promoting leadership globally through scholarship, knowledge and technology to improve the health of the world's people. There are chapters of Sigma Theta Tau throughout the world. The Sigma Theta Tau International Leadership Institute (ILI) focuses on the development and advancement of nurses as exceptional healthcare leaders. The ILI assists nurses internationally to develop leadership skills by creating and sharing knowledge.

Increasingly, professional nursing organisations are playing a role in terms of social advocacy and also mentoring and supporting nursing colleagues in developing countries. Particularly in situations of social disadvantage, nurses can play an important role in advocacy. What is increasingly apparent in a variety of settings is that a united voice can be a powerful force (Kraus 2008). For example, the International Council of Nursing has taken strategic stances on issues such as ethical recruitment and women's health.

Take the time to view the information and resources on the following professional nursing organisation websites, particularly in respect of professional development and the ongoing evaluation and development of nursing practice. These sites can also provide an opportunity to reach out to other nursing colleagues.

- the Australian College of Critical Care Nurses: www.acccn.com au
- the Australian College of Midwives: www.acmi.org.au
- the Australasian College of Cardiovascular Nurses: www./acnc.net.au
- the Australian Nurse Practitioner Association: www.nursepractitioners.org.au
- the Australian and New Zealand College of Mental Health Nurses: www. healthsci.utas.edu.au/nursing/college/index.html
- the College of Nursing: www.nursing.aust.edu.au
- the Royal College of Nursing, Australia: www.rcna.org.au
- Sigma Theta Tau International: www.nursingsociety.org
- the International Council of Nursing: www.icn.ch/

LEADERSHIP IN EVIDENCE-BASED PRACTICE

The appraisal of the cost-effectiveness and efficacy of nursing interventions and the relationship to patient outcomes is becoming increasingly important. Patient outcomes are largely dependent on implementing the best available evidence. You will hear a lot of discussion about evidence-based practice. This term refers to the implementation of the best available evidence within the context of the patient's needs, knowledge and belief systems, and using the clinician's expertise (Sackett et al 1996). As a consequence, nurse leaders have to be increasingly focused not only on assessing the needs of the patients and their families, but also on measuring outcomes. Outcome evaluation continues to be an important way in which nurses demonstrate their influence, not only to others but also to each other. This underscores that to be an effective clinical leader, beyond the charismatic attributes, nurses need to not only interpret and implement clinical evidence, but also evaluate the efficacy of nursing interventions (Davidson et al 2006b). Clinical leaders recognise that strategies to support research and scholarship are important to develop the evidence base for supporting nursing practice.

Significance of expert clinical practice

Expert clinical practice remains the foundation of the nursing profession's standing in communities. Clinical practice, informed by nursing science, is what makes nursing exceptional and unique, and is the key to our autonomous, professional practice (Porter-O'Grady & Malloch 2008, Stanley et al 2008). This underscores the importance of emphasising expert nursing within models of professional practice, education and research. Nursing roles such as clinical nurse specialists, clinical nurse consultants and nurse practitioners are crucial in advocating for expert nursing care. Internationally and even nationally, the names for these roles may differ, but the fundamental attributes are similar. Nurses who function as leaders in these roles carry not only the privilege but also the professional responsibility to direct healthcare practices to optimise the health of the populations they serve and also to foster the professional development of their colleagues. This is achieved through promoting evidence-based practice, nursing scholarship, and developing and delivering care that is tailored to the needs of patients and their families. Take the time to review the code of conduct of peak nursing organisations, such as the Australian Nursing and Midwifery Council.

CONCLUSION

In this chapter we have discussed the challenges, strategies and progress for clinical leadership. Contemporary health systems are facing considerable challenges because of the increasing burden of chronic conditions, population ageing and fiscal constraints. Yet never before has the importance of nursing care and the evidence to support nursing interventions been so strong. It is an exciting time to be embarking on a nursing career. Never before has leadership been so crucial. As you begin your nursing career, it is important to try to turn challenges into opportunities. You will be working in rapidly evolving settings, and the practice environments you enter in the next few years are likely to be radically different on the tenth anniversary of your graduation. Focusing on the needs of patients and their families is important in shaping care models for the future and also in setting your compass.

The test remains to influence nursing practice through positive and enabling leadership strategies and to develop innovative approaches to dealing with challenges facing current clinical environments. In order to achieve this, a system of mentoring, career progression and succession planning in the clinical setting needs to be created and nurtured. Clinical and academic settings require a culture that develops innovation and fosters leadership potential (Donaldson & Fralic 2000). It is important to realise that at every level of an organisation, and regardless of whether nurses work in clinical, education and management streams, they have the potential to influence and direct patient care by exemplary leadership and excellence in clinical practice. The potential for nursing practice to influence clinical outcomes is an empowering and motivating concept. As you embark upon your nursing career, seek enabling clinical environments and mentors who will guide you along your professional journey.

REFLECTIVE QUESTIONS

1 How can clinical leadership influence clinical outcomes?

2 What are nurse-sensitive patient outcome indicators? Identify an indicator from one of your clinical practice settings and consider how nursing leadership can influence the capacity to achieve optimal outcomes.

3 Identify a professional nursing organisation, and review their activities relating to leadership. This exercise may require review of journals, websites or other publications.

4 What are the important elements of fostering leadership from what you have read in this chapter?

RECOMMENDED READINGS

Aiken L, Havens DS, Sloane DM 2000 The magnet nursing service recognition program: a comparison or two groups of magnet groups. American Journal of Nursing 100(3):26–36

Daly J, Speedy S, Jackson D (eds) 2004. Nursing leadership. Churchill Livingstone, Sydney

Davidson PM, Elliott D, Daly J 2006 Clinical leadership in contemporary clinical practice: implications for nursing in Australia. Journal of Nursing Management 14(3):180–188

Porter-O'Grady T, Malloch K 2008 Beyond myth and magic: the future of evidence-based leadership. Nursing Administration Quarterly 32(3):176–187

REFERENCES

Aiken L, Havens DS, Sloane D 2000 The magnet nursing service recognition program: a comparison or two groups of magnet groups. American Journal of Nursing 100(3):26–36

Aldrich R, Kemp L, Williams JS, Harris E, Simpson S, Wilson A, McGill K, Byles J, Lowe J, Jackson T 2003 Using socioeconomic evidence in clinical practice guidelines. British Medical Journal 327(7426):1283–1285

Allan HT, Smith PA, Lorentzon M 2008 Leadership for learning: a literature study of leadership for learning in clinical practice. Journal of Nursing Management 16(5):545–555

Astley C, Portelli L, Whalley G, Davidson P 2007 Coming of age: affiliate member profile and articipation in the Annual Scientific Meeting of the Cardiac Society of Australia and New Zealand. Heart, Lung and Circulation 16:447–451

Atsalos C, O'Brien L, Jackson D 2007 Against the odds: experiences of nurse leaders in clinical development units (nursing) in Australia. Journal of Advanced Nursing 58(6):576–584

Australian Commission on Safety and Quality in Health Care 2008 Submission to the National Health and Hospitals Reform Commission on the beyond the blame game: accountability and performance benchmarks for the next Australian Healthcare Agreements, NHRC, Canberra. Online. Available: www.nhhrc.org.au/internet/nhhrc/publishing.nsf/Content/commission-1lp

Australian Institute of Health and Welfare (AIHW) 2007 Older Australia at a glance. AIHW, Canberra

Beaglehole R, Ebrahim S, Reddy S, Voute J, Leeder S 2007a Chronic disease action: prevention of chronic diseases: a call to action. Lancet 370(9605):2152–2157

Beaglehole R, Reddy S, Leeder SR 2007b Poverty and human development: the global implications of cardiovascular disease. Circulation 116(17):1871–1873

Ben-Shlomo Y, Kuh D 2002 A life course approach to chronic disease epidemiology: conceptual models, empirical challenges and interdisciplinary perspectives. International Journal of Epidemiology 31(2):285–293

Berry A, Davidson P 2006 Beyond comfort: oral hygiene as a critical nursing activity in the intensive care unit. Intensive and Critical Care Nursing 22:318–328

Cicatiello JSA 2000 A perspective of healthcare in the past: insights and challenges for a healthcare system in the new millennium. Nursing Administration Quarterly 25(1):18–29

Clark RA, Inglis SC, McAlister FA, Cleland JG, Stewart S 2007 Telemonitoring or structured telephone support programmes for patients with chronic heart failure: systematic review and meta-analysis. British Medical Journal 334(7600):942–945

Cook MJ 2001 The renaissance of clinical leadership. International Nursing Review 48:38–46

Cooper PG 2008 A call for a paradigm shift in nursing and healthcare leadership. Nursing Forum 43(1):1

Cummings GG, Olson K, Hayduk L, Bakker D, Fitch M, Green E, Butler L, Conlon M 2008 The relationship between nursing leadership and nurses' job satisfaction in Canadian oncology work environments. Journal of Nursing Management 16(5): 508–518

Cunningham G, Kitson A 2000 An evaluation of the RCN Clinical Development Programme: part 2. Nursing Standard 15(13–15):34–40

Daly J, Chang E, Jackson D 2006 Quality of work life in nursing: some issues and challenges. Collegian 13(4):2

Davidson P, Daly J, Meleis A, Douglas M 2003 Globalization as we enter the 21st century: reflections and directions for nursing research, science and practice. Contemporary Nurse 15(3):161–174

Davidson PM, Elliot D, Daly J 2006 Clinical leadership in contemporary clinical practice: implication for nursing in Australia. Journal of Nursing Management 14:180–187

Davidson P, Halcomb E, Hickman L, Phillips J, Graham E 2006b Beyond the rhetoric: what do we mean by a model of care? Australian Journal of Advanced Nursing 23(3):47–55

Donaldson SK, Fralic MF 2000 Forging today's practice–academic link: a new era for nursing leadership. Nursing Administration Quarterly 25(1):95–101

Driscoll A, Worrall-Carter L, O'Reilly J, Stewart S 2005 A historical review of the nurse practitioner role in Australia. Clinical Excellence for Nurse Practitioners 9(3):141–152

Dunn S, Yates P 2000 The roles of Australian chairs in clinical nursing. Journal of Advanced Nursing 31:165–171

Fedoruk M, Pincombe J 2000 The nurse executive: challenges for the 21st century. Journal of Nursing Management 8(1):13–20

Gardner A, Gardner G 2005 A trial of nurse practitioner scope of practice. Journal of Advanced Nursing 49(2):135–145

Grady KL, Dracup K, Kennedy G, Moser DK, Piano M, Warner Stevenson L, Young JB 2000 Team management of patients with heart failure. A statement for healthcare professionals from the Cardiovascular Nursing Council of the American Heart Association. Circulation 102:2443–2456

Hall P, Weaver L 2001 Interdisciplinary education and teamwork: a long and winding road. Medical Education 35:867–875

Harris MD 2000 Challenges for home healthcare nurses in the 21st century. Home Healthcare Nurse 18(1):38–44

Heller R 1999 Achieving excellence. DK Publishing, New York

Hinshaw A 2000 Nursing knowledge for the 21st century: opportunities and challenges. Journal of Nursing Scholarship 32(2):117–124

Jackson D 2008 Servant leadership in nursing: a framework for developing sustainable research capacity in nursing. Collegian 15(1):27–33

Jackson D, Daly J 2008 Nursing and pre-registration nursing education under the spotlight again. Collegian 15(1):1–2

Kraus K 2008 What's at stake for women and global AIDS? A new platform seeks signers: health rights = healthy women. Journal of Ambulatory Care Management 31(3):282–283

Lett M 2002 The concept of clinical leadership. Contemporary Nurse 12(1): 16–21

McAlister FA, Stewart S, Ferrua S, McMurray JJ 2004 Multidisciplinary strategies for the management of heart failure patients at high risk for admission. Journal of the American College of Cardiology 44(4):810–819

Marshall DR 2008 Evidence-based management: the path to best outcomes. Journal of Nursing Administration 38(5):205–207

Morgan BS 2000 Testing leadership and management concepts: the relevancy factor. Nurse Educator 25(4):181–185

Needleman J, Buerhaus P, Mattke S, Stewart M, Zelevinsky K 2002 Nurse-staffing levels and the quality of care in hospitals. New England. Journal of Medicine 346(22):1715–1722

O'Rourke M 2001 Building organizations to succeed beyond 2000 takes conviction. Seminars for Nurse Managers 9(1):16–32

Pascoe T, Foley E, Hutchinson R, Watts I, Whitecross L, Snowdon T 2005 The changing face of nurses in Australian general practice. Australian Journal of Advanced Nursing 23(1):44–50

Porter-O'Grady T, Alexander DR, Blaylock J, Minkara N, Surel D 2006 Constructing a team model: creating a foundation for evidence-based teams. Nursing Administration Quarterly 30(3):211–220

Porter-O'Grady T, Malloch K 2008 Beyond myth and magic: the future of evidence-based leadership. Nursing Administration Quarterly 32(3):176–187

Poulin-Tabor D, Quirk RL, Wilson L, Orff S, Gallant P, Swan N, Manchester N 2008 Pioneering a new role: the beginning, current practice and future of the clinical nurse leader. Journal of Nursing Management 16(5):623–628

Ramanujam R, Abrahamson K, Anderson JG 2008 Influence of workplace demands on nurses' perception of patient safety. Nursing and Health Sciences 10(2):144–150

Rogers AE, Dean GE, Hwang W, Scott LD 2008 Role of registered nurses in error prevention, discovery and correction. Quality and Safety in Health Care 17(2):117–121

Rycroft-Malone J 2008 Evidence-informed practice: from individual to context. Journal of Nursing Management 16(4):404–408

Sackett DL, Rosenberg WMC, Gray JAM, Haynes RB, Richardson WS 1996 Evidence based medicine: what it is and what it isn't. British Medical Journal 312(7023):71–72

Sheer B, Wong FKY 2008 The development of advanced nursing practice globally. Journal of Nursing Scholarship 40(3):204–211

Siela D, Twibell KR, Keller V 2008 The shortage of nurses and nursing faculty: what critical care nurses can do. AACN Advanced Critical Care 19(1):66–77

Sorensen R, Iedema R, Severinsson E 2008 Beyond profession: nursing leadership in contemporary healthcare. Journal of Nursing Management 16(5):535–544

Stanley D 2008 Congruent leadership: values in action. Journal of Nursing Management 16(5):519–524

Stanley JM, Gannon J, Gabuat J, Hartranft S, Adams N, Mayes C, Shouse GM, Edwards BA, Burch D 2008 The clinical nurse leader: a catalyst for improving quality and patient safety. Journal of Nursing Management 16(5):614–622

Tzeng H 2004 Roles of nurse aides and family members in acute patient care in Taiwan. Journal of Nursing Care Quality 19(2):169–175

Weber J 2007 Creating a holistic environment for practicing nurses. Nursing Clinics of North America 42(2):295–307

Wilson V, McCormack B 2006 Critical realism as emancipatory action: the case for realistic evaluation in practice development. Nursing Philosophy 7(1):45–57

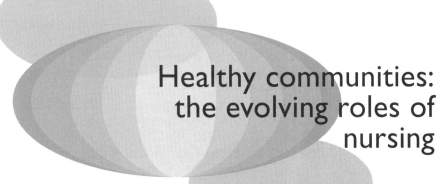

CHAPTER 18

Healthy communities: the evolving roles of nursing

Gay Edgecombe and Ray Stephens

LEARNING OBJECTIVES

When you have completed this chapter, you will be able to:

- identify key determinants of a healthy community
- recognise the role of public health in Australia
- understand the importance of early intervention throughout the life span
- describe the role of nurses involved in healthy community programs, and
- recognise nursing's role in policy development and implementation.

KEY WORDS

Community nursing, public health, early intervention, healthy communities, health promotion, social support

INTRODUCTION

The majority of nurses and midwives employed today spend limited time in the community. For many, their only experience is their clinical placement as a student. But for those who do decide on a career as a community nurse, they are rewarded by the expanded scope of practice. For example, community nursing can involve delivering services to populations of families with infants and young children, school children, marginalised groups, and individuals with acute and/or chronic conditions living at home. These universal public health services are designed to facilitate and support healthy communities.

A key strategy used by such services is a strength-based approach. Strengths-based approaches focus on identifying and building on the existing strengths of individuals, families and communities. Deficit-based approaches of the past focused on single issues, people's gaps and inadequacies, and community problems. Such approaches can reinforce perceptions of loss, low self-esteem and failure. This change of approach in public health signalled a shift in thinking from the 'old' public health to a 'new' public health. In the former, public health agencies usually decided what was best for communities. In the latter, communities are actively engaged to decide on priorities and preferences for health (Baum 2008, Keleher & Murphy 2004, McMurray 2007). The five action strategies from the Ottawa Charter (World Health Organization 1986:i–v) illustrate this change:

1. the development of healthy public policy
2. the creation of supportive environments
3. strengthening community action
4. the development of personal skills, and
5. reorientation of health services.

Marshall (2004:175) has taken the five action areas of the Ottawa Charter and developed a useful table (Table 18.1) to illustrate examples under each action. Table 18.1 provides an example from a local government's maternal and child health service initiative that was begun by two maternal and child health nurses (Higgins & Jones 2004).

1. Build healthy public policy	2. Create supportive environments	3. Strengthen community action	4. Develop personal skills	5. Reorient health services
Infant nutrition. Support for breastfeeding in public places	Pram walking groups. Stops at supportive coffee shops	Pram walking groups established by mothers	Education sessions about breastfeeding and exercise	Multidisciplinary teams in health services, local government planning team, and parents

Table 18.1 Ottawa Charter health promotion action areas
Source: Adapted from Marshall (2004) and Higgins and Jones (2004).

The public health movement began in the nineteenth century with the goal to keep nations well across the life span through providing direct public health services to populations (universal maternal and child health services), enacting government legislation (e.g. to provide safe water, milk and food; to set standards for housing) and nationwide programs (e.g. immunisation, chest X-ray screening for tuberculosis) (Baum 2008, Duckett 2004). Early public health service providers included public health nurses, school health nurses, maternal and child health nurses, health visitors and occupational health nurses. Each of these nursing specialties focused on a section of the population and provided a universal service to that population. The generalist public health nurse provided a range of services to local communities and worked with the specialist nurses and other members of the public health team to provide school and maternal and child health services.

Public health nursing has been developing along with the public health movement for the last 100 years under the auspices of national, regional and/or local government public health departments. Although the range and scope of this development varies greatly between countries, the main reasons worldwide for the development of public health nursing have been crushing poverty, inequity, lack of basic health services, environmental pollution and infectious disease. The strong, informed leadership capacity of public health nurses has been vital in ensuring that innovative programs are developed, implemented and evaluated, and receive ongoing funding.

HEALTHY COMMUNITIES

Terms such as 'healthy settings', 'community health' and 'community wellness' have evolved through public health initiatives over the last century. The Healthy Cities projects were developed in response to the Ottawa Charter, which called for the creation of 'supportive environments' (World Health Organization 1986:2). Most work by the World Health Organization (WHO) to date has related to WHO Healthy Cities projects initiated by the WHO Regional Office for Europe (Baum 2008, World Health Organization 2003). Many countries, including Australia, have initiated a range of healthy community projects (Baum 2008). The WHO Healthy Cities project has four overarching actions:

1. action to address the determinants of health and the principles of health for all
2. action to integrate and promote European and global public health priorities
3. action to put health on the social and political agendas of cities, and
4. action to promote good governance and partnership-based planning for health (World Health Organization 2003:1).

If you are just beginning to work as a community nurse in any setting, it is very useful to find out exactly what other healthcare providers and agencies are doing in your area to support healthy communities.

COMMUNITY ASSESSMENT

In order to develop an understanding of the community, a community nurse will need to investigate the issues and resources related to the health of the community (Jackson & Edgecombe 2008). A community assessment is one strategy used to provide current information on local services and programs that may be useful for clients (Stanhope & Lancaster 2008).

There are a number of methods you can use to assess your local community. These may include:

• interviews with key stakeholders
• attendance at local health forums

- monitoring of local media
- observing the geographical area and being aware of any issues or new projects (e.g. new transport, housing estate or need for a recreational centre), and
- reviewing available data (e.g. immunisation status, annual reports).

Evidence-based Healthcare (Muir Gray 2001) is a very useful background text for community assessment. It also contains lists of key websites. The Australian Institute of Health and Welfare offers current data on a wide range of health-related issues. The data cubes contained on this website allow easy access to up-to-date information. The following websites are useful for community assessment:

- Australian Bureau of Statistics: www.abs.gov.au/
- Australian Institute of Health and Welfare:
  www.aihw.gov.au/publications/index.cfm/series/13 (Australia's health)
  www.aihw.gov.au/dataonline.cfm (searchable data)
- Communicable Disease Network of Australia and New Zealand: www.health. gov.au/internet/main/publishing.nsf/Content/cda-cdna-index.htm
- Australian Indigenous HealthInfoNet: www.healthinfonet.ecu.edu.au/

It is useful to use a conceptual model to guide your community assessment. Bronfenbrenner's (1979) ecological model of human development is being revisited by leaders in child health (Australian Research Alliance for Children and Youth 2006, Australian Institute of Family Studies 2002:xi, Keating & Hertzman 1999, Scott 1992) because of the growing interest in how families relate to their local communities and larger social systems (Scott 1992: 204). This model can be helpful for community-based nurses undertaking a community assessment when considering the complexity of the influences impacting on any family or community.

Another useful document to consider for guiding a community assessment is 'Social determinants of health: the solid facts' (Wilkinson & Marmot 2003). This document is based on evidence supporting the impact of the ten main social determinants on our health:

1. **The social gradient**. Life expectancy is shorter and most diseases are more common further down the social ladder in each society. Health policy must tackle the social and economic determinants of health.
2. **Stress**. Stressful circumstances, making people feel worried, anxious and unable to cope, are damaging to health and may lead to premature death.
3. **Early life**. A good start in life means supporting mothers and young children: the health impact of early development and education lasts a lifetime.
4. **Social exclusion**. Life is short where its quality is poor. By causing hardship and resentment, poverty, social exclusion and discrimination cost lives.
5. **Work**. Stress in the workplace increases the risk of disease. People who have more control over their work have better health.
6. **Unemployment**. Job security increases health, wellbeing and job satisfaction. Higher rates of unemployment cause more illness and premature death.
7. **Social support**. Friendship, good social relations and strong supportive networks improve health at home, at work and in the community.
8. **Addiction**. Individuals turn to alcohol, drugs and tobacco, and suffer from their use, but their use is influenced by the wider social setting.

9. **Food**. Because global market forces control the food supply, healthy food is a political issue.
10. **Transport**. Healthy transport means less driving and more walking and cycling, backed up by better public transport.

Any assessment of a community must include an understanding of cultural diversity. McMurray (2004:16–17) also points out the need for evidence-based nursing practice that is culturally sensitive. The Department of Human Services (2004b), Victoria, has published a useful 'Cultural diversity guide'. The policy statement's core principles are: valuing diversity; reducing inequity; encouraging participation; and promoting the social, cultural and economic benefits of cultural diversity.

PUBLIC HEALTH

Community health nursing takes place within the context of public health considerations. Public health is a population-based approach to healthcare. Community health nurses will integrate their knowledge of the community with knowledge about the entire population of the country (i.e. Australia) to formulate understandings of the health and illness experiences of individuals and families within the population they serve. Last (1988) states that public health is:

> … one of the efforts organized by society to protect, promote, and restore the people's health … Public health activities change with changing technology and social values but the goals remain the same: to reduce the amount of disease, premature death, and disease-produced discomfort and disability in the population. Public health is thus a social institution, a discipline, and a practice (Last 1988:107).

A feature of public health programs is the concept of universal service provision. Universal health services are usually free at the point of access and are intended to promote equal access to all individuals and families. Such services provide scope for more intensive services for those who need extra support (Elkan et al 2001). Examples in Australia include Homeless Outreach Psychiatric Services (HOPS), Victoria's Maternal and Child Health Service, school nursing programs, the QUIT program, and drug and alcohol services (Duckett 2004:167, Keleher 2004:102). In the past, many more services were provided in this manner to people on the basis of their need, but a growing number now have a fee or co-payment requirement (Hopkins & Speed 2005).

'OLD' AND 'NEW' PUBLIC HEALTH

'Old' and 'new' public health are terms used to describe the change in approach to public health. Table 18.2, adapted from Baum (2008:37), is very useful when trying to compare the changes that are still taking place. Many of the strategies of the 'old' public health are still very important in the 'new' public health. This can be very confusing for new community nurses to unravel and understand.

POPULATION-FOCUSED PRACTICE VERSUS INDIVIDUAL-FOCUSED PRACTICE

Population health, rather than the health of the individual, is the focus of public health departments (Baum 2008, Duckett 2004, Keleher 2004, Stanhope & Lancaster 2008). Population-focused practice in nursing includes interventions such as providing an immunisation program or developing a health campaign for a defined population

'Old' public health	'New' public health
Improving infrastructure (e.g. adequate housing, clean water and sanitation)	Improving infrastructure and social determinants of health (e.g. social support and lifestyle)
Legislation and key policy mechanisms (such as green and white papers), especially in nineteenth century championed by healthcare reformers such as Florence Nightingale	Legislation and policy reaffirmed as critical tools for public health intervention/action
Medical-profession-dominated decision making for public health. Public health nursing developed with close links to medical profession	Multidisciplinary team central to the development and delivery of public health
Top-down development with little community involvement	Community involvement valued and incorporated through wide distribution of discussion papers and town-hall meetings. Level of community involvement variable
Epidemiology-dominant research method	A range of research methodologies accepted
Health is viewed as absence of disease or illness. Programs designed to prevent disease	Health is viewed as a state of wellbeing. Programs include a focus on positive aspects of health
Focus on infectious and contagious threats to human health	Concern with all threats to health and increasingly with changes to the physical environment
Conditions of the poor and special needs groups considered	Equity an explicit aim of new public health philosophy

Table 18.2 'Old' and 'new' public health
Source: Adapted from Baum (2008:37).

or subpopulation. Most professional health education is aimed at increasing proficiency in attending to the health needs of individuals. Individual-focused practice relates to objectives for an individual client, such as the need to link the client into as many resources as possible. Community nurses need to be very familiar with population-focused practice and individual-focused practice because they work with both models simultaneously (i.e. they need to be mindful of population and individual needs in their practice).

In addition to the competencies required for the care of the individual, work by US public health nurses over the last decade identified competencies for the care of populations. These included:

- analytic/assessment
- policy development/program planning
- communication
- cultural competencies
- community dimensions of practice

- basic public health services (e.g. immunisation)
- financial planning and management, and
- leadership and systems thinking (Stanhope & Lancaster 2008:8).

Awareness of and responding to the changing needs of the population will also allow the community nurse to provide benefits to individuals. Government-supported public health services will give priority to population-focused approaches and expect the community health nurse to be competent in managing both approaches. An example of this may be the community nurse wanting to see additional clients for a longer consultation when the answer may be establishing and developing a multidisciplinary support group. The community nurse will monitor and support the group and also attend to the needs of individuals that may occur.

EARLY INTERVENTION

A key strategy for nurses working in the community is early intervention. Early intervention can mean intervening early through working with parent(s) during pregnancy and infancy, or it can mean intervening early during a key transition point or pathway in an individual's life. Through early intervention and referral, issues can be dealt with before they become entrenched problems.

There has been a renewed interest in early intervention early in life as a result of new research on brain development, particularly during the first 3 years of life (Keating & Hertzman 1999). Early intervention has always been a feature of public health programs. But the success of early intervention is dependent on the skills of front-line health workers, such as community health nurses and their integrated referral and follow-up systems.

HEALTHY COMMUNITIES: NURSING INITIATIVES

There are numerous examples of new initiatives being designed and implemented by nurses and midwives in the community that support healthy community development. Three such projects are briefly described to illustrate how nurses and midwives are embracing the 'new' public health.

Initiative 1: alcohol and drug nurses develop a harm minimisation model

The response of the Victorian home-based withdrawal nurses to promote equity and wellbeing is an example of nurses acting in a 'new' public health framework.

Withdrawal from alcohol and other drugs can be a complex and arduous process for some people. The Victorian Alcohol and Drug Treatment System includes the provision of nurses to care for people undertaking withdrawal. These nurses work in a range of services including home-based and outpatient withdrawal services.

The Victorian home-based withdrawal service offers nursing support for clients undertaking withdrawal from alcohol or other substances in their own home. To receive support from a home-based withdrawal service, the nurse must assess the client for eligibility for the service. Specific contraindications that would render a client ineligible for home management of withdrawal include:

- current dependence on other drugs
- previous seizures

- current acute psychiatric condition
- unstable home environment
- inadequate support available, and
- geographical isolation (Furler et al 2000).

We know that many clients who are substance dependent also have mental health issues or are homeless or transient (SANE Australia 2005). These contraindications would leave these clients ineligible for support from the home-based nursing team.

In 1998, home-based withdrawal nurses from the Turning Point Alcohol and Drug Centre in Melbourne, Victoria, collected statistics on the number of clients they were assessing for withdrawal who did not meet the eligibility requirements for home-based support. They found that between 70% and 97% of clients who required support for their withdrawal were ineligible for assistance (McPherson & Doreian 1998). The nurses were able to demonstrate:

> … a state-wide problem with the delivery of home-based services and an obvious need to develop a complementary model of care to adequately address the issues and needs of people who did not meet the current guidelines for home-based withdrawal (McPherson & Doreian 1998).

Rather than refuse care for these clients, the home-based withdrawal nurses developed a new model of service that they called the Harm Minimisation Model. The home-based withdrawal nurses also utilised the Non-Residential Withdrawal Nurses State Network to provide a forum to gather data to support the establishment, development and peer review of the model.

The aims of the Harm Minimisation Model are to:

- effect the discontinuation of a pattern of heavy and regular drug use that cannot be sustained within the client's physical, psychological and social resources (for some clients this may be a reduction in substance use)
- provide education and information based on a harm minimisation philosophy
- provide linkages with internal and external agencies that appropriately address the client's drug use and physical, psychological and social needs
- support, educate and inform the family and/or significant others of the client and, where appropriate, facilitate referral
- ensure that service delivery is appropriately informed by, and responsive to, review and evaluation of service delivery within the context of best practice developments, and
- facilitate coordination, accountability and continuity of service delivery where clients are managed from point of entry into the service system to case closure through the process of case management.

New care pathways, assessment and consent forms, referral documentation and client information were developed to support the new model of care and the Department of Human Services, Victoria, expanded the definition of a treatment episode of care to include clients supported under the Harm Minimisation Model.

This necessary change to the approach of home-based withdrawal in Victoria has allowed alcohol and drug nurses in Victoria to deliver appropriate responses to drug and alcohol requests that could not have otherwise been accommodated by the previous models of service delivery. It was recognised with a Victorian Public Health Award for Excellence and Innovation in 1999.

Initiative 2: the Secondary School Nursing Program

Victoria's Secondary School Nursing Program is a useful service to examine as it also follows the principles of the 'new' public health. The Department of Human Services, Victoria, employed the first 20 secondary school nurses during April 2000. The next 80 nurses were employed and orientated to their new role during May, June and July 2001. The goals of the program are to:

- play a key role in reducing negative health outcomes and risk-taking behaviours among young people, including drug and alcohol abuse, tobacco smoking, eating disorders, obesity, depression, suicide and injuries
- focus on prevention of ill health and problem behaviours by ensuring coordination between the school and community-based health services
- support the school community in addressing contemporary health and social issues facing young people and their families
- place nurses in areas of greatest health needs and socioeconomic disadvantage
- provide appropriate primary healthcare through professional clinical nursing, including assessment, care, referral and support, and
- establish collaborative working relationships between primary and secondary school nurses to assist young people to deal with any difficulties in their transition from primary to secondary school (Department of Human Services 2000:3).

The role of the secondary school nurse was designed to be in line with government policy and was summarised by the Department of Human Services in July 2000 (Department of Human Services 2000:3):

- **Primary care/health education**. Nurses will provide health-related counselling, information, education and advocacy to individuals and groups within the school community.
- **Community liaison**. Nurses will help to establish links between students, parents, school staff and relevant primary health services in their local community.
- **School welfare team participation**. Nurses will work within the school as a professional member of the school welfare team, and this may include liaising with relevant primary school welfare staff to support the transition from primary to secondary school, particularly for vulnerable students.
- **School team participation**. Where appropriate, nurses will participate in the broader school community by attending relevant staff and committee meetings, attending in-service programs for school staff and contributing to the school's planning, evaluation and review processes.

A study by Edgecombe et al (2004) followed the new secondary school nurses from July 2001 until the end of 2002 as they implemented the new program. One aim of the study was to 'improve understanding of the issues involved in implementing new nursing programs in Victoria, including an examination of public policy processes'.

Figure 18.1 illustrates the policy processes secondary school nurse participants were involved in. Key themes to emerge from findings included the speed at which the program was implemented and the care taken by policy makers and nurses alike to implement the policy on the ground in the way it was intended. Orientation of new school nurses was viewed by all participants as essential to ensure uniform policy implementation across the state. Barriers encountered by nurse participants were many and related to school structure, school policy, school staff, lack of Department of Human Services policy for some situations and lack of adequate space in some schools.

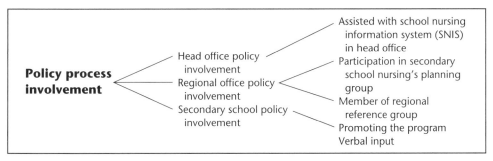

Figure 18.1 Policy process involvement of secondary school nurse participants
Source: Survey Question 47 in Edgecombe et al (2004).

Initiative 3: Midwives and Maternal and Child Health Nurses Continuity of Care Protocols

Nurses working in the community have many opportunities to become involved in policy development and policy implementation (Hennessy & Spurgeon 2000:ix). Not all take up these opportunities. Hennessy asks, 'Do nurses understand how to use the political and economic processes so that their extensive first-hand knowledge of patients, and their needs, is related in policy developments?' Many community-based nurses get these opportunities in Australia through state health departments, nurses' boards and national professional organisations. There are many examples of nurses' and midwives' involvement in policy development and implementation. A useful example is the 2003–04 team of policy makers, maternal and child health nurses, and midwives who worked together to develop protocols for midwives and maternal and child health nurses to ensure women receive continuity of care through pregnancy and childbirth. The protocols were launched in 2004 and are being used across the state (Department of Human Services 2004a:1). The aims of the protocol are to:

- enhance continuity of care for mothers and their babies from pregnancy through early parenthood by maternity services and Maternal and Child Health Services
- promote and strengthen professional partnerships between maternity services and Maternal and Child Health Services
- clarify processes to identify and engage families, with emphasis on those who are vulnerable or at risk
- promote mutual understanding of the respective roles and responsibilities of Maternal and Child Health Services and maternity services, and
- promote standardised and complementary approaches to the transfer of information between maternity services and Maternal and Child Health Services.

The principles underpinning the protocol are:

- effective continuity of care provided by maternity and Maternal and Child Health Services within the local community supports mothers and their babies during the first weeks following birth
- shared philosophical basis and common focus between services supports more effective service provision
- coordinated service to recent mothers and babies is dependent upon maternity services and Maternal and Child Health Services working collaboratively and with a clear understanding of each other's role and responsibilities
- provision of preventive services or early intervention through collaborative care planning is usually more effective than the later provision of targeted or statutory services; the best interests of new mothers and babies are usually met through family-centred practice
- information provided to families should be accessible and culturally sensitive, including use of interpreter services, and
- information exchange between maternity services and Maternal and Child Health Services should occur with the knowledge and consent of the mother, unless this action would put the baby at significant risk of harm; in this instance, the welfare of the baby takes precedence.

This initiative is very important because midwives and maternal and child health nurses have had ad hoc connections for more than 100 years. Let's hope they begin to coordinate their universal services to ensure parents and their new babies receive integrated care from the hospital to the home.

Summary

These three examples are focused on facilitating healthy community development across an entire state. Wherever you work in Australia or overseas, there will be some programs similar to the ones discussed here.

CONCLUSION

The role of nurses and midwives in supporting healthy communities is as important today as it was in the nineteenth century. Their leadership and social support roles are vital for individuals, families and communities. There are many examples of innovative practice that embrace the 'new' public health and which build social capitol. Examples of nurses' impact on community health and empowerment are to be found across the life span in places where communities live, work and play.

REFLECTIVE QUESTIONS

1 Describe the role of nurses in establishing and sustaining healthy communities.
2 What are the key aspects of a community assessment? What local, national and international databases will you utilise?
3 What strategies will you utilise in supporting healthy communities?

RECOMMENDED READINGS

Baum F 2008 The new public health, 3rd edn. Oxford University Press, Melbourne
Hennessy D, Spurgeon P 2000 Health policy and nursing. Macmillan Press, London
McMurray A 2007 Community health and wellness: a socioecological approach, 3rd edn. Mosby Elsevier, Sydney
Muir Gray JA 2001 Evidenced-based healthcare. Churchill Livingstone, London
Stanhope M, Lancaster J (eds) 2008 Public health nursing: population-centered health care in the community, 7th edn. Mosby, St Louis

REFERENCES

Australian Institute of Family Studies 2002 Introducing the longitudinal study of Australian children. Australian Institute of Family Studies, Melbourne
Australian Research Alliance for Children and Youth (ARACY) 2006 ARACY topical paper: school readiness. Centre For Community Child Health, Royal Children's Hospital, Murdoch Children's Research Institute, Melbourne
Baum F 2008 The new public health, 3rd edn. Oxford University Press, Melbourne
Bronfenbrenner U 1979 The ecology of human development. Harvard University Press, Cambridge, Massachusetts
Department of Human Services (DHS) 2000 Victorian Secondary School Nursing Program: consultation paper DHS, Melbourne
Department of Human Services (DHS) 2004a Continuity of care: a communication protocol for Victorian maternity services and the Maternal and Child Health Service. Community Care Division, DHS, Melbourne. Online. Available: health.dhs.vic.gov.au/commcare/
Department of Human Services (DHS) 2004b Cultural diversity guide. Policy and Strategic Projects Division, Victorian Government, DHS, Melbourne. Online. Available. www.dhs.vic.gov.au/multicultural/html/cultdivguide.htm
Duckett SJ 2004 The Australian health care system, 2nd edn. Oxford University Press, Melbourne
Edgecombe G 2004 Child and family nursing and early intervention. Contemporary Nurse 18(1):143–144
Edgecombe G, Hope M, Ward M 2004 Because you're a nurse—I thought I would come and see you: a participatory action research project of Victoria's Secondary School Nursing Program. RMIT University, Melbourne
Elkan BA, Robinson J, Williams D, Blair M 2001 Universal verus selective services: the case of British health visiting. Journal of Advanced Nursing 33(1):113–119
Furler J, Patterson S, Clark C, King T, Roeg S 2000 Shared care: specialist alcohol and drug services and GPs working together. Turning Point Alcohol and Drug Centre, Melbourne
Hennessy D, Spurgeon P 2000 Health policy and nursing. Macmillan Press, London
Higgins Y, Jones C 2004 Baby take a walk in the park. City of Darebin, Melbourne. Online. Available: www.darebin.vic.gov.au
Hopkins S, Speed N 2005 The decline in 'free' general practitioner care in Australia: reasons and repercussions. Health Policy 73(3):316–329
Jackson D, Edgecombe G 2008 Caring for a child and adolescent in the community. In: Kralik D, van Loon A (eds) Community nursing in Australia: context, issues and applications. Blackwell Publishing, Melbourne
Keating DP, Hertzman C (eds) 1999 Developmental health and the wellbeing of nations: social, biological and educational dynamics. Guildford Press, New York

Keleher H 2004 Public and population health: strategic responses. In: Keleher H, Murphy B (eds) Understanding health: a determinants approach. Oxford University Press, Melbourne

Keleher H, Murphy B (eds) 2004 Understanding health: a determinants approach. Oxford University Press, Melbourne

Last JM 1988 (ed.) A dictionary of epidemiology, 2nd edn. Oxford University Press, Oxford

McMurray A 2004 Culturally sensitive evidence-based practice. Collegian 11(4):14–18

McMurray A 2007 Community health and wellness: a socioecological approach, 3rd edn. Mosby Elsevier, Sydney

McPherson S, Doreian M 1998 Duty of care model: implementing appropriate responses to drug and alcohol requests that cannot be accommodated by Victorian models of service delivery. Victorian Public Health Awards for Excellence and Innovation, Melbourne

Marshall B 2004 Health promotion in action: case studies from Australia. In: Keleher H, Murphy B (eds) Understanding health: a determinants approach. Oxford University Press, Melbourne

Muir Gray JA 2001 Evidenced-based healthcare. Churchill Livingstone, London

SANE Australia 2005 Factsheet 21: drugs and mental illness. Online. Available: www.sane.org/information/factsheets/drugs_and_mental_illness.html Aug 2008

Scott D 1992 The ecology of the family and family functions. In: Clements A Infant and family health in Australia. Churchill Livingstone, Melbourne

Stanhope M, Lancaster J (eds) 2008 Public health nursing: population-centered health care in the community, 7th edn. Mosby, St Louis

Wilkinson R, Marmot M 2003 Social determinants of health: the solid facts, 2nd edn. WHO Regional Office for Europe, Copenhagen. Online. Available: www.euro.who.int/InformationSources/Publications/Catalogue/20020808_2

World Health Organization (WHO) 1986 Ottawa Charter for health promotion. Health Promotion 1(4):i–v. Online. Available: www.euro.who.int/AboutWHO/Policy/20010827_2

World Health Organization (WHO) 1998 Geneva. Health promotion glossary. Online. Available: www.wpro.who.int.hpr/docs/glossary.pdf

World Health Oganization (WHO) 2003 Phase IV (2003–2007) of the WHO Healthy Cities network in Europe: goals and requirements. WHO Regional Office for Europe, Copenhagen. Online. Available: www.euro.who.int/healthy-cities

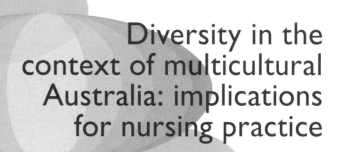

Diversity in the context of multicultural Australia: implications for nursing practice

Akram Omeri and Lynette Raymond

LEARNING OBJECTIVES

Upon completion of this chapter, the student should be able to:

- outline the cultural and linguistic demographic characteristics of Australia's diverse population groups
- describe the evolution of Australia's immigration and multiculturalism policy for all Australians
- explore the major multiculturalism policy directions and their impact on the healthcare system and practice domains in Australia
- examine how the diverse cultural and social structural influences impact on health access and outcomes for multicultural Australia
- understand the importance of addressing the inequities in the provision of healthcare services in Australia and in contemporary nursing practice, and
- examine the impact of evidenced-based transcultural nursing knowledge as it relates to the promotion of health and wellbeing of people from culturally and linguistically different backgrounds in Australia.

KEY WORDS

Australia's multiculturalism, cultural diversity, poverty, rural–remote, refugees, age, disability, culturally competent and congruent care

---

INTRODUCING MULTICULTURAL AUSTRALIA

Cultural and social structures, such as race, religion, language, education, ethnicity and economic status, are major influences on people's health and wellbeing. The Australian people represent a wealth of cultural diversity. The term culture in this chapter is used in the broad sense to mean the cultural and social structural dimensions or institutions in the environment that influence the development of an individual's beliefs, values and behaviour patterns.

In addition to the Indigenous population, Australia's cultural diversity has increased through immigration. Australia has one of the largest proportions of immigrant populations in the world, with an estimated 24% of the total population (4.96 million people) born overseas (Commonwealth of Australia 2008c). Well over half of these, one in seven Australians, were born in a non-English-speaking country (Australian Institute of Health Welfare 2008). In excess of 200 cultural and linguistic groups are represented in today's Australian population (Commonwealth of Australia 2008a, 2008c).

Diversity exists too in the wide range of contexts and environments in which people live. Variations in land, climate and settings compound diversity in social and cultural characteristics of people, as reflected in the diversity of settings in which healthcare is delivered. Healthcare is delivered in rural–remote areas, in community health settings, in the home, and in a number of acute settings within or outside hospitals in urban settings.

The purpose of this chapter is to inform student nurses and to develop in them an awareness of the benefits and challenges of diversity, with the aim of promoting the delivery of nursing care to diverse populations in culturally meaningful and safe ways. The desired outcomes are to:

- create an incentive for nurses to pursue transcultural nursing studies in order to further their sense of knowing about diversity beyond multiculturalism
- build upon the existing transcultural nursing knowledge through research and to understand the implications of culture-specific knowledge for improving nursing practice, and
- develop sensitivity and self-awareness towards cultural diversity that brings unity, respect for the other person, fairness for each other, and benefits for all.

Issues on Indigenous communities are not discussed in this chapter as this topic is addressed elsewhere in this book.

The term multicultural is used by the Australian Government to describe the cultural and linguistic diversity that exists in Australian society (Commonwealth of Australia 2003, 2007a). From an historical perspective, Australia's policies on immigration have evolved in response to social changes and a commitment to the development of society as a whole (see Table 19.1). Since 1947, Australia's immigration policies have shifted between phases of assimilation, integration, multiculturalism and mainstreaming, to inclusiveness and being united in diversity.

Years	Policy	Features	Health policy implication
1945–70	Assimilation	Predominantly White Australian Anglo-Saxon policies	Absence of government assistance
1970–80	Integration	White Australia policy relaxed and gradually abandoned Some cultural characteristics tolerated	Relevant services provided Welfare needs of migrants being addressed
1980–89	Multiculturalism	Pluralistic approach to immigration Policies to limit discrimination on racial and ethnic grounds Cultural and ethnic diversity becoming more accepted in Australian society Cultural identity, social justice and economic efficiency were adopted	Provision of various health services Equality of access to culturally appropriate services
1983	Mainstreaming	Redirecting service delivery from marginal to a central base Concern of government institutions based on social equity and access; economic efficiency and cultural identity	Promotion of culturally sensitive health services Equality of access to health services by immigrants
1999	Inclusiveness	Diversity Multicultural policies built upon civic duty, cultural respect, social equity and productive diversity The term multiculturalism to remain Inclusiveness	Promotion of culturally sensitive health services Equality of access to health services by immigrants
2000–08	United in diversity	National agenda for a multicultural Australia Policy framework including: all Australians are expected to have a 'loyalty to Australia and its people, and to respect the basic structures and principles underpinning our democratic Society. These are: Constitution, Parliamentary democracy, freedom of speech and religion, English as the National language, the rule of law, acceptance and equality' (Commonwealth of Australia 2003:6). The current Rudd Labor Government has reaffirmed its support for the relevance and constitution of Australia's Multiculturalism Policy	Main components of 'Multicultural Australia: united in diversity policy 2003–06': responsibility, respect, fairness and benefits for all

Table 19.1 Periods in immigration policy development
Source: Commonwealth of Australia (1999, 2003, 2007b, 2008b).

The principles of Australia's multiculturalism emphasise the importance of valuing differences, and utilising the cultural knowledge and skills of people from different backgrounds (Commonwealth of Australia 2003, 2007b). The policy is intended for all Australians, not just for those people from non-English speaking backgrounds. The 'Multicultural Australia: united in diversity policy 2003–06' is based on four principles:

1. **Responsibility for all**. All Australians have a civic duty to support those basic structures and principles of Australian society that guarantee us our freedom and equality and enable diversity in our society to flourish.
2. **Respect for each person**. All Australians have the right to express their own culture and beliefs and have a reciprocal obligation to respect the right of others to do the same.
3. **Fairness for each person**. All Australians are entitled to equality of treatment and opportunity. Social equity allows us all to contribute to the social, political and economic life of Australia.
4. **Benefits for all**. All Australians benefit from the significant cultural, social and economic dividends arising from the diversity of our population. Diversity works for all Australians (Commonwealth of Australia 2003:6).

To gain a deeper understanding of the historical perspectives of multicultural policies, students are encouraged to refer to the many recommended references provided throughout this chapter.

CHARACTERISTICS OF DIVERSITY

The remainder of this chapter will explore a number of Australia's diversity characteristics, along with the implications they have both individually and collectively for nursing practice.

Economic status: impact of poverty on health

As a welfare state, Australia prides itself on meeting the health needs of all Australians, not just those economically advantaged. This approach to health services is based on the belief that a healthy society is a wealthy society. The International Council of Nurses (2004) states that poverty and health are linked in four ways:

1. ill health leads to poverty
2. poverty leads to ill health
3. good health is linked to higher incomes, and
4. higher incomes are linked to good health.

Income is a key factor in relation to poverty, but other factors are also significant for good health. In a broader definition of poverty, such things as access to health services, clean water, sanitation, literacy levels and infant mortality are included (United Nations Development Programme 2002–03). Poverty and disease are inextricably linked in a direct correlation with wealth; the poorer the person the greater the incidence of ill health, the richer the person the less frequent the incidence of ill health. Disease often further impoverishes the poor (McMurray 2007). In addition, cultural factors in combination with poverty are recognised as having a significant impact upon health (Australian Institute of Health and Welfare 2000, Commonwealth of Australia 2004, Fuller et al 2004, International Council of Nurses 2004, Royal College of Nursing Australia 2004, Sacs 2005).

Socioeconomic and environmental factors, such as low income, poor housing, overcrowding, job insecurity, unemployment, few community resources, poor education, social exclusion, reduced social approval and self-esteem, are known to have an impact upon health. While government policy can have a significant impact upon health by redistributing wealth and ensuring access to health services, poor social and economic circumstances contribute to disempowerment and hopelessness among the poor and serve to keep the poor in ill health (McMurray 2007).

Language diversity

Culture is a shared experience that is mediated through language and other symbols. Australia's national language is English, with a further 200 languages spoken among the more than 200 diverse cultural and linguistic groups they represent (Commonwealth of Australia 2008a, 2008c). Spradley (1979) states that language is an important cultural expression and the major means for humans to share, construct and understand the world around them. He goes on to say that the decoding of cultural symbols and identification of meaning involves the discovery of relationships between the symbols, their usage and the cultural context in which they are expressed. Accordingly, language needs to be understood in relation to the cultural and social structures that influence the development of an individual's beliefs, values and behaviour patterns (Spradley 1979).

In response to the diversity of languages that exist in Australia, a number of both government and non-government interpreter and translator language support services and resources are currently available for both healthcare workers and clients of healthcare services. There are benefits to accrue from a heathcare workforce that is either bilingual or multilingual, particularly one that reflects the demographic language characteristics of Australia's population as a whole (Commonwealth of Australia 2008a).

Education

Educational attainments are known to influence an individual's lifestyle choices, employment opportunities, and perceptions of health and wellbeing.

Given the diverse knowledge and skill levels that exist in Australia's population, healthcare workers when planning, developing and delivering educational programs and services need to take into consideration the age, language, culture and educational background of the target population. Working in collaboration with the intended recipients of resources and services during the planning, development and delivery stages enhances the effectiveness of the information provided and health outcomes for all population groups (McMurray 2007).

Religion

The religious, spiritual and philosophical beliefs adopted by people influence the way that individuals, families and community groups respond to significant life events such as birth, illness, death and dying, as well as their behaviours to maintain health and wellbeing.

There is diversity in the religious affiliations of Australians. They comprise 26% Catholic, 19% Anglican and 19% other Christian denominations. Major non-Christian religions comprise 6% and include Buddhism (2.1%), Hinduism (0.8%), Islam (1.7%) and Judaism (0.5%) (Commonwealth of Australia 2008c).

Religious diversity has enormous implications for the planning, development and delivery of mainstream health services. Religious ceremonies may involve family members, requests for religious representatives or prayer sessions during hospitalisation or procedures. In compliance with the codes of ethical and professional nursing practice (Australian Nursing and Midwifery Council 2008a, 2008b) and competency standards for nurses (Australian Nursing and Midwifery Council 2006), nurses are required to demonstrate respect for the beliefs and values of diverse cultural groups in their care. Knowledge of different cultural rites and ceremonies and accommodation of such requests is one example of how a nurse can demonstrate respect for diverse beliefs, values and lifeways.

Health and wellbeing

The World Health Organization (WHO) defines health as a state of complete physical, mental and social wellbeing, not merely the absence of disease or infirmity (McMurray 2007). The degree to which a society experiences health and wellbeing is largely dependent upon the social and cultural structures in place to support the nation's most vulnerable population groups.

Groups such as the very young, the very old, and the very poor, newly arrived refugees, and people living with a disability, are undeniably a nation's most vulnerable and in need of support at a far greater level than other population groups. Compared with those who have social and economic advantages, disadvantaged Australians are more likely to have shorter lives, higher levels of disease risk factors and lower use of preventive health services (Australian Institute of Health Welfare 2000).

Research has found that most immigrants enjoy health that is at least as good as, if not better than, that of the Australian-born population and that they often have lower death and hospitalisation rates, as well as lower rates of disability and lifestyle-related risk factors (Australian Institute of Health Welfare 2002, cited in Australian Institute of Health Welfare 2008). This effect is believed to result from two main factors. First, a self-selection process includes those who are willing and economically able to migrate, and excludes those who are sick or disabled. Second, the government selection process involves certain eligibility criteria based on health, education, language and job skills.

Age

Australia's 2006 census findings reported that 13% of the population are aged 65 years and over, and 2% are 15 years of age or younger. Based on current birthing and immigration trends, the Australian Bureau of Statistics (ABS) projects that aged persons will comprise 26–28% of the population by 2051, whereas those people under the age of 15 years will decrease to represent 13% of the population. At 30 June 2006, older people from non-English-speaking countries numbered over 583,200, compared with 370,000 from the main English-speaking countries and 1,780,400 who were born in Australia. In 2004, approximately 300,000 people were found to be aged 85 years and over, comprising 1.5% of the population (Commonwealth of Australia 2008c). In 2006, the most common countries of birth for non-English-speaking older people were Italy (113,900) and Greece (57,200) (Commonwealth of Australia 2008c).

Definitions of ageing among different cultural groups can be vastly different from mainstream and dominant cultures in Australia and elsewhere; hence, the nurse needs to include cultural assessment in their practice in order to provide culturally congruent, safe and competent care. Older people often have to contend with negative stereotypes, prejudice and discrimination. Such attitudes are forms of ageism (i.e. the systematic devaluing of a group of people on the basis of a characteristic in common). Ageism is similar to racism or sexism; generalised judgments are made about people as a group rather than as individuals. Ageism can be challenged by nurses as we become conscious of the need to eliminate discrimination (Clark McCann 2004). Australia's Department of Health and Ageing (2006–09) 'Corporate plan' expresses a vision for better health and active ageing for all Australians. Top priorities for achieving this vision can be summarised as:

- focusing on prevention and early intervention
- ensuring choice and access to quality aged care services, and
- improving health of Indigenous Australians.

Refugees and asylum seekers

Between 1998 and 2002, over 600,000 refugees and displaced people resettled in Australia. The quota resettled in the Humanitarian Program in 2002–03 was 12,000. Four thousand of these places were reserved for the refugee category (Commonwealth of Australia 2007b). In January 2004, the Australian Government announced that it would seek to increase migrant and humanitarian settlement in regional Australia. In 2004–05 the department-funded Integrated Humanitarian Settlement Strategy assisted the settlement of refugees in regional Australia (Commonwealth of Australia 2007b). As a result, the Australian Government's Refugee and Special Humanitarian Programme increased the annual intake of refugees to 13,500 per annum. In 2007–08 the top five countries of origin of offshore refugee and Special Humanitarian Program entrants were Burma, Iraq, Afghanistan, Sudan and Liberia (Refugee Council of Australia 2008).

Refugees may have experienced severe deprivation, trauma and torture that can lead to post-traumatic stress disorder (PTSD), a condition that can profoundly affect a person's health and capacity to resettle. There is a body of literature on the medical and psychological responses of people to war and conflict that includes Afghan refugees in Australia (Harris Telfer 2001, Silove et al 1998, Steel & Sil 2001, Sultan & O'Sullivan 2001, Omeri et al 2004, 2006, Procter 2004a, 2004b). The specific factors that impact on resettlement of refugees are poorly understood outside of relief agencies (Summerfield 2000). In their study of Afghan refugees in New South Wales, Omeri et al (2006) identified a number of issues of central concern to this group, including: emotional responses to trauma; migration and resettlement experiences; culture-specific health maintenance strategies; and barriers impeding access to and appropriateness of Australian healthcare services. The findings have relevance for improving the quality of culture-specific healthcare for the Afghan community in Australia.

Disability status

The way disability is defined and understood has changed in the last decade. Disability was once assumed as a way to characterise a particular set of largely stable limitations. The World Health Organization has moved towards a new international classification system known as the International Classification of Functioning, Disability and Health (ICF) (Commonwealth of Australia 2008c). The ICF system emphasises functional status over diagnosis. It focuses on analysing the relationship between the person's capacity and their performance ability. If capacity is greater than performance, then the gap is addressed by removing barriers and identifying facilitators that could improve the individual's performance. The ICF system specifically promotes 'universal design', a concept that serves to identify facilitators that can benefit all people.

Disability is now seen as a contextual variable, that is dynamic and changes over the person's lifetime and in relation to their personal circumstances. In 2003, one in five (20%) people in Australia reported having a disability (SDAC 2003, cited in Commonwealth of Australia 2008c). The rates were found to be the same for men as women (see Fig 19.1). The number of people indicating that they had a disability increased with age. Furthermore, a survey by the Australian Bureau of Statistics revealed that 6% of Australia's population was reported as having a profound or severe core activity limitation that required assistance with self-care, mobility or communication (Commonwealth of Australia 2008c).

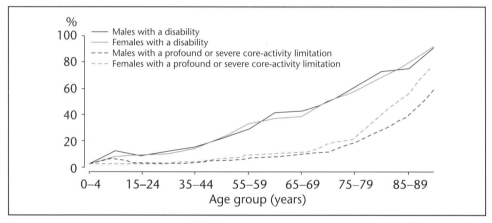

Figure 19.1 Disability rates: 2003
Source: Commonwealth of Australia (2008a).

The change in defining disability calls for a change in the provision of healthcare services and nursing practice and services. It requires a shift from preventive and enabling services to promoting and developing the level of functioning of people who were initially classified differently. Nurses need to be aware that different cultural groups respond differently to a person living with a temporary or permanent disability.

Rural–remote inequalities

People living in rural and remote areas tend to have shorter lives and higher levels of illness and disease risk factors than those in major cities (Australian Institute of Health Welfare 2008). The problem of poverty and disadvantage for people in many rural and regional areas across Australia is evidenced by generally lower incomes, reduced access to services such as health, education and transport, as well as declining employment opportunities. These factors are compounded by the problems of distance and isolation (Australian Institute of Health Welfare 2008, Royal College of Nursing Australia 2004).

The provision of services to rural and remote areas is problematic due to distance, low service density and the social and cultural adaptation needed to make them effective (Jong et al 2005). Jong et al (2005) highlight the need for improved primary healthcare, and access to expert multidisciplinary services in a coordinated fashion for rural and remote populations. These authors called for cooperation between governments for the successful development of pathways with innovative information systems, to improve interaction between services to address inequalities in care in rural Australia. The 'Review of settlement services for migrants and humanitarian entrants report' outlined in recommendation 29 a proposal that the department seek further opportunities to settle humanitarian entrants in regional Australia (Commonwealth of Australia 2007c). The report recommendation 29 also highlighted the need for the department to liaise more closely with stakeholders regarding regional locations where employment opportunities exist and where appropriate community services and support currently exists or may be developed.

As a result of this recommendation, many newly arrived immigrants and refugees now transfer to country locations for employment and affordable housing (Commonwealth of Australia 2007c). However, social support networks and access to culturally appropriate services are reduced in regional areas, in comparison to urban and metropolitan regions in Australia.

CULTURALLY COMPETENT NURSING CARE FOR CULTURALLY DIVERSE POPULATIONS

Culture reflects the values, beliefs, customs, thoughts, actions, communications and belief systems of racial, ethnic, religious or social groups. Competence, on the other hand, implies a capacity to function within the cultural context and pattern of behaviour, of a designated group, community or an institution. Combining these concepts enables a system, community, institution or group of professionals to develop a congruent set of behaviours and policies to function effectively in a culturally diverse situation.

Cultural competence has been defined as a set of congruent behaviours, practices, attitudes and policies related to embracing cultural differences that are integrated into a system or agency or among professionals (Mays et al 2002:139). Cultural competence also means having the knowledge, awareness and sensitivity of culture sufficient to meet the culture care needs of individuals, families, groups and communities. It involves respect for difference and a desire to learn from and accept diversities.

Having discussed diversity and its implications for culturally competent nursing care, the following description includes a summary of skills needed for the planning, development and delivery of culturally competent nursing care. These guidelines have been adapted from Andrews and Boyle (2008). They are:

- **Cultural self-assessment**. This enables nurses to develop an awareness of their own cultural values, attitudes, beliefs and practices. These insights enable one to overcome ethnocentric tendencies and cultural stereotypes, which are often vehicles for perpetuating prejudice and discrimination. Cultural self-assessment is the foundation for culturally competent and culturally congruent nursing care.
- **Cross-cultural communication**. This is identified as one of the most important landmarks in cultural assessment in establishing a culturally congruent care plan. Therefore, it is necessary to examine the ways in which people from various cultural backgrounds communicate with one another. In addition to oral and verbal communication, messages are conveyed

non-verbally through gestures, body movements, posture, tone of voice and facial expressions.

- **Non-verbal communication**. Non-verbal communication patterns vary widely across cultures. Therefore, nurses must be alert for cues that convey cultural differences in the use of silence, eye contact, touch, space, distance and facial expressions. Cultural influences on appropriate communication between individuals of different genders also need to be considered. Non-verbal behaviours are culturally significant and failure to adhere to cultural norms of behaviour may be viewed as a serious transgression. Violating norms that relate to appropriate male–female relationships among various cultural groups may jeopardise nurses' therapeutic relationship with patients and their families.

- **Touch**. This deserves careful consideration. While we recognise the often-reported benefits in establishing rapport with clients through touch, including the promotion of healing through therapeutic touch, physical contact with clients conveys various meanings cross-culturally.

- **Space and distance**. These are significant in cross-cultural communication. The perception of appropriate distance zones varies widely among cultural groups. In the early 1960s, Edward Hall pioneered the study of proxemics, which focuses on how people in various cultures relate to their physical space. Although there are intercultural variations, the intimate distance in interpersonal interactions ranges from 0–0.5 metre. At this distance, people experience visual detail and each other's odour, health and touch. Personal distance varies from 0.4–1.2 metres, the usual space within which communication between friends and acquaintances occurs. Nurses frequently interact with clients in the intimate or personal distance zones. Socially acceptable personal distance between people refers to approximately 1 metre, whereas anything greater than 1.5 metres is considered public space (Hall 1963, cited in Andrews & Boyle 2008:26).

IMPLICATIONS FOR PROVISION OF CULTURALLY COMPETENT NURSING AND HEALTHCARE

Based on an internet survey, Andrews and Boyle (2008) reported on two major categories of cultural competence: organisational cultural competence and individual cultural competence. Organisational competence requires:

> … a defined set of values and principles and demonstration of behaviours, attitudes, policies and structures that enable people to work effectively cross-culturally. Individual cultural competence refers to a complex integration of knowledge, attitudes, beliefs, and encounters with those from cultures different from one's own (Andrews & Boyle 2008:16).

Cultural competence in nursing has been defined as a process, as opposed to an end point, in which nurses continuously strive to work effectively within the cultural context of an individual, a family or community with diverse cultural backgrounds (Andrews & Boyle 2008, Campinha-Bacote 2003). Campinha-Bacote (2003:14) suggests that 'the process involves the integration of cultural desire, cultural awareness, cultural knowledge, cultural skill and cultural encounter'.

Assuring culturally competent nursing and healthcare is the responsibility of systems, agencies and institutions (Omeri 2003). There is a growing understanding revealed in the literature that organisations providing culturally and linguistically appropriate services (i.e. culturally competent services) have the potential to reduce cultural and ethnic health disparities (Anderson et al 2003). The nursing profession is responsible for developing cultural competence in its practitioners, not only in its novitiates, but also on a continuing basis as measured by the demonstration of requisite skills, knowledge and attitudes. However, there is no agreement as to how continuing competence should be monitored, nor is there any provision for continuing education in transcultural nursing for faculty and nurse administrators.

CONCLUDING REMARKS

Meeting the healthcare needs of diverse populations in Australia is one of the greatest challenges faced by nurses and healthcare professionals. This chapter has provided an overview of population trends relating to cultural and linguistic diversity and the ways it impacts on the role and function of nurses and healthcare professionals. It has highlighted issues relating to globalisation and the impact of poverty on health and subsequent disadvantage of some populations in accessing health and other services. Furthermore, the impact of policy directions on healthcare and education were discussed. Culturally congruent, safe and competent nursing and healthcare were proposed as a way to improve nursing practice and health outcomes for diverse population groups. This chapter also highlighted the importance of transcultural nursing knowledge and its application for nursing practice in an attempt to improve the health and wellbeing of the diverse populations in Australia.

REFLECTIVE QUESTIONS

1 What are some of the factors influencing healthcare of diverse populations in Australia? Reflect upon those discussed in this chapter.

2 How can poverty be defined? How is it linked to health and wellbeing outcomes?

3 Take some time to think about your own cultural beliefs in relation to health and healthcare. How might your own beliefs be similar or different from someone from another culture?

4 How can nurses embrace diversity to enhance workplace practices?

RECOMMENDED READINGS

Andrews M, Boyle J 2008 Transcultural concepts in nursing care, 5th edn. Lippincott Williams Wilkins, Philadelphia

Leininger M, McFarland M 2002 Transcultural nursing concepts, theories, research and practices, 3rd edn. McGraw Hill, New York

Omeri A 2003 Meeting diversity challenges: pathway of advanced transcultural nursing practice in Australia. Contemporary Nurse 15(3):175–187

Omeri A 2006 Transcultural nursing: the way to prepare culturally competent
practitioners in Australia. In: Papadopoulos I (ed.) Transcultural health and social
care: development of culturally competent practitioners. Churchill Livingston,
Elsevier, Edinburgh

REFERENCES
Anderson L, Scrimshaw S, Fullilove M, Fielding J, Normand J 2003 Culturally
competent healthcare systems: a systematic review. American Journal of
Preventative Medicine 24(3S):238–246

Andrews M Boyle J 2008 Transcultural concepts in nursing care, 5th edn. Wolters
Kluwer/Lippincott Williams & Wilkins, Philadelphia

Australian Institute of Health and Welfare (AIHW) 2000 International health: how
Australia compares: social and economic environment. Online. Available: www.
aihw.gov.au/publications/phe/ihhac/ihhac-c07f-2000-09-04

Australian Institute of Health and Welfare (AIHW) 2008 Australia's health 2008: the
eleventh biennial health report of the Australian Institute of Health and Welfare.
Online. Available: www.aihw.gov.au/publications/index.cfm/title/10585 15 Aug
2008

Australian Nursing and Midwifery Council (ANMC) 2006 National competency
standards for the registered nurse. Online. Available: www.anmc.org.au 2 Sept
2008

Australian Nursing and Midwifery Council (ANMC) 2008a Code of ethics for nurses
in Australia. Online. Available: www.anmc.org.au 2 Sept 2008

Australian Nursing and Midwifery Council (ANMC) 2008b Code of professional
conduct for nurses in Australia. Online. Available: www.anmc.org.au 2 Sept 2008

Camphina-Bacote J 2003 The process of cultural competence in the delivery of health
care services: a culturally competent model of care, 4th edn. Transcultural CARE
Associates, Cincinnati

Camphina-Bacote J 2008 Cultural desire 'caught' or 'taught'. Contemporary Nurse
28(1–2):141–148

Clark E, McCann T 2004 Ageing and health. In: Grbich C (ed.) Health in Australia:
sociological concepts and issues, 3rd edn. Pearson Longman, Sydney, pp 152–72

Commonwealth of Australia 1999 Australian multiculturalism for a new century:
towards inclusiveness. Online. Available: www.immi.gov.au/fact-sheets/06evolution.
htmlhttp://www.immi.gov.au/fact-sheets/06evolution.html 23 Aug 2008

Commonwealth of Australia 2003 Multicultural Australia: united in diversity.
Updating the 1999 new agenda for multicultural Australia: strategic directions for
2003–06. Online. Available: www.immi.gov.au/media/fact-sheets/06evolution.
htm 23 Aug 2006

Commonwealth of Australia 2004 A hand up not a handout: renewing the fight
against poverty. Report on poverty and financial hardship. Senate Community
Affairs References Committee, Canberra. Online. Available: www.aph.gov.au/
senate/commitee/clac_ctte/poverty/report/index.htm 20 Jan 2004

Commonwealth of Australia 2007a Fact sheet 6: the evolution of Australia's
multicultural policy. Canberra National Communications Branch, Department
of Immigration and Citizenship. Online. Available: www.immi.gov.au/media/
factsheets/06evolution.htmwww.immi.gov.au/media/fact-sheets/06evolution.htm
23 Aug 2008

Commonwealth of Australia 2007b Fact sheet 66: integrated humanitarian settlement strategy. Department of Immigration and Citizenship. Online. Available: www.immi.gov.au/media/fact-sheets/66ihss.htm 25 Aug 2008

Commonwealth of Australia 2007c Fact sheet 97: humanitarian settlement in regional Australia. Department of Immigration and Citizenship. Online. Available: www.immi.gov.au/media/fact-sheets/66ihss.htm 25 Aug 2008

Commonwealth of Australia 2008a 2008 International year of languages. Online. Available: www.minister.immi.gov.au/parlsec/media/media-releases/2008/lf08001.htm 23 Aug 2008

Commonwealth of Australia 2008b A new lease of life for multicultural Australia. Online. Available: www.minister.immi.gov.au/parlsec/media/media-releases/2008/lf08004.htm 23 Aug 2008

Commonwealth of Australia 2008c Year book Australia. Australian Bureau of Statistics (ABS), Canberra. Online. Available: www.abs.gov.au 23 Aug 2008

Department of Health and Ageing 2006–09 Corporate plan: better health/better care/better life. Online. Available: http://www.health.gov.au/internet/main/publishing.nsf/Content/corporate -plan/10 Aug 2008

Fuller J, Harris E, Nutbeam N, Harris M 2004 UK health inequalities: the class system is alive and well. Medical Journal of Australia 181(10):583–584

Harris M, Telfer B 2001 The health needs of asylum seekers living in the community. Medical Journal of Australia 175:589–592

International Council of Nurses (ICN) 2004 ICN on health and human rights: nursing matters fact sheet. Online. Available: www.icn.ch/matters humanrights-print.htm 18 Mar 2008

Jong K, Vale P, Armstrong B 2005 Rural inequalities in cancer care and outcome. Medical Journal of Australia 182(1):13–14

McMurray A 2007 Community health and wellness: a socio-ecological approach, 3rd edn. Mosby Elsevier, Sydney, pp 85–102

Mays R, De Leon Siantz M, Viehweg S 2002 Accessing cultural competence of policy organisations. Journal of Transcultural Nursing 13(2):139–144

Omeri A 2003 Meeting diversity challenges: pathway of advanced transcultural nursing practice in Australia. Contemporary Nurse 15(3):175–187

Omeri A, Lennings C, Raymond L 2004 Hardiness and transformational coping in asylum seekers: the Afghan experience. Diversity in Health and Social Care 1(1):21–30

Omeri A, Lennings C, Raymond L 2006 Beyond asylum: implications for nursing and health care delivery for Afghan refugees in Australia. Journal of Transcultural Nursing 17(1):30–39

Procter N 2004a Beyond asylum: the significance of supportive counselling in the process of seeking asylum. Nursing Review March:5

Procter N 2004b Retraumatization, fear and suicidal thinking: a case study of 'boat people' to Australia. Migration Letters: An International Journal of Migration 1(1):42–49

Refugee Council of Australia (RCOA) 2008 Australia's refugee program overview. Online. Available: www.refugeecouncil.org.au/arp/overview.htmlhttp://www.refugeecouncil.org.au/arp/overview.html 14 Sept 2008

Royal College of Nursing Australia (RCNA) 2004 Issues paper: poverty profile of Australia. Online. Available: www.rcna.org.au 20 Jan 2004

Sacs J 2005 The end of poverty: how we can make it happen in our lifetime. Penguin Books, London

Silove D, Steel Z, McGorry P et al 1998 Trauma exposure, post-migration stressors and symptoms of anxiety, depression and post-traumatic stress in Tamil asylum seekers: comparisons with refugees and immigrants. Acta Psychiatry Scand 97:175–181

Spradley JP 1979 The ethnographic interview. Harcourt Brace Jovanovich, Fort Worth

Steel Z, Sil D 2001 The mental health implications of detaining asylum seekers. Medical Journal of Australia 175:596–604

Sultan A, O'Sullivan K 2001 Psychological disturbances in asylum seekers. Medical Journal of Australia 175:593–596

Summerfield 2000 Childhood war refugeedom and trauma: three core questions for mental health professionals. Transcultural Psychiatry 37:417–433

United Nations Development Programme 2002–03 Human development report. Online. Available: www.hdr.undp.org/does/publications/background_papers/2004/HDR2004-Will_Kamolica.Pd8 20 Dec 2004

CHAPTER 20

Cultural awareness: nurses working with Indigenous Australian people

Isabelle Ellis, Christine Davey and Vicki Bradford

LEARNING OBJECTIVES

After completing this chapter, readers will be able to:

- outline the cultural diversity of Australia and identify where Indigenous people live
- recognise the effect of racism and social class on the health of Indigenous people
- differentiate between the terms cultural awareness, cultural safety and cultural competence
- assess the healthcare environment through the lens of cultural competence, and
- develop a plan to increase personal cultural competence, particularly in relation to working with Indigenous people.

KEY WORDS

Indigenous health, Aboriginal health, cultural competence, racism, social class

INTRODUCTION

Aboriginal and Torres Strait Islander culture is said to be the oldest living culture in the world, spanning more than 40,000 years. Prior to colonisation, there were more than 200 language groups and a higher number of dialects (Aboriginal and Torres Strait Islander Commission 1998:8).

Since colonisation, Australia has developed into a multicultural society with 23.8% of its population born overseas, with 43% of those from just four countries: the United Kingdom, New Zealand, Italy and Vietnam (Australian Bureau of Statistics 2005b). Prior to colonisation the population of Australia was predominantly Aboriginal and Torres Strait Islander peoples; however, there have been many claims that trading was strong between Aboriginal and Torres Strait Islander people and the neighbouring countries. This has changed dramatically since colonisation, with the population changed to being predominantly Anglo-Celtic by 1900. Aboriginal and Torres Strait Islander people make up 2.5% of the population (Australian Bureau of Statistics & Australian Institute of Health and Welfare 2008:xxi), Anglo-Celtic 74%, other European 19%, and Asian 4.5% (Australian Bureau of Statistics 2005a). So although we consider ourselves multicultural, we are predominantly from an English-speaking coloniser background.

Australia as a nation has attained a degree of longevity, which is used as an indicator of a robust and effective health system for all groups except Indigenous Australians. The difference in life expectancy between Indigenous and non-Indigenous people is a stark reminder that there is a need for urgent action to 'close the gap' (Aboriginal and Torres Strait Islander Social Justice Commissioner 2005) and nurses, wherever they work, have a role to play.

In this chapter, we will explore some of the issues involved in working with Indigenous people as consumers, clients, patients, families and communities. We will identify why cultural competence is as important as clinical competence to improving the health of Aboriginal and Torres Strait Islander people for whom we care. We will also touch on some of the rewards and challenges of working cross-culturally with Aboriginal and Torres Strait Islander people.

WHAT DOES IT MEAN TO BE INDIGENOUS IN AUSTRALIA?

Being an Indigenous person means that a person identifies as an Indigenous person and acknowledges their Indigenous heritage. The United Nations has rejected the need for a definition for Indigenous people; however, it endorses the notion of a description of the concept of Indigenous, particularly the one put forward by José R Martínez Cobo in his famous study on the problem of discrimination against Indigenous populations.

> Indigenous communities, peoples and nations are those which, having a historical continuity with pre-invasion and pre-colonial societies … consider themselves distinct from other sectors of the societies now prevailing in those territories … They form at present non-dominant sectors of society and are determined to preserve, develop and transmit to future generations their ancestral territories, and their ethnic identity, as the basis of their continued existence as peoples, in accordance with their own cultural patterns, social institutions and legal systems (Cobo 1983:379–382).

The Department of Aboriginal Affairs published a report in 1981 with the working definition of Aboriginal and Torres Strait Islander, which has been tested in the courts in relation to Indigenous land claims, the jurisdiction of the Royal Commission into

Aboriginal Deaths in Custody and clarifying elements of the Constitution (Gardiner-Garden 2000).

> An Aboriginal or Torres Strait Islander is a person of Aboriginal or Torres Strait Islander descent who identifies as an Aboriginal or Torres Strait Islander and is accepted as such by the community in which he (she) lives.

This working definition has been adopted by government departments and organisations to determine eligibility for some programs and services. Although this three-part working definition, which comprises descent, self-identification and community recognition and acceptance, is in line with the concept of Indigenous accepted by the United Nations, it has been criticised as not originating from Indigenous people. However, it should be noted that many Indigenous people prefer to be referred to as being Aboriginal or Torres Strait Islander people rather than by the term Indigenous.

The history of recognition as an Indigenous person or community has not been straightforward in Australia. Early definitions used family tree mapping as a way of defining people's Aboriginality and alluded to notions of dilution of Aboriginality through mixing of blood with the colonisers. These definitions were regularly used by the government to develop and implement policies from 1788 to the 1960s, and led to descriptions of people as full blood, half caste or quarter caste, based mainly on the description of skin colour by those wishing to describe, exclude or implicate the Aboriginal person in question (Eckermann et al 2006). These terms are no longer used and it is inappropriate to do so; as described by Eckermann et al (2006), it is considered to be a form of scientific racism.

THE EFFECT OF CULTURE, RACE AND CLASS ON HEALTH

Stratification of society exists in all countries. In Australia, the strata are not only between rich and poor suburbs in our major cities, but also between urban and remote areas and between non-Indigenous and Indigenous Australians. Social class, according to Walter and Saggers (2007:88), is a 'broad concept which encapsulates both objective material position and subjective understandings and incorporates the important notion of differential access to power'. Social class also relates to social mobility, which refers to an individual's opportunity to move up or down the social class structure. This is often leveraged through access to education, employment and health services, resulting in a sustainable standard of living. The further from the major capital cities you go, the poorer you are likely to be; and being Indigenous also makes you more likely to be poor.

Social class structures are maintained or strengthened by the process of 'othering' (Cahoone 2003), whereby the dominant culture, structure or class maintains its hierarchy by creating a duality and then actively excluding or opposing the other. Difference is highlighted and accentuated. The classic Dr Zeus story about the Sneetches on the beaches is a wonderful example of othering; the only difference between the two groups is whether they have a star on their belly or not. The star-bellied Sneetches create and maintain their privileged position by highlighting this difference. Othering can be expressed as bullying, social exclusion and excessive vigilance by authority figures, such as when young people are followed in shops in case they shoplift. When expressed as racism, the effects on the health of individuals and communities can be profoundly negative (Larson et al 2007).

Defining racism is not easy. In his recent systematic review on self-reported racism, Paradies (2006) found that, of the 138 studies included in the review, only 34 gave a definition of racism. Paradies proposes that racism is a form of:

> … oppression/privilege which exists in a dialectical relationship with antiracism … a societal system in which people are divided into races, with power unevenly distributed, or produced based on their racial classifications (Paradies 2006:68).

Interpersonal racism is experienced as emotional upset (anger, sadness or frustration)—when a person perceives that they have been treated unfairly or have been demeaned in some way on the basis of their race. It can also be experienced as physical upset (headaches, an upset stomach, tensing of the muscles or a pounding heart). The study by Larson et al (2007) that examined the experiences of 639 residents of a town, of whom 183 identified as Aboriginal, found that Aboriginal people reported that they had received 3.6 times the amount of negative racially based treatment than non-Aboriginal people. They were more than twice as likely to report their heath as fair to poor.

In line with other research (Coffin 2007, Eades 2000, Paradies 2006), the stress experienced has a negative impact on the mental and physical health of individuals. The researchers concluded that racially based negative treatment was so common in this group that 40% of Aboriginal respondents reported it. The research found no association of negative racially based treatment for gender, education or employment status, and they concluded that all Aboriginal people may equally experience perceived racism as part of daily life.

Interpersonal racism can be overt or covert. Covert racism is unintentional, with the perpetrator not being aware (Henry et al 2004), whereas overt racism is intentional and can be perpetrated in many ways, such as: commenting on the dress or smell of a person and linking those observations to race; treating people in unequal ways based on race, such as making people wait while others are attended to straight away; speaking to adults as if they are children, such as simplifying explanations and using a tone of voice that sounds scolding or patronising.

Organisations are also able to create an atmosphere of 'othering'. When service organisations do not recognise the need for and provide culturally safe services, they can be accused of institutional racism (Henry et al 2004). Henry et al provide several examples of institutional racism within the healthcare system, such as cultural barriers, insufficient funding, and the inequities in addressing overspending (e.g. an Aboriginal Medical Service had funding cut for overspending, while a government service was given an additional $100 million to address the overspend).

Institutional racism occurs when the policies of an organisation or institution result in Aboriginal people receiving less benefit from the same policies. This can occur in intentional or non-intentional ways (e.g. when the visiting times of a hospital do not coincide with the public transport schedules, or when the policy of the hospital states only immediate family members are able to visit an inpatient (Coffin 2007)).

Where do Aboriginal and Torres Strait Islander people live?

Indigenous people make up 2.5% of the total Australian population, with 32% living in major cities, 43% in regional areas and 25% in remote areas (Australian Bureau of Statistics & Australian Institute of Health and Welfare 2008:xxi). This distribution does not match that of the non-Indigenous population. The percentage of the total population who live in very remote areas of Australia is only 1%, as classified by the Australian Standard Geographic Classification (ASGC). Of those, Indigenous people make up 45%. In contrast, 89% of non-Indigenous people live in the major capital cities and regional areas of Australia and only 3% live in remote or very remote areas. Fifty per cent of Indigenous people live in the major capital cities, 23% live in regional areas and 27% live in remote and very remote areas.

Larson's analysis of the migration patterns and fertility trends for remote Australia point to a continuing increase in the remote Indigenous population, as a result of both a higher fertility rate and an increase in total numbers of Indigenous people due to a lower out-migration trend. This is in contrast to a higher out-migration of non-Indigenous people, which leads to increasing Indigenisation of remote Australia (Larson 2006). It has been proposed that the remote Indigenous population will increase by 22% between 2001 and 2016, and that this reflects a similar rate of growth between 1981 and 1996 (Larson 2006).

In 2006, an Aboriginal or Torres Strait Islander woman was expected to have 2.1 babies in her lifetime, while a non-Indigenous woman would have 1.8 as an average Australia wide (Australian Bureau of Statistics & Australian Institute of Health and Welfare 2008). The age of Aboriginal and Torres Strait Islander women having babies is much younger than non-Indigenous women, with the highest number of births recorded between the ages of 20 and 24 years. Aboriginal and Torres Strait Islander babies having higher incidences of low birth weight and perinatal (foetal and stillbirth) deaths (Australian Bureau of Statistics & Australian Institute of Health and Welfare 2008).

The health of Aboriginal and Torres Strait Islander people

The neverending story about Australian Indigenous people's health is and should be alarming to all healthcare professionals. The median age for an Indigenous person at the 2006 census was 21 years of age compared to non-Indigenous people, which is 36 years of age (Australian Bureau of Statistics & Australian Institute of Health and Welfare 2008). It is well recognised that there is a fundamental flaw in the population data collection methods that measure the health of the Indigenous population, with the Australian Institute of Health and Welfare (Australian Bureau of Statistics & Australian Institute of Health and Welfare 2008:5) noting that there was an undercount of 11.5%, but this was not distributed equally within the states and territories.

The census data is reliant on people completing the form accurately. The Australian Bureau of Statistics offers support to people who may have difficulty in completing the form. There are still many Indigenous people who are suspicious about the reason for the information and how it will be used because of past government policies and practices. There is a requirement to tick the box to identify as an Indigenous person on the national census, or Aboriginality must be recorded by a health professional in many state-based registers. The Australian Bureau of Statistics and the Australian Institute of Health and Welfare both acknowledge that there are major gaps in the Indigenous data, and many reports that appear to be national only account for some of the states, often excluding the large states of Queensland and New South Wales where 69% of the Indigenous population live.

Acknowledging these methodological problems, according to the Australian Bureau of Statistics (2003) and the Australian Institute of Health and Welfare (Standing Committee on Aboriginal and Torres Strait Islander Health and Statistical Information

Management Committee 2006), Aboriginal and Torres Strait Islander people were twice as likely as other Australians to report their health as fair to poor. Indigenous Australians were twice as likely to die from cardiovascular disease, and it is the major cause for Indigenous men dying 21 years younger than non-Indigenous men. In Central Australia, Aboriginal people had the highest incidence of diabetes in the world (Australian Bureau of Statistics 2003). In remote Australia, the incidence of end-stage renal failure is up to 30 times that of non-Indigenous Australians. In 2004, Indigenous patients accounted for 85% of all newly registered dialysis patients in the Northern Territory, 20% in Western Australia and 12% in Queensland (Australian Bureau of Statistics 2005a). The story of Indigenous health inequality does not end with chronic disease. The Western Australian Child Health Survey identified that children suffer from skin, ear and respiratory infections at a significantly higher rate than non-Aboriginal children (Zubrick et al 2004).

The statistics paint a bleak picture of the physical health of Indigenous Australians. They paint a picture of increasing disadvantage starting from conception that spirals through a childhood marred by acute infection and illness, to early onset of chronic disease and rapid deterioration in health status and early death. Identifying the causes of poor health is the first step in trying to address poor outcomes. We are constantly reminded in the media that if we eat less, drink less alcohol, exercise more and do not smoke we will be less likely to suffer chronic disease, become healthier and live longer. This puts responsibility for improving health status squarely at the feet of individuals.

However, there is a growing body of research that has looked at the social determinants of health and tried to identify their impact on health outcomes (Marmot & Wilkinson 1999, Turrell & Mathers 2000, Saggers & Gray 2007). It is clear that income, environmental issues and education have a profound impact on health across the lifespan for all people, but the stories of Indigenous people describe a specific group of social determinants that impact on their health. Indigenous people describe their health in terms of culture, community, access to land and sacred sites, access to resources and key services, and involvement in the political, economic and social life of post-colonised Australia (Hunter 1993).

USE OF HEALTH SERVICES BY ABORIGINAL AND TORRES STRAIT ISLANDER PEOPLE

Indigenous Australians visit their general practitioner (GP) and are hospitalised for circulatory diseases, diabetes, respiratory diseases, musculoskeletal conditions, kidney disease, eye and ear problems and mental and behavioural disorders (Australian Bureau of Statistics 2005a). However, they are less likely to visit their GP, use private health services or residential aged care than non-Indigenous Australians. They are more likely to use public hospitals for a range of care needs and are twice as likely to be hospitalised (Australian Bureau of Statistics 2006).

In his 2005 Social Justice report, Tom Calma, Aboriginal and Torres Strait Islander Social Justice Commissioner, made recommendations for equity in health within a generation culminating in the Close the Gap Campaign in March 2006 (Aboriginal and Torres Strait Islander Social Justice Commissioner and the Steering Committee for Indigenous Health Equality 2008). As a result of this, the Steering Committee for Indigenous Health Equality was formed and has worked tirelessly since to gain a commitment from government and non-government stakeholders to work collaboratively to 'close the gap'.

On 13 February 2008, the Prime Minister, Kevin Rudd, apologised to Aboriginal and Torres Strait Islander peoples for the wrongdoings by governments of the past. In his speech, not only did the Prime Minister apologise, but he also committed to develop partnerships with Indigenous people to close the gap in life expectancy, employment and educational opportunities (Aboriginal and Torres Strait Islander Social Justice Commissioner and the Steering Committee for Indigenous Health Equality 2008).

In March 2008, a Close the Gap Indigenous Health Equality summit was held in Canberra. On the final day of the summit, a Statement of Intent to work in partnership to reduce the gap in life expectancy of Indigenous people within a generation was produced. The statement was signed by the Prime Minister, Minister of Health, Minister of Indigenous Affairs, Leader of the opposition, the Aboriginal and Torres Strait Islander Social Justice Commissioner, Leaders of National Aboriginal Community Controlled Health Organisation (NACCHO), Congress of Aboriginal and Torres Strait Islander Nurses (CATSIN), Australian Indigenous Doctors Association (AIDA) and the Indigenous Dentists Association of Australia. During the three-day summit, targets were developed to address disparities in the morbidity and mortality of Indigenous people.

The targets are addressed under five broad categories:

1. partnerships
2. health status
3. primary healthcare and other health services
4. infrastructure, and
5. social determinants.

In his speech on 20 March 2008, Tom Calma highlighted the importance of working together to achieve the health targets; this has been further supported more recently with the Australian government allocation of funds to address inequities (Aboriginal and Torres Strait Islander Social Justice Commissioner and the Steering Committee for Indigenous Health Equality 2008).

Access to health services

Accessibility of health services is widely acknowledged as a major factor determining their use. The Australian Institute of Health and Welfare website notes:

> Overall, Indigenous Australians experience lower levels of access to health services than the general population, attributed to factors such as proximity, availability and cultural appropriateness of health services, transport availability, health insurance and health services affordability and proficiency in English (Aboriginal and Torres Strait Islander Health and Welfare Unit 2006).

The availability of transport and the distance to the nearest health service is a factor in accessibility of health services. In 2001, only 60% of Indigenous people over the age of 18 had access to, and a licence to drive, a car compared with 85% of non-Indigenous people. In rural and remote areas, 78% of discrete Indigenous communities are located more than 50 kilometres from the nearest hospital and 50% are located more than 25 kilometres from the nearest community health service (Aboriginal and Torres Strait Islander Health and Welfare Unit 2006).

Although English is the official language of Australia, many Indigenous people, particularly from very remote areas, do not speak it as their primary language. State hospitals and health services do have interpreter services available for a range of languages, but there are very few trained interpreters for Indigenous languages and there is very little written material that has been translated into Indigenous languages. Aboriginal and Torres Strait Islander health workers, liaison officers or extended family members are the key resources for providing translation services.

Aboriginal and Torres Strait Islander health services

Aboriginal and Torres Strait Islander health services have been set up to improve access to comprehensive primary healthcare services for Indigenous people. Services are funded by the Australian Government Office of Aboriginal and Torres Strait Islander Health Services (OATSIH). These comprehensive primary healthcare services can be general practice medical services, or offer a range of services to meet the social and mental health needs of Aboriginal and Torres Strait Islander people. They often work in partnership with other government and non-government organisations. Many of these services work very hard to address accessibility by providing transport services and training local Aboriginal and Torres Strait Islander people for health careers. They also place a high value on the cultural competence of their employees as a strategy to address the lack of cultural safety experienced by Aboriginal and Torres Strait Islander people when accessing mainstream services.

CULTURALLY COMPETENT NURSING PRACTICE

Nursing competency standards have developed over the last two decades to better inform the public and the profession of what can be expected from nurses in a range of practice settings. The Australian Nursing and Midwifery Council competency standards are the basis for all nursing education in Australia leading to registration with one of the state-based and territory-based Boards of Nursing and Midwifery. In addition to competency standards, nursing practice is governed by a code of ethics and a code of professional conduct. The revised code of ethics for nurses in Australia was released in August 2008 by the Australian Nursing and Midwifery Council. It clearly recognises that nurses have a responsibility to consider human rights in their care for individuals and communities.

The code of ethics outlines the profession's view of the 'critical relationship between health and human rights' and the importance of reconciliation between Aboriginal and Torres Strait Islander peoples and non-Indigenous Australians. It also states that the model of care for Aboriginal and Torres Strait Islander peoples must include physical, spiritual and cultural wellbeing as an 'expected whole'. The code of ethics explicitly states that nurses have a responsibility to provide 'just, compassionate, culturally competent and culturally responsive care to every person requiring or receiving nursing care' (Australian Nursing and Midwifery Council et al 2008). Cultural competence has been defined as a set of 'congruent behaviours, attitudes and policies that come together in a system, agency or among professionals to enable that system, agency or that group of professionals to work effectively in cross cultural situations' (National Health and Medical Research Council 2005).

CULTURAL SAFETY

Cultural safety is a term that originated in New Zealand in the 1980s (Ramsden 1992, 2002). It supports a social justice approach to healthcare and, unlike cultural competence which is generic, pertains to all cross-cultural situations. Cultural safety is specific to working in a cross-cultural context with Indigenous peoples, which is endorsed by CATSIN as being essential when providing healthcare to Aboriginal and Torres Strait Islander peoples (Indigenous Nurse Education Working Group 2002). It is a philosophy of healthcare that 'aims to improve the health of all Indigenous peoples in First World Colonised Countries, by providing culturally appropriate healthcare services' (Edwards et al 2007:62). The development of culturally safe practice requires openness, honesty, commitment and respect. It is achieved by personal reflection and understanding your own culture and values before you can meaningfully interact with Indigenous people (Ramsden 2002). There are three principles that underpin cultural safety: partnership, participation and protection.

Partnership and participation require the development of responsive service delivery models in partnership with the Indigenous people who are expected to use the service. This may be a service designed specifically for Indigenous people to reduce inequity or it may be a mainstream service. Protection is against individual, structural and institutional racism. There needs to be a recognition that Indigenous people may have had past negative experiences with the system, both as recipients of care and observers of others receiving care. There needs to be acknowledgment that language and cultural barriers may prevent meaningful exchanges and that there are variances between the concepts of health and wellness between cultures (Edwards et al 2007). Some authors identify three clearly defined steps to cultural safety: cultural awareness, cultural sensitivity and finally with a growing knowledge base, increased experience and reflection on practice, cultural safety (Eckermann et al 2006). When a health service institutes policies and protocols to ensure that consumers receive a culturally safe service, then the service is considered culturally secure (Coffin 2007).

Cultural awareness

Cultural awareness is about acknowledging that we do not all have a shared history—nor a shared understanding of the present. The culturally aware nurse is able to question the source of information and recognise the filter through which information is presented. It may be information in the news or popular press. It may be organisational or policy documents. The culturally aware nurse recognises the importance of listening. Most health services in rural and remote Australia and some government and non-government health services in urban areas have a requirement for health professionals to attend cultural awareness training on commencement of employment. This needs to be meaningful and presented by Aboriginal or Torres Strait Islander people, preferably people who are Indigenous to the area in which the health service is provided.

Cultural awareness does not develop from a generalised summary about Aboriginal and Torres Strait Islander culture, which often serves no greater function than to reinforce stereotypes. Where health services have engaged the services of an appropriate Aboriginal or Torres Strait Islander facilitator, you will find you learn most by listening. Edwards et al (2007) suggest that the first principle for working effectively with Australian Indigenous people is to 'stand back, be quiet, listen, hear and wait'. If you adopt this from your first encounter, you will find that you will learn much more than by asking to have your questions answered.

Cultural sensitivity

Cultural sensitivity is a process—a dawning. By reflecting on what you have learnt about the local Aboriginal or Torres Strait Islander community and about how your own life experiences impact on others and therefore your practice as a health professional, you gradually come to the realisation that your actions and interactions have an effect on the health of the people for whom you are caring. The culturally sensitive nurse will work to get to know the community and be respectful at all times, being open to different understandings, beliefs, values, practices and norms. In time, you may even enjoy a joke at your own expense, particularly as you realise how you have been and are perceived by others (Eckermann et al 2006, Edwards et al 2007).

PLANNING YOUR OWN JOURNEY TOWARDS CULTURAL COMPETENCE AND SAFETY

Developing into a culturally safe practitioner requires leadership on your part. It requires you to reflect on your own values and culture. It requires you never to participate in racist behaviour; it requires you to lead others around you to build a culturally safe health service, which is participative and works in partnership with Aboriginal and Torres Strait Islander people. It requires you to actively engage with the social justice agenda.

The exercise in the box on the next page is a self-assessment tool you can use to examine your cultural competence. It has been adapted from the Multicultural Disability Advocacy Association of New South Wales (MDAA) at www.mdaa.org.au/faqs/workers-mdaa.doc.

CONCLUDING REMARKS

Providing appropriate holistic nursing care to Aboriginal and Torres Strait Islander people needs to be a priority for all nurses. The health status of Indigenous Australians is negatively impacted by interpersonal and institutional racism. Developing your own cultural safety and working to make your healthcare organisation culturally secure will have a positive impact.

In this chapter, we have provided a snapshot of what it means to identify as an Aboriginal or Torres Strait Islander and where Indigenous people live. We have highlighted some of the health inequities and provided insight into the complexity of the causes. We recognise that it would be preferable to have a 'quick fix' to some of the worst problems faced by Aboriginal people living in very remote areas, and to be able to address some of the social and emotional wellbeing issues caused by racism, but in our experience there is no recipe book or instant solution. We hope you see this personal leadership journey of becoming culturally safe as a way that you can impact positively on the health of all of the Aboriginal and Torres Strait Islander people that you come across in both your personal and professional life.

REFLECTIVE QUESTIONS

1 Where would you find out who are the traditional owners of the land where you live?

2 How might you learn about the history of colonisation and the impact of past government policies on the Aboriginal or Torres Strait Islander peoples in the state or territory in which you live?

3 Write down a list of words that you would like to learn in the language of the traditional owners of the land where you live.

CULTURAL COMPETENCE SELF-TEST

Read each statement and record a number from 1 to 3 that most closely reflects what you do, or would do, when caring for someone from a culturally or linguistically different background from your own.

1 I frequently do this.   2 I occasionally do this.   3 I rarely or never do this.

MY COMMUNICATION

For people who speak languages other than English, I attempt to learn basic greetings.	1	2	3
I am competent and confident in determining the language used and in using accredited interpreters.	1	2	3
When interacting with people who have limited English proficiency, I always keep in mind that:			
• limited English does not equate with limited intellectual functioning	1	2	3
• limited English has no relation to the ability of a person to communicate in their first language.	1	2	3

OUR WORKPLACE

I seek information from people and other community contacts to assist me in adapting my practice to the diverse needs/preferences of people.	1	2	3
I attend training sessions that enhance my cultural competence.	1	2	3
All over the work environment there are posters, pictures and other materials that reflect the cultural diversity of the communities my agency serves.	1	2	3

MY VALUES

I explore my own values, beliefs, assumptions and attitudes about cultural diversity and how they impact on how I work with people using the service.	1	2	3
I avoid imposing my values.	1	2	3
In every situation, I discourage colleagues, service users and others from using racial and ethnic slurs by helping them understand the impact their language can have on others.	1	2	3

If you frequently responded 1, you are engaged in practices that recognise and promote cultural diversity and you aim to deliver a culturally competent service to people. If you found you frequently responded 2 or 3 to any of the statements, you may need to change your practices to respond more effectively to the needs of people from culturally or linguistically different backgrounds from your own. For all of the questions where you responded 2 or 3, you may want to consider how you can change your practices to be more culturally competent.

RECOMMENDED READINGS

Eckermann A-K, Dowd T, Chang E, Nixon L, Gray R, Johnson S 2006 Binan Goonj: bridging the cultures in Aboriginal health, 2nd edn. Elsevier, Sydney

Edwards T, Dade Smith J, Smith R et al 2007 Cultural perspectives In: Dade Smith J (ed.) Australia's rural and remote health: a social justice perspective, 2nd edn. Tertiary Press, Melbourne

Larson A, Gilles M, Howard PJ, Coffin J 2007 It's enough to make you sick: the impact of racism on the health of Aboriginal Australians. Australian and New Zealand Journal of Public Health 31(4):322–329

Walter M, Saggers S 2007 Poverty and social class. In: Carson B, Dunbar T, Chenall R, Baille R (eds) Social determinants of Indigenous health. Allen & Unwin, Sydney, pp 87–94

REFERENCES

Aboriginal and Torres Strait Islander Commission (ATSIC) 1998 As a matter of fact: answering the myths and misconceptions about Indigenous Australians. ATSIC, Canberra

Aboriginal and Torres Strait Islander Health and Welfare Unit 2006 Access to health services. AIHW, Canberra. Online. Available: www.aihw.gov.au/indigenous/health/access.cfm

Aboriginal and Torres Strait Islander Social Justice Commissioner 2005 Social Justice Report, 3/2005. HREOC, Canberra

Aboriginal and Torres Strait Islander Social Justice Commissioner and the Steering Committee for Indigenous Health Equality 2008 Close the gap: national Indigenous health equality targets. HREOC, Sydney

Australian Bureau of Statistics (ABS) 2003 The health and welfare of Australia's Aboriginal and Torres and Strait Islander peoples. AIHW, Canberra

Australian Bureau of Statistics (ABS) 2005a The health and welfare of Australia's Aboriginal and Torres Strait Islander peoples. ABS, Canberra

Australian Bureau of Statistics (ABS) 2005b Year book Australia 2005. 1301.0. ABS, Canberra

Australian Bureau of Statistics (ABS) 2006 National Aboriginal and Torres Strait Islander health survey 2004–05. ABS, Canberra

Australian Bureau of Statistics (ABS), Australian Institute of Health and Welfare (AIHW) 2008 The health and welfare of Australia's Aboriginal and Torres Strait Islander peoples 2008. AIHW, Canberra

Australian Nursing and Midwifery Council (ANMC), Royal College of Nursing Australia (RCN), Australian Nursing Federation (ANF) 2008 Code of ethics for nurses in Australia. ANMC, RCN and ANF, Canberra

Cahoone L 2003 From modernism to postmodernism: an anthology, expanded 2nd edn. Blackwell, Cambridge

Cobo JRM 1983 Study of the problem of discrimination against Indigenous populations. United Nations, Geneva

Coffin J 2007 Rising to the challenge of Aboriginal health by creating cultural security. Aboriginal and Islander Health Worker Journal 31(3):22–24

Eades SJ 2000 Reconciliation, social equity and Indigenous health. Medical Journal of Australia 172:468–469

Eckermann A-K, Dowd T, Chang E, Nixon L, Gray R, Johnson S 2006 Binan Goonj: bridging the cultures in Aboriginal health, 2nd edn. Elsevier, Sydney

Edwards T, Dade Smith J, Smith R et al 2007 Cultural perspectives. In: Dade Smith J (ed.) Australia's rural and remote health: a social justice perspective, 2nd edn. Tertiary Press, Melbourne

Gardiner-Garden J 2000 Research policy note 18: 2000–01. The definition of Aboriginality. Social Policy Group, Canberra

Henry B, Houston S, Mooney G 2004 Institutional racism in Australian health care: a plea for decency. Medical Journal of Australia 180(10):517–520

Hunter E 1993 Aboriginal health and history. Cambridge University Press, Melbourne

Indigenous Nurse Education Working Group (INEWG) 2002 Getting 'em 'n' keepin' 'em: report of the Indigenous Nursing Education Working Group to the Commonwealth Department of Health and Ageing Office for Aboriginal and Torres Strait Islander Health, September 2002 INEWG, Canberra

Larson A 2006 Rural health's demographic destiny. Rural and Remote Health 6(551):1–8

Larson A, Gilles M, Howard P et al 2007 It's enough to make you sick: the impact of racism on the health of Aboriginal Australians. Australian and New Zealand Journal of Public Health 31(4):322–329

Marmot M, Wilkinson RG 1999 Social determinants of health. Oxford University Press, New York

National Health and Medical Research Council (NHMRC) 2005 Cultural competency in health: a guide for policy, partnership and participation. NHMRC, Canberra

Paradies Y 2006 A systematic review of empirical research on self reported racism. International Journal of Epidemiology 35(4):888–901

Ramsden I 1992 Kawa Whakaruruhau: guidelines for nursing and midwifery education. Nursing Council of New Zealand, Wellington

Ramsden I 2002 Cultural safety and nursing education in Aotearoa and Te Waipounamu. Victoria University, Wellington

Saggers S, Gray D 2007 Defining what we mean. In: Carson B, Dunbar T, Chenall R (eds) Social determinants of Indigenous health. Allen & Unwin, Sydney

Standing Committee on Aboriginal and Torres Strait Islander Health and Statistical Information Management Committee 2006 National summary of the 2003 and 2004 jurisdictional reports against the Aboriginal and Torres Strait Islander health performance indicators. AIHW cat. no. IHW16. AIHW, Canberra

Turrell G, Mathers C 2000 Socioeconomic status and health in Australia. Medical Journal of Australia 172:434–438

Walter M, Saggers S 2007 Poverty and social class. In: Carson B, Dunbar T, Chenall R, Baille R (eds) Social determinants of Indigenous health. Allen & Unwin, Sydney, pp 87–94

Zubrick SR, Lawrence DM, Silburn SR, Blair E, Milroy H, Wilkes T, Eades S, D'Antoine H, Ishigushi P, Doyle S 2004 The Western Australian Aboriginal child health survey: the health of Aboriginal children and young people. Telethon Institute for Child Health Research, Perth

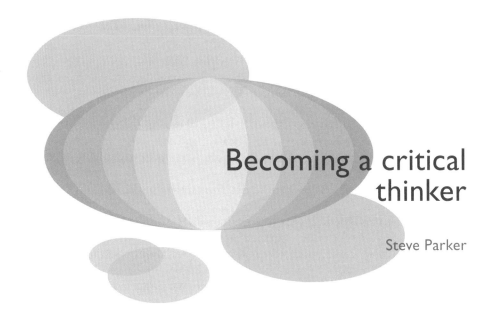

CHAPTER 21

Becoming a critical thinker

Steve Parker

LEARNING OBJECTIVES

At the completion of this chapter, the student will be able to:

* describe the essential nature of critical thinking
* describe the main characteristics of a critical thinker
* explain the basic structure of an argument
* apply the basic structure of an argument to various areas of nursing practice, and
* identify resources for further reading and the study of critical thinking.

KEY WORDS

Thinking, reflection, action, evaluation, argument, induction, premise, nursing process, decision making

WHAT IS CRITICAL THINKING?

There are a variety of definitions of critical thinking and no consensus on any one of them (Riddell 2007). This situation means we need to be careful about relying on any one definition. In essence, however, critical thinking refers to the activity of *questioning what is usually taken for granted*.

Whether we are aware of it or not, all behaviour is based on certain values, assumptions and beliefs. These form the basis for our decisions to act in certain ways. In a professional context such as nursing practice, everything that we think, say or do is the result of a complex web of beliefs, values and assumptions that have formed as a result of our life experiences. As we grow up in our family, attend school, participate in religious communities, associate with friends, watch television, read newspapers, and work for various employers, we develop a 'pair of spectacles' through which we understand and interpret the world and all that happens in it. Just as a person who wears glasses eventually becomes unaware that they are even wearing them, so too each of us adjusts to our worldview 'spectacles' until, often, we are completely unaware what values, beliefs and assumptions are influencing us in a specific situation.

Critical thinking means stopping and reflecting on the reasons for doing things the way they are done or for experiencing things the way they are—focusing on what is frequently taken for granted and evaluating the values, beliefs and assumptions that are held, and asking whether or not what is done and thought is justifiable or not. These characteristics of critical thinking imply a self-consciousness of what, how and why we are thinking, with the intention of improving thinking. In short, 'critical thinking is thinking about your thinking while you're thinking in order to make your thinking better' (Paul 2008). Improving thinking is essential because it is intimately related to the many decisions that need to be made each day. The quality of our lives is determined by the quality of our decisions, and the quality of our decisions is determined by the quality of our reasoning (Schick & Vaughn 1995). In particular, '[i]f nurses are to deal effectively with complex change, increased demands and greater accountability, they must become skilled in higher level thinking and reasoning abilities' (Simpson & Courtney 2002:89).

An important aspect of critical thinking is healthy scepticism. This scepticism is necessary because there are many attempts to persuade people to accept various claims. These attempts to persuade also occur in professional contexts. For example, research reports suggest changes to practice; peers argue that their way of acting is the right one; therapists promote various interventions; administrators argue that certain changes need to be made to the workplace; and so on. Often these claims are contradictory, so they cannot all be acceptable.

Practitioners need to sort through all these, often competing, claims. To accept them all without question will, at best, be highly confusing and, at worst, may endanger the lives of others if actions are based on wrong information or conclusions. To adopt an attitude of healthy scepticism means to cautiously listen to or read the claims that others make, carefully evaluating their legitimacy, and not rushing to accept a conclusion without careful thought.

The same rigorous thinking needs to be done about our own nursing practice. We make decisions every moment, which we assume are of benefit to our patients. Asking questions about the practices we engage in, including what evidence is available to support their efficacy, is essential if our nursing practice is to produce positive outcomes for those for whom we care.

It is possible, of course, to become too pedantic, resulting in inaction because we are not prepared to accept anything unless it is 100% proven. This is why the scepticism needs to be healthy. There is a limit to what can be known for certain. And part of critical thinking is knowing these limits and making the best evaluation under the circumstances.

THE RELATIONSHIP BETWEEN CRITICAL AND CREATIVE THINKING

Critical thinking is not the same as creative thinking. According to Miller and Babcock (1996:117), creative thinking is, among other things, more divergent, messy, unpredictable, provocative, spontaneous and playful than critical thinking. They describe critical thinking as selective, orderly, predictable, analytical, judgmental and evaluative.

Creative thinking, although different from critical thinking, is an essential, complementary process to critical thinking. As a practitioner, there are many situations that arise that do not fit with the ideal or that are not predictable. No individual person for whom nurses care ever fits the 'average' because each person and situation is unique. In order to solve problems for these unique situations and individuals, the practitioner needs to be able to develop new approaches and solutions so that all parties have their needs met. Miller and Babcock suggest that:

> Creative thinking is very useful when what we know and what we know how to do are not working, including the rules of reason, common sense, gravity, and routine. The creative thinker is willing to think wildly, without having any idea where her or his path of thinking may lead. Deliberative cognition is temporarily held in abeyance (Miller & Babcock 1996:120).

Because creative thinking is so 'chaotic' it means that it needs to be evaluated to ensure that any conclusions that are reached are appropriate. In this regard, Ruggiero understands the mind to have two phases:

> It both produces ideas and judges them. These phases are intertwined; that is, we move back and forth between them many times in the course of dealing with a problem, sometimes several times in the span of a few seconds (Ruggiero 1998:81).

In the past, critical thinking has often been presented apart from creative thinking. However, in practice, creative and critical thinking go hand-in-hand. Without creative thinking, critical thinking would be dry and mechanical. Without critical thinking, creative thinking would be chaotic and inefficient. As Ruggiero (1998:81) asserts, '[t]o study the art of thinking in its most dynamic form [where creative and critical thinking are intertwined] would be difficult at best'. Consequently, in practice, we need to consider them separately. However, although critical thinking and creative thinking are distinct from each other, they should never be separated.

THE CHARACTERISTICS OF CRITICAL THINKING

So what are the characteristics that a critical thinker will demonstrate? Jacobs et al (1997) have developed a set of observable skills that indicate the presence of critical thinking. These are grouped into categories, as described below.

First, a critical thinker needs the ability to integrate information from all relevant sources by being able to distinguish between relevant and irrelevant data, validate data that are obtained, recognise when data are missing, predict multiple outcomes, and recognise the consequences of actions.

Second, to think critically means to be able to examine assumptions by recognising them when they are present, detect bias, identify assumptions that are not stated, recognise the relationships of action or inaction, and transfer thoughts and concepts to diverse contexts, or develop alternative courses of action.

Third, it is important for the critical thinker to be able to identify relationships and patterns. This includes recognising inconsistencies or fallacies of logic, working out generalisations, developing a plan of action consistent with a model, and, where appropriate, seeking out alternative models.

Jacobs et al offer a definition of critical thinking that incorporates all these characteristics:

> Critical thinking is the repeated examination of problems, questions, issues, and situations by comparing, simplifying, synthesizing information in an analytical, deliberative, evaluative, decisive way (Jacobs et al 1997:20).

Many more examples of various ways of describing the characteristics of critical thinking could be offered. One way of summarising these is to focus on critical thinking as reasoning. The heart of reasoning is the argument. In what follows, the nature of argument will be described, followed by a survey of the ways in which arguments 'appear' in nursing. Suggestions will then be offered regarding the way in which the principles of critical thinking might be applied in these areas. By doing so, the way in which this approach synthesises the skills of critical thinking will become obvious.

WHAT IS AN ARGUMENT?

In colloquial language the word 'argument' is often used for a shouting match between two people who are having a disagreement where the participants are very angry, abusive or physically aggressive. There may be shouting, pointing of fingers, threats, crying, name-calling, and so on.

However, in critical thinking, the term 'argument' does not apply to these situations. In fact, these situations are the very opposite of critical thinking. In critical thinking, an argument consists of a conclusion and one or more reasons that are intended to support the conclusion. Figure 21.1 shows the relationship between these parts of an argument. Each reason may or may not have evidence that is intended to support the reason or reasons.

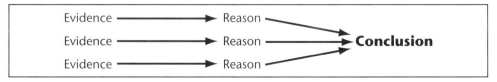

Figure 21.1 Components of an argument

Here is an example of an argument:

Every person has the right to choose how they live their lives. Therefore, a person has the right to choose to practise life-threatening behaviours if they wish.

This is an argument because it has a conclusion ('A person has the right to choose to practise life-threatening behaviours if they wish') and a reason intended to support that conclusion ('Every person has the right to choose how they live their lives'). At this stage, we are not concerned whether this is a good argument or not, only with what makes something an argument. If it were desirable, a person presenting this argument could provide some evidence for the first statement by drawing attention, for example, to various statements of human rights, the constitutions of countries, or discussions about ethics. So an argument needs to have the following:

- a conclusion, and
- one or more reasons intended to support the conclusion.

WHAT MAKES A SOUND ARGUMENT?

For an argument to be sound, three criteria need to be met. First, the reasons need to be acceptable to the person evaluating the argument. Second, the reasons need to be relevant. And, third, the reasons need to provide adequate grounds for accepting the conclusion. Govier (1992) offers a useful way to remember these three criteria, which she calls the conditions of argument. If the first three letters of the word argument (ARG) are taken on their own, each letter stands for one of the conditions of argument. That is:

A   Acceptability
R   Relevance
G   Grounds

Govier's definitions of each of these conditions are also useful:

- **Acceptability**: The premises [reasons] are acceptable when it is reasonable for those to whom the argument is addressed to believe these premises. There is good reason to accept the premises—even if they are not known for certain to be true. And there is no good evidence known to those to whom the argument is addressed that would indicate either that the premises are false or that they are doubtful.
- **Relevance**: [Premises are relevant to the conclusion] when they give at least some evidence in favor of the conclusion's being true. They specify factors, evidence, or reasons that do count toward establishing the conclusion. They do not merely describe distracting aspects that lead you away from the real topic with which the argument is supposed to be dealing or that do not tend to support the conclusion.
- **Grounds**: The premises provide sufficient or good grounds for the conclusion. In other words, considered together, the premises give sufficient reason to make it rational to accept the conclusion. This statement means more than that the premises are relevant. Not only do they count as evidence for the conclusion, they provide enough evidence, or enough reasons, taken together, to make it reasonable to accept the conclusion (Govier 1992:68–69).

The following example illustrates these criteria:

Nurses must have a practising certificate to be employed as a nurse.
Sue does not have a practising certificate.
Therefore, Sue is not permitted to be employed as a nurse.

Statements 1 and 2 are both reasons, which are intended to support the conclusion in Statement 3. If this is a sound argument, then the reasons must be relevant and acceptable, and they must provide adequate grounds for accepting the conclusion.

Statement 1 is certainly acceptable. Most countries have a requirement that nurses need to be licensed to practise. Statement 2 is hypothetical, so we will assume that it is true for the sake of the discussion. All the reasons, then, are acceptable. The two reasons are also relevant to the issue under consideration.

The next question is whether these reasons provide adequate grounds for accepting the conclusion. We can test this by asking:

Is it possible to reject the conclusion and still believe the reasons to be true? Or, in other words, even though the reasons are true, is there a legitimate way that we can escape accepting the conclusion?

In other words, could one believe that Sue could practise and still believe that the two reasons offered are true? In this case, the answer is no. If it is true that a nurse must have a practising certificate to practise, and Sue does not have one, we are 'compelled' to accept the conclusion that Sue cannot practise. This argument, then, is a sound one.

Another example will illustrate a poor argument:

Everyone's hair falls out when undergoing chemotherapy.
Jo is undergoing chemotherapy.
Therefore, Jo's hair will fall out.

First, are the reasons acceptable? Does a person's hair fall out when they are undergoing chemotherapy? Sometimes it does, but not necessarily everyone's. So this reason is not acceptable because, although some people's hair falls out, not everyone's does. For the sake of this discussion, the second reason can be accepted (that Jo is undergoing chemotherapy).

Both of the reasons are relevant, and so the final question is whether the reasons offered provide adequate grounds for accepting that Jo's hair will fall out. The answer is no because the first reason was false. Although it might be true that Jo's hair will fall out, it is not possible to predict it because not everyone's hair does when they are undergoing chemotherapy.

To summarise:

- An argument consists of a conclusion, with one or more relevant reasons that are intended to support the conclusion.
- Evidence may or may not be offered to support each reason.
- A sound argument is one in which the reason(s) are acceptable and provide adequate grounds for accepting the conclusion.

There are a few technical terms that need to be remembered in regard to what has been covered so far.

- A *reason* can also be called a *premise*.
- The question of whether reasons provide grounds for the conclusion is a question of *validity*. In everyday conversation, the word validity often has a broader meaning. In critical thinking, it is used to refer to the logical relationship between the reasons and the conclusion.
- When an argument has reasons that are acceptable and is valid (i.e. the reasons provide adequate grounds for accepting the conclusion), then the argument is said to be *sound*.

It is important to note that an argument can be valid but unsound. For example, the following argument is valid but unsound:

All nurses are female.
Jo is a nurse.
Therefore, Jo is female.

Statement 1 is not true, of course. Some nurses are male. Statement 2 can be assumed to be true. Because Statement 1 is false, we already know that this argument is unsound. But is it valid? Yes it is. If Statement 1 were true, the acceptance of Statement 3 would be unavoidable. This means that the argument is logically valid, but it is not sound—that is, it is not a sound argument.

CRITICAL THINKING IN NURSING

Critical thinking, in essence, means being able to identify the presence of an argument in any form and evaluate it. Once what makes a sound argument, and the questions needed to be asked to evaluate it, are known, it is possible to assess any argument that is encountered. Critical thinking means applying to this task thinking that has the characteristics discussed above.

This basic approach can be applied to many areas within nursing. In the following sections, some examples of these areas will be surveyed, how the basic framework introduced above applies to that area will be discussed, and some guidelines for thinking critically about issues in the respective area will be offered. The overlaying of the structure of argument onto the various areas in nursing builds on the work of Mayer and Goodchild (1995) in their discussion of critical thinking in psychology.

Clinical practice

In clinical practice, decisions are constantly being made to act in certain ways for the benefit of clients. These actions can be beneficial or have serious consequences for the health and wellbeing of the people a nurse is working for or with. It is essential that these interventions be considered critically. Figure 21.2 illustrates the application of the basic argument framework to clinical practice.

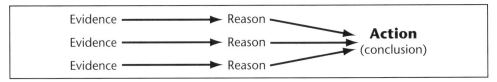

Figure 21.2 The basic argument framework applied to clinical practice

As can be seen, very little alteration is necessary. The equivalent of the conclusion is the particular action that has been, or will be, performed. Each of a nurse's actions should be able to be justified by appealing to an appropriate set of reasons. These reasons, in turn, must be based on high-quality evidence.

In the past, many of the actions and interventions of nurses have been based on tradition, folklore, or no evidence at all. In recent years, however, the developing professional status of nursing has resulted in more concern about the basis for nursing action. There is a growing and strengthening movement called evidence-based practice, which promotes an attitude of thinking critically about what is done by nurses and asking on what basis can actions be justified.

The increasing interest of consumers in their own healthcare has also had an effect. People are no longer willing to allow health professionals to make all the decisions for them and are demanding higher quality care. The increasing incidence of litigation has also motivated a concern for basing nursing action on high-quality evidence.

On an individual level, a nurse should be able to justify any action performed on behalf of a client. The reasons need to be based on solid evidence. The source of this evidence may take many forms, including personal experience, traditions handed down between 'generations' of nurses, and what is taught during nurse education. However, on their own, these sources of knowledge are not adequate. A formal process for exploring nursing knowledge is needed, which allows the testing of ideas and the validation of actions and interventions.

The activity of formal research provides this opportunity. Nursing research will be examined below from a critical thinking perspective. First, however, there are a number of questions that can be asked about practice, which will help nurses think critically about it. When reflecting on an action or intervention, ask the following questions:

- What are the reasons for acting or intervening in the way that is planned?
- What evidence is available that supports the reasons for acting in this way?
- Are the reasons relevant to the issue that is being considered?
- Are there other reasons that need to be considered?
- Is there any evidence that raises questions about the manner of acting or intervening?
- Do the reasons provide adequate grounds for acting in the planned way?
- Are there alternative actions or interventions that could be chosen and the reasons still be acceptable in these situations?

The nursing process

The nursing process is a common framework for making practice decisions in nursing; therefore, it will be briefly explored in relation to critical thinking. The steps of the nursing process are:

1. collection of subjective and objective data
2. arrival at a diagnosis of the client's problem(s)
3. planning of appropriate nursing interventions in response to the problem(s)
4. implementation of the planned intervention(s), and
5. ongoing evaluation of the effectiveness of the intervention(s) in relation to the client's problem(s).

The nursing process can be summarised in three 'phases':

1. diagnosis
2. intervention, and
3. evaluation.

Each of these three phases can be understood as an argument (remember the technical meaning of the term argument). Figure 21.3 illustrates this.

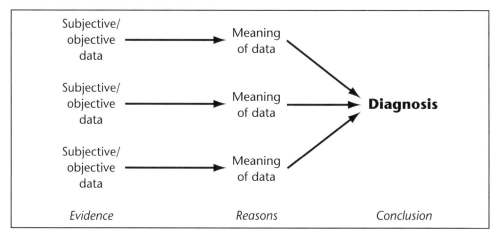

Figure 21.3 The three phases of nursing represented as an argument

The diagnosis is the equivalent of the conclusion in an argument. The data that are collected come from observations of the patient, as well as information provided by the client, relatives, friends, history, and so on. These raw data need to be interpreted and take on meaning in the context of developing a diagnosis. Finally, on the basis of the meaning of the data, a conclusion is arrived at in the form of a diagnosis.

Of course, the description here is somewhat simplistic. The actual process is much richer and more complex than this. However, understanding the process of diagnosis as an argument leads us to ask questions such as the following:

- Are the data collected accurate? If not, how reliable are they?
- Have the data been understood and interpreted correctly?
- Are the data and their interpretation relevant to the diagnosis that has been chosen?
- Does the interpretation of the data provide adequate grounds for arriving at the diagnosis?
- Are there any other diagnoses that could possibly fit the data that have been collected? Are any of these more consistent with the data?

A similar process applies to the intervention and evaluation phases. Interventions and evaluation criteria must be justified to support claims of improvement, deterioration or preservation of the status quo. Figures 21.4 and 21.5 illustrate the structure of argument related to these two phases.

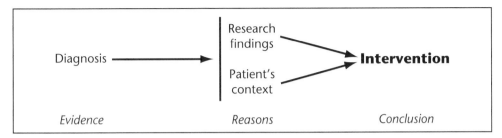

Figure 21.4 The structure of argument: intervention

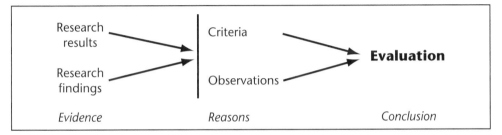

Figure 21.5 The structure of argument: evaluation

Thinking critically about research

The need for nursing research and the current focus on evidence-based practice has been described above. Nursing research provides the evidence nurses need to evaluate the appropriateness of nursing practice, helps to raise new questions for nurses to explore, and provokes new ways of looking at what nurses do.

Nurses may relate to research in three ways. A nurse may be a 'consumer' of research, a researcher, or both. In this discussion, we will be focusing particularly on the role of research consumer.

It has already been argued that nurses must base their practice on high-quality evidence. The results of nursing research form the most significant source of this evidence for nurse practitioners. Nurses must avail themselves of the latest research in their area of practice, and this means that some understanding of the process is important.

Every research project suffers from limitations and flaws of some sort or another. So nurses cannot take a research report and automatically assume that it provides them with the best guidance for practice. The nurse needs to think critically about research reports. Understanding a research report to be an argument assists in thinking critically about the conclusions it draws (Mayer & Goodchild 1995). Mayer and Goodchild (1995) discuss the way in which any research can be understood as an argument. Figure 21.6 illustrates this approach.

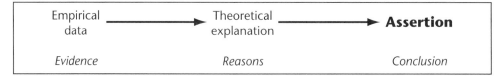

Figure 21.6 Understanding research as an argument

Given this understanding, it is possible to formulate a number of questions to help think critically about research:

- What is the assertion that is being made in the research report? What type of assertion is it? What type of evidence would be needed to be convinced of the truth of the assertion?
- What sort of evidence is offered to support the assertion being made? Is the evidence relevant to the assertion being made? Is adequate information provided to convince the reader that the evidence has been collected rigorously?
- Does the evidence offered provide adequate grounds for accepting the assertion that is being made? Is it possible to think of any other conclusions that could be drawn from the evidence offered? Are these alternative solutions more reasonable than the assertion made in the report?
- Does the theoretical explanation make sense? Are there alternative explanations that make more sense? Does the application of Occam's Razor (the principle that the simplest explanation is most likely to be the right one) make any difference to the likelihood of the explanation being correct?

Asking these questions in relation to any research report heightens one's awareness that the conclusions of research are not always correct, nor is the process in arriving at that conclusion automatically sound. This promotes a careful assessment of new nursing practice proposals and consequent higher levels of safety in practice.

Thinking about ethics

Another essential area of which nurses need to be aware is ethics. Thinking ethically means to be able to justify what is done in terms of ethical principles. All behaviour needs to be ethical. Although there are high-profile issues such as euthanasia, abortion and organ transplantation that demand a great deal of attention, they are, perhaps, not the most important issues for nurses.

Issues such as the style of communicating with a patient, the facilitation of the signing of a consent form, communication with other professional colleagues and patients, the management of work rosters, the provision of childcare for employees, the influencing of clients in choosing treatment options—all need to be considered in ethical terms if the individual nurse is to practise with integrity and fulfil his or her obligations to clients.

Most professional bodies have documented codes of ethics and the nursing profession is no different. For example, the Code of Ethics for Nurses in Australia (Australian Nursing & Midwifery Council 2008) contains eight value statements for nurses to use as 'a guide when reflecting on the degree to which their clinical, managerial, educational or research practice demonstrates and upholds those values'. As the code points out, however:

> [A] code does not provide a formula for the resolution of ethical issues, nor can it adequately address the definition and exploration of terms, concepts and practical issues that are part of the broader study of nursing, ethics and human rights. Nurses have a responsibility to develop their knowledge and understanding of ethics and human rights in order to clarify issues relevant to their practice and to inform their response to the issues identified.

Because of this, nurses need to develop skills to be able to think through these issues and evaluate various options for practice. Understanding ethical thinking as an argument can help in this task. Figure 21.7 illustrates the components of an ethical argument. Each of these components will now be examined in relation to critical thinking.

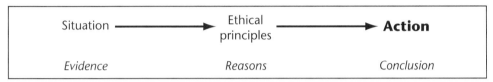

Figure 21.7   The components of an ethical argument

The situation

Ethical thinking is often taught using highly controversial case studies that involve an often unresolvable dilemma between competing principles. However, a number of false impressions may be gained from this. One possible false impression is that 'the continued use of controversial examples serves to exaggerate the extent to which morality, as distinct from moral theory, is controversial' (Coope 1996).

In reality, ethical thinking should pervade all activities, and ethical questions about practice should be continually asked. Ethical thinking should be an everyday activity, which may not always be about problems.

We usually find ourselves in situations where a decision needs to be made about how to act towards another person. These situations continually occur for nurses. For example, a patient might require a sponge in bed. This may not appear to be a situation where ethical thinking needs to take place. But, as this example is explored below, it will be seen that ethical thinking is fundamental to ensuring that the best care is provided.

The first thing to do when thinking ethically is to be aware of as much about the situation as is possible. Too often assumptions are made on the basis of past experience; but every person is different and has unique needs.

The principles

Everyone has a system of principles (values) which guide their lives and how they act. Some of these will be conscious; others may be unconscious. In healthcare, four principles have been identified as an essential starting point for ethical thinking. They are:

1. **Autonomy**: the right a person has to direct their own life and make their own decisions.

2. **Beneficence**: the responsibility of actively doing good.
3. **Non-maleficence**: the responsibility to actively avoid doing harm.
4. **Justice**: the responsibility to be fair in the way we treat others.

After gaining a knowledge of the situation, the next step is to ask which of the principles (values) are relevant to consider in the particular situation in which the nurse finds themselves. In the example of the person who needs to be washed in bed, the issue of autonomy is clearly relevant. How is autonomy to be ensured in this particular situation? How will the patient be empowered to make their own decisions about their hygiene and the way they wish to maintain it?

The principle of beneficence is also relevant. The whole reason for instituting the patient washing in bed is because it is believed it is good to promote hygiene. It is possible, however, that beneficence may spill over into a denial of the person's autonomy. When this happens, nurses are acting paternalistically—doing what they think is best for the patient—even if the patient does not agree with the nurse. Paternalism needs to be rigorously justified because it overrides a person's fundamental right to autonomy.

Many examples can be found of situations where paternalism occurs: imposing medication on a psychotic individual; or legally enforcing a blood transfusion for a child of a Jehovah's Witness parent. Unfortunately, on many occasions paternalistic attitudes prevail without adequate ethical justification.

Action
Once the situation is understood and the implications of the relevant ethical principles have been thought through, it is necessary to make a decision about how to act. Often this will not be easy. Sometimes, ethical principles conflict with each other (such as when beneficence and autonomy conflict). Nurses do not live and practice in an ideal world, and so it is necessary to be satisfied with the best decision that can be made under the circumstances. The point is not that perfect decisions have to be made; that is never possible. It is rather that whatever decisions are made and whatever actions are performed, they have been carefully thought through and can be justified by appeal to accepted ethical principles.

The ethics of critical thinking
Often, when people learn the tools of critical thinking, they become highly critical of others. It is important that critical thinking be viewed primarily as a set of tools applied to one's own thinking. When evaluating the ideas of others, critical thinking skills are used to decide whether an idea is acceptable or should be rejected. Who the other person is, is usually irrelevant. And when critical thinking skills undermine or attack other people, then the purpose of critical thinking is lost. One of the most important distinctions to remember is that between an idea and the person who presents the idea.

The critical thinker always needs to think critically within the framework of well-developed interpersonal relationship skills. Critical thinking skills are not weapons to be wielded to cut another person down to size. They are tools of personal growth, which allow one to travel through an often confusing landscape and keep one's bearings, while providing the best possible quality care for those to whom one is responsible and accountable.

USING SOFTWARE TO PRACTISE REASONING

It takes considerable practice to become accomplished at reasoning and evaluating arguments. There are quite a few software packages available that can help visualise arguments and aid in the process of analysis. One of the best of these is Rationale, which allows you to create diagrams of arguments and your evaluation. Figure 21.8 shows a diagram, produced by Rationale, of the argument about hair loss following chemotherapy described above.

You can download a trial version of this software from http://rationale.austhink.com.

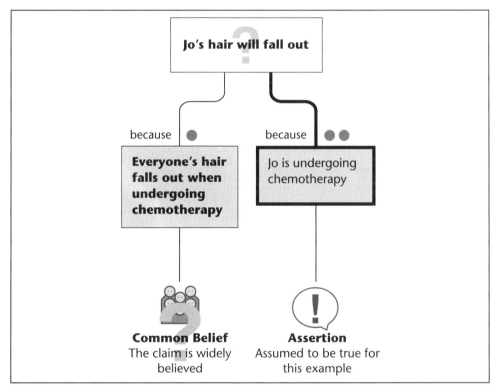

Figure 21.8 The argument about hair loss following chemotherapy

DEVELOPING CRITICAL THINKING SKILLS

There is no magical solution to actually developing critical thinking skills. An awareness of what critical thinking is and where it can be applied is an appropriate start. Like anything, it requires continual practice. Ultimately, it is about developing a conscious attitude of reflection during daily and professional life. Halpern (1998) suggests a number of attitudes and dispositions that support the development of critical thinking. They are: willingness to plan; flexibility; persistence; willingness to self-correct; being mindful ('the habit of self-conscious concern for and evaluation of the thinking process'); and consensus-seeking. As Halpern says:

No one can become a better thinker just by reading a book. An essential component of critical thinking is developing the attitude and disposition of a critical thinker.

Good thinkers are motivated and willing to exert the conscious effort needed to work in a planful manner, to check for accuracy, to gather information, and to persist when the solution is not obvious or requires several steps (Halpern 1998:10–11).

Although it is hard work to develop new skills in critical thinking, the time and energy are well worth the rewards that come with the ability to think clearly.

CONCLUDING REMARKS

Critical thinking is a vital skill to have as a nurse. Nurses are engaged in providing care to people who have a right to high-quality professional conduct and health services. Nurses have a responsibility to make sure that their actions are based on rigorous evidence and can be justified with acceptable reasons. Although developing the skills to think critically may at times be difficult and demanding, thinking critically provides a greater level of confidence and satisfaction as nurses interact with colleagues, and it promotes high-quality, safe practice.

REFLECTIVE QUESTIONS

1 How has your understanding of thinking changed as a result of reading this chapter?

2 What areas of your professional life would benefit from applying the principles of critical thinking to them?

3 What will you do now to further develop your skill in critical thinking?

RECOMMENDED READINGS

Bandman EL, Bandman B 1998 Critical thinking in nursing, 2nd edn. Appleton & Lange, Norwalk, Connecticut

Browne MN, Keeley SM 2006 Asking the right questions, 8th edn. Prentice Hall, New Jersey

Miller A, Babcock DE 1996 Critical thinking applied to nursing. Mosby, St Louis (currently out of print but check your library)

Paul RG, Elder L 2002 Critical thinking: tools for taking charge of your professional and personal life. Prentice Hall, New Jersey

Rubenfeld MG 2006 Critical thinking in nursing: an interactive approach. JB Lippincott, Philadelphia

REFERENCES

Australian Nursing and Midwifery Council (ANMC) 2008 Codes of professional conduct and ethics for nurses and midwives. ANMC, Canberra

Coope C 1996 Does teaching by cases mislead us about morality? Journal of Medical Ethics 22(1):46–52

Govier T 1992 A practical study of argument, 3rd edn. Wadsworth, Belmont, California

Halpern D 1998 Critical thinking across the curriculum: a brief edition of thought and knowledge. Lawrence Erlbaum Associates, Mahweh, New Jersey

Jacobs P, Ott B, Sullivan B, Ulrich Y, Short L 1997 An approach to defining and operationalizing critical thinking. Journal of Nursing Education 36(1):19–22

Mayer R, Goodchild F 1995 The critical thinker, 2nd edn. Brown & Benchmark Publishers, Madison

Miller M, Babcock D 1996 Critical thinking applied to nursing. Mosby, St Louis

Paul R 2008 Critical thinking: basic questions and answers. Foundation for Critical Thinking. Online. Available: www.criticalthinking.org/aboutCT/CTquestionsAnswers.cfm 18 Oct 2008

Riddell T 2007 Critical assumptions: thinking critically about critical thinking. Journal of Nursing Education 46(3):121–126

Ruggiero V 1998 The art of thinking: a guide to critical and creative thought, 5th edn. Longman, New York

Schick T, Vaughn L 1995 How to think about weird things: critical thinking for a new age. Mayfield Publishing Company, Mountain View, California

Simpson E, Courtney M 2002 Critical thinking in nursing education: a literature review. International Journal of Nursing Practice 8:89–98

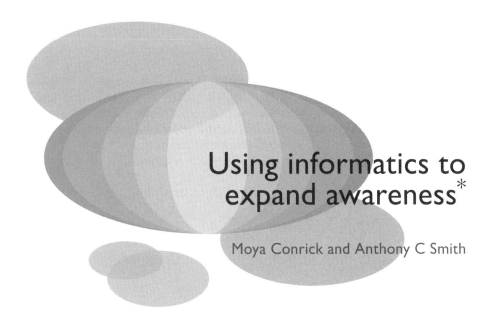

CHAPTER 22

Using informatics to expand awareness*

Moya Conrick and Anthony C Smith

LEARNING OBJECTIVES

At the completion of this chapter, the reader should be able to:

- articulate and discuss the major concepts underpinning informatics
- critically reflect on informatics as a tool of nursing practice
- assess and critically reflect on the automation of nursing and health data
- critically evaluate the infostructure requirements for nursing information systems, and
- appreciate the importance of knowledge management in nursing at a beginning level.

*I was most grateful for the opportunity to co-author this book chapter alongside an author renowned for her passion and vision in the area of nursing informatics. Dr Moya Conrick was one of the founders of health informatics in Australia, a pioneer in nursing informatics and a leader internationally. Sadly, Dr Conrick passed away on 30 January 2008. This book chapter is dedicated in her honour.

KEY WORDS

Health informatics, e-health, nursing informatics, knowledge management, current awareness, electronic health records, infostructure

---

NURSING AND INFORMATION TECHNOLOGY

The health industry faces many challenges—because the health sector is complex and fragmented, involves multiple levels of government, numerous individuals and a large number of private sector organisations. Health services are becoming more expensive, and the demand on health services is growing due to factors such as the ageing population, the increasing burden of chronic disease, and the costs of new methods of diagnosis and treatment (Armstrong et al 2007, Conrick 2006).

In a report by the Australian Department of Finance and Administration (2006), national spending on information and communication technology (ICT) is about $5 billion a year, while ICT expenditure in the Australian healthcare industry is estimated at $2 billion per year, which seems to be an indication by government policy makers that ICT is a useful resource in efforts to improve patient care and deliver quality health outcomes (Conrick et al 2004). Automation has much to offer healthcare workers and, indeed, the last ten years have seen the beginnings of a transformation in healthcare, triggered by a rapid rise in the use of information technology across all areas of healthcare and the rapid increase in the sophistication of information systems. While health administration was an early adopter of information technology, and new technology for diagnostic and treatment purposes is becoming commonplace, investment in systems and strategies to support clinicians lags well behind. Clinicians usually have to navigate myriad paperwork and often make decisions based on fragmented and poor-quality data.

There is potential for information technology to be used for the storage and delivery of health information, especially between clinicians, which in turn may contribute to better patient outcomes and reduction in errors, by delivering timely clinical information quickly and at the point-of-care in a form that can be read and understood. It also empowers clinicians by providing them with the tools of evidence-based decision making, with the deployment of knowledge databases and information repositories. Leonard et al (2004) suggest that information technology has the ability to address the communication failures that account for approximately 70% of causes of sentinel events reported to the Joint Commission for Hospital Accreditation. In retrospect, however, caution should be taken with the use of ICT, as some reports have emerged which suggest that the risk of errors (such as in medication prescribing) could increase in some circumstances due to inaccurate data entry (Magrabi et al 2007).

Information technology eases the burden of gathering and manipulating large amounts of data and can reduce repetition. Provided that appropriate protocols and standards are in place, computers manipulate complex data quickly and are able to communicate seamlessly across the health system. This supports the efficient collection and sharing of comprehensive, quality health information that can be used to improve the delivery of health services across populations. One only has to look at the changes in communications since the development of the internet to realise that information technology has permanently transformed the way in which we communicate. A simple example is that of the telephone with alpha designations, which allow short message services (SMS) to be sent to other telephones. Communication via SMS has become so widespread it is estimated around 10 billion messages are sent each year in Australia.

The benefits of SMS in the healthcare sector are very promising. In the United Kingdom, the National Health Service sends routine SMS to patients to make them aware of visits, follow-up or changes to appointments. According to work reported in Australia by Downer et al (2005), SMS reminders sent to patients prior to their scheduled outpatient appointment has a similar impact to standard telephone reminders, but was much more economical due to the ability to send large volumes of customised messages in one instance.

This chapter expands health professionals' awareness of informatics as a tool for clinical practice and discusses the major issues for nursing in its uptake. It will expand readers' awareness of the use of technology in the collection, use and sharing of digitised health information. There are many branches of health informatics, but it is predominantly nursing informatics that will be perused in this chapter. In such a complex discipline, it is not surprising for confusion in nomenclature to arise and it is pertinent here to discuss the common terms of e-health and health informatics.

HEALTH INFORMATICS OR E-HEALTH

The term nursing informatics was introduced into the nursing profession in the late 1980s in alliance with the many technical advances that have been reported to date. Among the definitions, a widely accepted definition is that of the Nursing Informatics Specialist Group of the International Medical Informatics Association (IMIA–NI). According to the IMIA–NI, nursing informatics is 'the integration of nursing, its information, and information management with information processing and communication technology, to support the health of people world-wide' (Conrick 2006:5). Other terms that are also sometimes associated with informatics but are used to describe the use of communication technology in healthcare are telemedicine, telehealth and e-health.

Telemedicine refers to the delivery of 'medical' services across a distance using a range of communication techniques, such as telephone, email and videoconferencing (Smith 2007). With recent advances in all areas of healthcare, including medical, nursing and allied health, a more general term 'telehealth' has often been adopted (see Ch 16). Despite this, there are always new terms being introduced that are often a cause for confusion. The introduction of yet another term (i.e. 'e-health') seemed to be in response to the growth of internet (web-based) services and exploitation of information technology in the healthcare sector.

'E-health' is defined by the World Health Organization (2008) as the use, in the health sector, of digital data—transmitted, stored and retrieved electronically— in support of healthcare, both at the local site and at a distance. It refers to the healthcare components delivered, enabled or supported through the use of information and communications technology. Examples include clinical communication systems such as online referrals, e-prescribing and electronic health records. E-health is identified as a platform for remote health service delivery, patient-centred care, supported self-care, remote access and monitoring, and health system sustainability.

Health informatics is an evolving sociotechnical and scientific discipline that deals with the collection, storage, retrieval, communication and optimal use of health-related data, information and knowledge. The discipline utilises the methods and technologies of the information sciences for the purposes of problem solving and decision making— thus, assuring quality healthcare in all basic and applied areas of biomedical sciences for the community it serves (Health Informatics Society of Australia 2007).

In healthcare, the use of information technology has caused some debate, some of which has been quite passionate. In time, we suspect that parallels will be drawn with the following quote, and healthcare workers might then wonder what the fuss was all about:

> That it will ever come into general use, notwithstanding its value, is extremely doubtful because its beneficial application requires much more time and gives a good bit of trouble, both to the patient and to the practitioner because its hue and character are foreign and opposed to all our habits and associations (*The London Times*, 1834, commenting on the stethoscope).

INFORMATICS AS A TOOL FOR NURSING

Nurses focus on patients' responses to illness, injury, treatment and care within the context of the patients' family, social structure and location (Conrick et al 2004). In addition, their services are guided by patient risk assessments, which form the basis of preventative nursing interventions. These assessments and interventions include the broader health context of psychosocial, environmental and family/carer considerations, and are crucial to the ongoing health of our community. Nurses are the only professionals who work across health transitions and therefore the continuum-of-care. To effectively and efficiently engage with patients and clients across such diverse practice areas, nurses must use the most efficient and effective tools available to them, and technology is able to provide many of these.

Nurses are found in a diversity of practice areas and geographical settings supporting an increasingly transient community. This is an increasing challenge, particularly in rural and remote Australia, where they (nurses) are often isolated from other practitioners and must, by necessity, practise alone. The fragmented records of care and inadequate methods of communication are a major issue. Information technology has the potential to support clinicians by providing timely, quality data, and to largely negate the tyranny of distance, through high-speed broadband and satellite access. This is the domain of nursing informatics.

Nursing informatics may be defined as:

> … a specialty area that integrates nursing science, computer science, and information science to manage and communicate data, information and knowledge in nursing practice settings. It facilitates the integration of data, information and knowledge to support patients, nurses and other providers in their decision-making in all roles and settings, by using information structures, information processes, and information technology (Staggers & Thompson 2002:262).

As information technology permeates nursing, all nurses must have a working knowledge of informatics and understand what it offers the profession. Nursing input is essential in the development of information systems, and anecdotal evidence suggests that it is a significant factor in the success or failure of these systems.

GATHERING EVIDENCE TO AID DECISION MAKING

It is crucial that robust and relevant electronic data are collected for use in clinical practice and professional collaboration, because these data are the basis for decision making and evidence-based practice in the healthcare sector. In informatics terms, the gathering of evidence for decision making actually begins with the most basic of language building blocks—that is, data.

The International Standards Organization defines data as the representation of real-world facts, concepts or instructions in a formalised manner suitable for communication, interpretation or processing by human beings or by automatic means (International Standards Organization 1999). Information builds on data and is the output of the data interpretation, organisation and structure (Standards Australia 2003). When information has been synthesised, interrelationships are identified and formalised knowledge is created (Standards Australia 2003). The evidence for use as clinical information and nursing knowledge result from the progressive cognitive or automated processing and manipulation of data, language and knowledge, and in turn governs it. Nurses are recognised as the key collectors, generators and users of patient/client data and information, and the delivery of good nursing care is dependent upon the quality and timeliness of the information available (Currell et al 2002, Hovenga & Hindmarsh 1996a).

THE COLLECTION OF DIGITISED HEALTH INFORMATION

According to Mercer (2003), there are three levels at which the collection of digitised health information can be used and shared. The first level is the service delivery level and most data are generated here (see Fig 22.1). At this level, computer systems capture initial patient care data, but may also exchange data between different systems (e.g. a referral could be generated from the hospital to a community service or from one program to another). Data from this level also form the basis of population surveys. National standards operate here to ensure quality and clean data collection. Mercer describes the second level as the intermediate level, saying that:

> ... data from the lowest level of the pyramid are often required to be reported, perhaps within a service delivery outlet (total activity counts for a day), or to a regional or area agency or authority (total activity counts for a week, or agency expenditure totals for a financial year) (Mercer 2003:16).

The volume of data reported to the intermediate level will normally be less than the data generated at the service delivery level because not all data that are generated need to be reported. Data may also be aggregated for reporting, or may be reported in the form of individual records for each patient or client.

In the final level, or the national level, data from intermediate levels, or at times directly from the service delivery level, may be reported to national data collection agencies. Alternatively, data from census or surveys may be collected at this level, using data captured from the service providers, patients/clients or the general population (Mercer 2003). Data from intermediate levels, or at times directly from the service delivery level, may be reported to national data-collection agencies, the third level of use and sharing. Alternatively, data from census or surveys may be collected at this level, using data captured from the service providers, patients/clients or the general population. From this it is easy to realise that a breakdown of data collection in any stage has far-reaching ramifications for health.

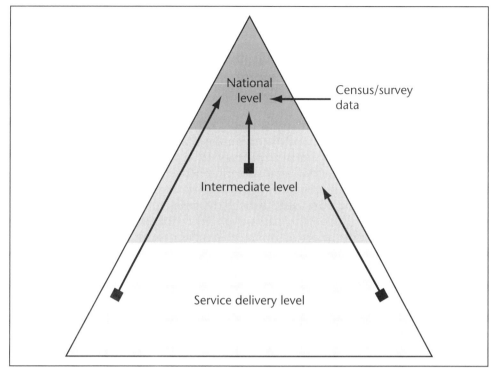

Figure 22.1 Pyramid of reporting activity
Source: Based on Mercer N 2003 Redevelopment of the AIHW knowledgebase—stage
1: scope and issues paper. AIHW, Canberra.

Data input processes must be rapid and intuitive, without placing any additional burden on the user, or mistakes will follow. While it is unlikely that any method of data collection, other than voice, will be faster than handwritten notes, the benefits of an electronic clinical information system far outweigh any minimal change in work process that might be required.

The most obvious benefits are those of legibility, error reduction, reduced documentation of redundant data, completeness and cleanness of the data collected, and the ability to use the data for secondary purposes. By eliminating the duplication of services, improving communication and streamlining data collection, clinical information systems can improve care and the outcomes of care, reduce costs and help to offset the effects of a growing worker shortage that is especially hard-felt in nursing.

Nursing data, information, knowledge and evidence

It is acknowledged that whereas a medical practitioner may be seen as the major primary care provider, in longitudinal care, nurses embrace the concept of continuity of care as both an aim and a philosophy that affects the delivery of care (Conrick et al 2004). Continuity always involves transitions on the part of individuals, such as wellness to illness, home to hospital, and the gaps they may encounter along the way.

In nursing, these transitions usually involve practice that deals with populations who have complex health issues. During times of transition, the nurse is very often the health professional most involved in evaluation, planning and delivering the changes in care that may be required (Conrick et al 2004). If patient care is not consistently and accurately recorded, the possible adverse effects on patient care, nursing practice and the development of nursing knowledge may be quite significant (Currell et al 2002).

A key strategy to assist with continuity of care and efficient access to health information is the standardisation of terminology used by nurses, in relation to assessment and clinical management of patients. In Australia, an initiative called the HealthOnline strategy, emphasised that nurses must decide how the 'natural language' text and oral data that are used in nursing can be entered into a computerised documentation system and translated, through the design of the computer software, into a database capable of supporting nationally agreed, consistent terms (Walker et al 2003). Without some type of organisation or classification, differences in language can be quite marked from hospital to hospital, and this is, of course, increased between states and territories, resulting in inappropriate interpretation of the record and the key process of nursing care being measured in different ways (Conrick 2005).

The development of a health information infrastructure in electronic format must (ultimately) be capable of supporting machine-readable terminology, as this will ensure that data can be readily accessed electronically. Nursing must be active in determining how health concepts are defined by computer software to ensure standardisation and accurate communication, meaning that a computer used by a nurse in one area is using the same concept (with the same meaning) when interacting with a computer used by a health practitioner elsewhere.

The development of classifications and terminologies is a priority, because they enable the standardised collection of machine-readable health information to:

- provide for the measurement of clinical care outcomes and support an evidence-based approach to client assessment—evaluating care outcomes for individuals requires the capacity to organise patient-based information from a variety of service delivery settings in both public and private sectors
- flow into case management and decision support software
- facilitate coordinated care across sectors (acute care, emergency, other ambulatory and community health settings, non-acute settings)
- improve the monitoring of safety and quality in healthcare
- enable statistical analysis and reporting of health information for decision making, policy development, service administration and financial management, and health research, and
- enable standardised indicator development (Walker et al 2003).

Defining the language of practice is also necessary so that all care settings are using the same unique terms. These factors are critical if service providers are to continuously improve safety, enhance the quality of health and healthcare, and to base their practice on evidenced-based research (Walker et al 2003). If language collection and definition can be achieved, it will enable activities such as outcomes research and benchmarking based on valid, consistent and reliable data. It will also underpin the development of nursing archetypes (discussed later in this chapter).

The patient's health record, whether electronic or paper, should contain a complete record of nursing work. In fact, this is the only place that it can be captured, but frequently the care given and outcomes of nursing care are poorly reported. The lack of structure of nursing data also means that they are infrequently used to support nursing practice because retrieval from patients' records is very difficult (Conrick 2005). These problems have existed for a long time, but it is still sobering to read recent studies that indicate that fragmented, disorganised and inaccessible clinical information continues to adversely affect the quality of healthcare and compromises patient safety (Gahart et al 2004). To provide better care for patients, it is essential that all clinicians and others involved in a patient's care can accurately communicate treatment plans, assessments, patient diagnoses and symptoms.

Information technology enables the sharing and storage of data not possible with paper-based records and other current means of communication. However, it must be done in an appropriate, specific and accurate manner, and the only way to achieve this is the use of standard, accepted, relevant terminology or terminologies that both the senders and receivers of information can understand. In an electronic environment, standard reference terminologies are required, and nursing has developed an International Reference Terminology (IRT) for this purpose. Such terminologies communicate information well, but at a higher level, and they are not suited for counting information units for statistical purposes. In order to both communicate health information, and to count it accurately (for burden of disease studies, epidemiology, public health initiatives, resource planning and so forth), both classifications and terminologies are needed (Walker et al 2003).

While humans communicate with each other using 'natural language', computers cannot; they need to be told what things are and how they are related to each other, and this is achieved through use of terminologies. Despite the considerable terminologies work that is underway in Australia and internationally, little has been done to identify those that will be acceptable to Australian nurses. Nurses, as they should, have rejected language classification systems that were inadequate or inappropriate, but with the implementation of electronic health records, consensus on language classification must be achieved. One of the most difficult problems has been finding an appropriate terminology that represents the spectrum of nursing practice, while making sense to both the user and the computer. There are several datasets that appear to have some merit and that are in use elsewhere, and they must be trialled in Australia.

Workforce challenges

Other than the state of its data, there are a number of factors that have the potential to undermine the use of technology to support nursing. Nursing workflow issues are some of the most important of these and they must be understood if nurses' information requirements are to be realised. Consideration of these issues is also necessary for nurses to work seamlessly across the continuity-of-care with individual patients or groups of patients or in interdisciplinary care teams. Although substantial investment may be expended on technology, this will not necessarily guarantee success, as nurses will not willingly use tools incompatible with their work or communication processes. Imposing information systems is also futile, as this usually results in the collection of sporadic, poor-quality data, which may impact on clinical decisions made by nurses.

Investment in information technology infrastructure also requires an investment in the health workforce to ensure that nurses have the skills required to effectively use the information and technology, and to enter the technology debate. Few universities offer sufficient informatics education to their undergraduate or postgraduate students, and nurses not recently qualified are likely to have minimal 'training' at work or may have undertaken self-education because of a particular interest in the field. A comprehensive national health informatics education framework is required to address this crucial issue.

Computer skills are just as essential to nurses in the twenty-first century as pencil and paper were in the eighteenth and nineteenth centuries. However, as technology changes, computer skills must be updated and this requires a systematic program of ongoing education, training and skills development. It is important to appreciate the education and training needs of nurses in relation to e-health. Although nurses have access to basic to intermediate computer training, there appears to be very limited access to training courses which help nurses learn about communication technology and e-health applications relevant to their workplace. A Queensland-based survey which investigated the knowledge, experience and comprehension of e-health of undergraduate nursing students in Australia showed that, despite nursing students having good access to computers and the internet, very few (nursing students) knew what e-health was or how they could use e-health in their role as clinicians (Edirippulige et al 2007). This highlights an important need to develop practical courses in the area of e-health—ideally, in undergraduate (pre-registration) curriculums and professional nursing education programs.

If nurses cannot evaluate systems and define technology needs, then others will continue doing this for them. Indeed, there are many vendors currently implementing or developing nursing systems that are targeted specifically for local use and, in fact, this is a selling point for their product. Nursing is at risk of continuing service delivery in a fragmented manner that is unable to traverse locations or geographical settings. It will perpetuate and exacerbate funding and retention issues, and thwart nursing's ability to achieve quality, cost-effective patient outcomes on a state-wide or national basis. In terms of the Australian Health Information Council's (AHIC) vision for Australia's health and its perceived 'opportunity to create one of the world's best healthcare systems' (Coats 2004), these are major issues.

THE STORAGE AND USE OF DIGITISED HEALTH INFORMATION

Healthcare organisations will continue to invest heavily in clinical information systems because they envisage an improvement in patient safety, reduced variability of care, and increased staff efficiency. This is because of the quality of data available for decision making. Nursing work is information intensive, with nurses processing information for multiple purposes: to create a greater awareness of patient needs; to guide practice; to report observations; and to document patient care. Although it is estimated that nurses spend at least 20% of their time processing written information and up to a further 30% engaging in verbal communication (Hovenga & Hindmarsh 1996b), currently across practice the highest recording rate of outcomes documentation is just 13%, with some practice areas failing to capture outcomes at all (Kennedy 2004). This leaves a huge gap in the continuity of care, but it also has ramifications for nursing knowledge and evidence for nursing practice.

Electronic health records

Many anecdotal reports about the problems of paper health records abound, and the literature also documents many of these. The following list typifies some of these:

- fragmentation of information and data
- illegible
- no linkages to underlying data
- no information or data management
- no decision support capabilities
- competition for access
- inaccessibility of information, and
- missing data.

Electronic health records (EHRs) may help to negate most of these difficulties and create an awareness of the holistic needs of the patient because information is readily available from multiple sources. Appropriate and timely information at the point-of-care improves decisions about what type of care is provided and how it is delivered, reducing risk and improving the quality and outcomes of care (Conrick 2005). An EHR is defined as the longitudinal collection of personal health information concerning a single individual, entered or accepted by healthcare providers, and stored electronically. The information is organised primarily to support continuing, efficient and quality healthcare, and is stored and transmitted securely. The EHR contains information that is:

- **retrospective**: an historical view of health status and interventions
- **concurrent**: a 'now' view of health status and active interventions, and
- **prospective**: a future view of planned health activities and interventions (Standards Australia 2003).

Health records serve not only as archival records, but may be viewed as diaries of diagnostic discoveries, observations made and care provided (Conrick et al 2004). A by-product of the rigorous collection and recording of health status data, and nursing activity data into a point-of-care EHR, would be the capacity to perform post-hoc analyses on these data to determine the effectiveness and efficiency of nursing activity in real-world settings. It would also feed data into a quality improvement cycle and form the basis of evidence-based decision making in clinical practice.

It is for many of these reasons that, in 2001, the Commonwealth Government of Australia, in collaboration with the states and territories, commissioned a program called HealthConnect—an overarching national change management strategy to improve safety and quality in healthcare by establishing and maintaining a range of standardised electronic health information products and services for healthcare providers and consumers. Despite efforts to establish a standardised electronic health record, there is limited evidence to suggest that this work is nearing accomplishment. In 2005, the HealthConnect program was transformed to the National eHealth Transition Authority (NeHTA), with a focus on e-health informatics standards and the development of standards for the exchange of information (Conrick 2006).

To realise the potential benefits of an EHR, systems must be designed around best-practice workflow of the end user. They must be comprehensive in their scope, with all major components of the clinical process, including all clinical orders (medications, diagnostic orders and specialty consults), nursing care and outcomes documentation available in an electronic records format (Conrick et al 2004). Self-population of multiple components and fields in the record will then eliminate duplicate data entry. They must enable once only and point-of-care entry that eliminates transcription errors and clinical systems that provide decision support to aid in the decision making of all clinicians. This information made available through clinical decision support systems assists clinicians to gather evidence for decision making and to prevent adverse events.

Clinical decision support

Clinical decision support systems (CDSSs) are usually built around alerting systems, based on rules of logic. The alerting system can notify clinicians immediately or may generate alerts over time, after relating data from multiple sources (Lyons & Richardson 2003). Broad categories of decision support systems include formatting tools, decision modelling, advisory and knowledgebase systems. They provide strategies to analyse, evaluate, develop and select effective solutions to complex problems in complex environments. Nurses are able to quickly access sources of evidence to assist with the provision of quality care, as the evidence can be locally sorted in policy and procedure manuals, for example, or it can be retrievable from wide-ranging sources such as journal databases or professional collaborative networks (Conrick et al 2004).

To date, much of the development work on electronic decision support systems has been fragmented and uncoordinated, leading to problems of accessibility, scalability, duplication and lack of integration with existing systems. The Commonwealth has begun a nationally coordinated approach for developments in the area and is perusing a national governance structure to provide direction and coordination (Commonwealth of Australia 2003). In the United Kingdom, 'The Map of Medicine™', a fast and intuitive decision support system, has been trialled and demonstrates the capabilities of CDSSs.

The Map™ is a clinical knowledge system that visually combines specialist knowledge with best practice, making the resources of medical information available to all clinical staff. It is designed to support interaction across disciplines, help improve the use of clinical resources and underpin professional development (Medic to Medic 2004). Clinical knowledge is organised into more than 300 patient 'journeys' in all major diagnostic areas, and 'maps' clinical process throughout the healthcare system, starting from initial patient presentation in the general practitioner's surgery or the accident and emergency unit. The Map™ is customisable to local clinical needs in the healthcare organization, and is designed to integrate into every aspect of modern healthcare, from diagnosis through to education and training. The developers describe a virtual 'desktop consultant' for healthcare professionals to use when the patient's journey leads them into unfamiliar territory (Medic to Medic 2004). Nurses in this project have remarked on the ways that the system has changed their process of decision making, from isolation to shared decision making. They report a sense of empowerment and a vision for the future.

Regardless of the advances in decision support systems, the nurse must still exercise and use clinical judgment in the context of the problem, as well as the recommendations of the decision support tool, and nursing must be responsible for nursing needs. The Map™ represents just one example of electronic clinical decision support, but just as important to the clinician is awareness of potential errors, which can also be built into these systems. Another type of clinical decision support can be built into medications management systems, in which data from clinical systems provide an alerting service.

These systems demonstrate the worth of clinical decision support in very tangible ways.

Medications management

Medications management is an ongoing concern in most countries and medication errors are responsible for considerable morbidity. In Australia, according to the Australian Institute of Health and Welfare (2002), misuse, underuse, overuse, and reactions to therapeutic drugs results in about 140,000 hospital admissions every year, with the inappropriate use of medicines costing the Australian public health system about $400 million per year. In a review of Australian data sources, Runciman et al (2003) estimated that between 2% and 4% of all hospital admissions were medication-related; and up to three-quarters of these were potentially preventable.

Meadows (2002) has found that clinical information systems can assist in reducing medication errors through sophisticated medication management solutions. Apart from legibility, prescribing safety is enhanced with online access to decision support databases carrying patient drug history, scientific drug information guideline reference, and patient-specific information. Such specific information, according to Ong (2002), includes discharge summaries, surgical procedure summaries, laboratory data and investigation reports. In addition, decision support and prompts can be built in to catch errant orders.

Technology enables doctors, pharmacists and nurses to make prescribing, dispensing and administration decisions based on knowledge of previous prescriptions, the current medications regime and previous medication reactions. These types of medications systems also provide consumers with the opportunity to become active participants in their medication management, which has demonstrated to improve outcomes. The area for greatest gains, however, may be at the hospital interface, where quick access to a patient's medication record could be life saving. Barcode-enabled point-of-care medication management systems that can also combine with computerised provider-order-entry systems, replacing handwritten prescribing, are designed to improve efficiency and reduce medication and other errors in the clinical setting. Barcodes on inpatients' identification bands assist with administration tasks, with alerts warning of allergies or interactions. According to the Australian Council for Safety and Quality in Health Care (2002), 'the evidence suggests that careful implementation of computerised prescribing with clinical decision support systems should be a priority'.

Gathering and sharing information using e-health

E-health may be used as a generic term to describe the delivery of healthcare over a distance, using a range of communication techniques. In clinical practice, e-health includes but is not limited to: diagnosis from radiological images; reviewing laboratory findings; interviewing, assessing and monitoring patients in rural and remote locations; consulting with specialist health professionals; and the provision of training and professional education.

There are two main forms of e-health. The first is 'store-and-forward' (asynchronous), where information is packaged and sent for review. Common examples include the delivery of information via the post, fax or email. The storage of digital images such as X-rays in radiology, pathology and dermatology are good examples. These images may be accessed by the specialist at a time that is convenient. This application is best suited for non-urgent consultations due to the potential delay in response time.

The second form of e-health includes real-time (synchronous) communication. As the name implies, the interaction or exchange of information occurs simultaneously. The telephone would be one of the most common real-time methods of communication used in nursing, and telephone triage is well established in many countries. Videoconferencing is another real-time application, which is slowly gaining popularity.

Videoconferencing is useful when participants need to see and hear each other during a meeting. In certain situations, one or more peripheral medical devices may be connected to the videoconference unit to provide an extra source (input) of information. For example, an ultrasound machine might be used to send live ultrasound images via videoconference. While access to high bandwidth telecommunications is not critical for meetings and most general education sessions, some applications do require a certain transmission speed (bandwidth) for the transfer of high-resolution video images such as cardiac and fetal ultrasonography. E-health is a useful application for regional and remote communities, which often have limited access to specialist health services. Smith et al (2003) reported that consultations conducted via videoconference save many patients the expensive and time-consuming journey away from home, and ensure equity of access to services that are more easily accessible in metropolitan areas. In addition, Smith et al (2007) have shown the potential for major savings mainly related to reduced travel costs.

Gathering evidence with patient dependency systems

Patient dependency systems (PDSs) are commonly used and were adopted solely as administrative decision-making tools to provide appropriate staff expertise and staff-to-patient allocation. More recently, nurse managers have used PDSs to match patient needs with the available nursing resources. Although nursing acuity systems have been discussed for many years and there are several in use, Willis et al (2008) found that few studies evaluate their use in practice, and those that do focus on validity and reliability, and cross-checking the relationships between nursing dependency, diagnosis-related groups (DRGs) and length of hospital stay (LOS).

Donaldson and Conrick (2004) demonstrated the ability of value adding to a PDS system and for it to acquire a clinical function. The PDA Auto Installing System (PAIS) produces timely data that are important in understanding acuity profiles and specific activities associated with patients from homogenous DRGs. These data lend themselves to active variance analysis and the flagging of the indicators that might suggest variance, which, in turn, improves decision making, leading to more comprehensive care planning and may achieve a more optimal LOS. This method is applicable in developing or reviewing existing clinical pathways, and is effective for all DRGs where there is a sufficient patient population to validate the data (Donaldson & Conrick 2004). Although this is not an automated pathway production program for the clinician, it is invaluable for providing evidentiary support and an awareness of all issues when making decisions regarding the inclusion of particular tasks in the clinical pathway (Donaldson & Conrick 2004).

When this method is incorporated into information systems, it could also form the basis for clinical decision support. Using 'live' data analysis, instead of retrospective clinical audit, enables active variance analysis, and the flagging of specific indicators in patients' conditions might preempt variance during an episode of care. The availability of this information may prompt appropriate intervention earlier, rather than later, resulting in better care planning and possibly optimal LOS.

Using data in clinical practice improvement

The real value of the adoption and use of clinical systems, EHRs, intelligent decision support and care planning is the ability to share clinical nursing information between systems (Conrick et al 2004). This information needs to be processable by the receiving computer system so that it is understood at the level of formally defined nursing domain concepts. This requires four prerequisites: a standardised EHR reference model; a service interface model; terminologies; and domain-specific concept models (for open EHR). The latter requires the development and adoption of nursing-domain-specific archetypes (constraint models discussed later), templates and agreed terminologies.

This infostructure will enable nurses to engage in effectiveness research using techniques such as the clinical practice improvement cycle (CPIC), which is designed to develop data-driven, analytically based protocols to achieve desirable outcomes, at the lowest essential cost over the continuum of care (Horn 2001). Information technology provides nurses with the tools to gather evidence for evaluation, comparison and the improvement of nursing service delivery relative to patient outcomes. Nurses collect data on outcomes, treatments and care activities, as well as patient signs and symptoms based on nursing assessments. Ideally, this can be achieved as a secondary function of routine documentation of care via a clinical information system (Conrick et al 2004). The use of standardised data enables studies that compare different practices in any number of organisations for specific patient cohorts and leads to the development of evidence-based clinical guidelines. These in turn can be incorporated in decision support systems and positively influence future care and clinical decision making. The cycle is completed when the results of improved practices are again evaluated.

However, clinical and nursing systems that enable the use of data-mining software and the adoption of methods such as CPIC must include or have access to sufficient demographic data to enable data aggregation across systems for specific patient cohorts. This will enable the undertaking of 'virtual' randomised clinical trials to evaluate and assess homogeneous patients and their outcomes relative to treatment and care options provided (Conrick et al 2004).

A national strategic approach for involvement in relevant international research and development would be possible with the development of a nursing information framework that would provide appropriate data for nursing research and evaluation. As standardised data are collected and used, automation would enable consensus on admission health status and nursing-sensitive outcome measures that would facilitate the automation of practice evaluation. It would also provide a foundation for the development of clinical decision support systems that would enable patients to be provided with the best possible evidence-based nursing care.

SEARCHING FOR AND SHARING KNOWLEDGE

Information and knowledge are the currency of the information technology revolution, but in today's environment of evidence-based healthcare, it is not possible for any healthcare provider to absorb all the knowledge required to maintain best practice. Nurses are true knowledge workers, using information and knowledge to support and inform all areas of their practice. Although the knowledge is an individual cognitive process, and as such cannot be managed by external processes, information technology makes it possible for knowledge to be captured in forms that can be stored and shared.

The health record should be the vehicle for comparing information and sharing knowledge, but the lack of standardisation of the existing paper records makes nursing data almost impossible to abstract. The use of electronic data capture and storage will change this, provided nurses are responsible for the development of such systems. The exchange of digitised information across settings using electronic knowledgebases, and being able to research that knowledge, is extremely important to nursing and to the outcomes of patient care.

Managing evidence and knowledge

It is accepted that a distributed national EHR system needs to be underpinned by an appropriate, standardised architecture that defines how patient information is structured, stored and managed, so it can be securely stored and safely used by healthcare providers (Conrick et al 2004). The South Brisbane HealthConnect trial assessed the openEHR architecture for this task. Fundamental to openEHR was the use of 'archetypes', or electronically generated documents, that provided a relatively simple means for clinicians to specify the structure, content and context of clinical information, without becoming involved in how programmers might represent the information within an EHR system. When implemented with appropriate software, these archetypes are used to manage clinical information and knowledge in an EHR system. In other words, this technology will, for the first time, enable nursing to articulate what it is that nurses do and will store this knowledge in an accessible knowledgebase. Nursing archetypes must be based on evidence, and the content and upkeep of the database is something for which all nurses must take responsibility.

Another type of knowledgebase is one that stores evidence-based nursing information and resources that are used by nurses on a daily basis to inform their practice (Conrick et al 2004). Much of this is already available in the form of journals, books and other types of peer-to-peer communications. A cursory surf of the worldwide web reveals a broad range of electronic health information that is extremely difficult and time consuming to sift through, and is dynamic—forever changing, expanding and shifting (Conrick 2002). A well-developed knowledgebase could organise this knowledge into a searchable form, and perhaps facilitate interactive peer-to-peer exchange, collective intelligence networking, debate, smart sharing, learning and discussion to support individuals and their organisations.

The knowledgebase should have tools such as smart browsers that only search particular types of sites or those with particular content. Networks of nurses interested in specific clinical or management problems can form 'virtual communities' to exchange knowledge, enabling skills development and shared learning, promoting best practice ideals and more informed decisions. This would improve productivity, effectiveness and efficiency of practice, increase satisfaction in the clinical area, and the sharing of evidence-based decision-making resources and tools, information and experiences.

The Australian Institute of Health and Welfare (2004) developed another type of knowledgebase, which is also internet-based. This is a 'registries store' and provides the contents of the national health, community services and housing assistance data dictionaries. Various groups and their associated national information management groups develop the contents of the knowledgebase. It also stores details of national minimum data sets (or agreed national data collections) and national information models, and provides links between these metadata components.

The current knowledgebase is undergoing redevelopment because of the pressures and issues facing national data development. The redevelopment provides for an opportunistic expansion of the database beyond the scope of the national data dictionaries. It will, in future, include other national metadata content and reflect changes in user expectations and needs, the international standard used to underpin the knowledgebase structure, and changes in technology and web-browser software, and so forth (Australian Institute of Health and Welfare 2004). The redevelopment provides an opportunity to consider these issues and to determine how a national metadata registry can best support the national data development work programs, many of which are crucial to supporting nursing work and communications between nurses and others in an electronic world.

Current awareness tools

'Current awareness' is a topical subject with worker shortages, time restraints and information overload being facts of life. Dynamic resource tools for 'knowledge and awareness discovery' enable the user to use the internet to access, read and retrieve material from library catalogues, online databases and resources from millions of sites. The internet has an expansive range of quantity and quality of materials available to support nursing. It also has a great deal of rubbish, and accessing the material stored there can be difficult and frustrating because of the variable nature of the resources available, and the challenge in locating them (Conrick 2002).

Although the internet is referred to as 'the web', it really consists of two webs. The first is the surface web that can be accessed by regular search engines. The second is the deep web, which consists of a sizeable proportion of government resources, databases and similarly structured materials not written in hypertext mark-up language (html)— the language of the surface web. It is estimated that the deep web is 500 times larger than the surface web, it is highly specialised, 95% fee free and is the largest growth category on the web (Conrick 2002).

Awareness tools come in many forms, and offer many current awareness resources, including e-mail alerts, table of content alerts and e-mail, all of which arrive in a timely fashion and can be read either online or offline. There are custom alerting services that will monitor the internet for the latest information to be posted to the web, based on the user's customised search algorithm. These alerting systems enable immediate awareness of these new resources, as they send e-mail alerts to the subscriber's computer, mobile telephone or personal digital assistant (PDA). PDA products have potential in nursing, as a modality to store and provide access to a large library of up-to-date information—as needed. Compliance and exploitation of these systems will largely depend on a range of factors, including ease of use, download speed and cost to the user. Another similar product is the tablet personal computer (PC), which is a compact notebook that offers similar functions to a standard PC. Tablet PCs have been reported to be useful by nursing students for reflective writing and access to clinical learning resources. The overriding benefit of these portable data systems is the ability to access information when and where it is needed.

Specific subject-based mailing lists, bulletin boards, message boards and forums have been available for many years, and provide one of the easiest ways of remaining current. List finders such as CataList and Delphi Forum assist in finding the most appropriate of these. Weblogs (blogs) and news aggregators are perhaps the fastest growing tools on the internet and offer huge amounts of current information and knowledge. The internet provides easy access to health information on almost any topic imaginable that is evidence-based and maintains currency. Nurses have access to the latest developments in patient care, particularly for patients with complex or multiple problems; they also have timely access to a solid base of the most recent evidence on which to base decision making.

Decision making is only possible with high-quality communication and, characteristically, nurses working across the continuity of care or with complex patients do not have all the information on which to base decisions or an awareness of their patients to deliver seamless care. Nursing event summaries and nursing referrals are of critical importance to nursing communications, and the continuity of care.

Nursing event summaries

Nurses have never been good at communicating outside of the institution, and nursing discharge summaries, if provided, are often not timely and the content leaves much to be desired. Nursing event summaries should contain all the information required by the receiving clinician to enable seamless and continuous care and sufficient information for ongoing decision making. However, other pressures on the discharging clinician often mean that discharge summaries are given a low priority. Automated systems event summaries can be developed by a computer with no other involvement from the discharging clinician other than to press the 'go' button as part of the discharge. Anecdotal evidence suggests that this was one of the most positive aspects of a trial in the Katherine region of the Northern Territory, in which a number of health consumers trialled HealthConnect. However, on a larger scale, discharge summary systems are reliant on many different sources systems, feeding data to the clinical repository, and where these will come from remains unclear.

CONCLUDING REMARKS

The nursing profession is an amalgamation of diverse practitioners working in many settings. Information technology will significantly redefine the way in which nurses work and the boundaries of practice, as it provides access to quality, timely data, information and knowledge. Nurses are key participants and the largest stakeholder group in healthcare; therefore, nursing will be most impacted by the introduction of any technology.

As new technology is developed and implemented, personnel and organisations have to adjust, and sometimes the adjustment is major. Technology has much to offer the clinician, but the acceptance of informatics requires more than mere buy-in or passive agreement because change is inevitable. It demands ownership by leaders willing to accept responsibility for making change happen in all of the areas they influence or control and an atmosphere of ownership by all nurses. Substantial changes to health education are required in both course design and content, and incentives for informatics education must be tangible for this to occur. Without these structures, nursing's approach to informatics will continue to be fragmented, duplication of effort will continue, and the workforce capacity in informatics will remain very low. Systems will fail because of either apathy or ignorance, and the projected improvement in clinical care and health outcomes will not eventuate.

Underpinning the real value of the adoption and use of clinical systems, EHRs, intelligent decision support and automated care planning, is the ability to share clinical nursing information between clinicians and systems. The ability to access knowledge from formerly inaccessible places (in departments or the minds of staff and in information repositories) will greatly change healthcare delivery, the boundaries of healthcare and how decisions in healthcare are made. Nursing concepts must be valid, be embedded in evidence, exist in searchable knowledgebases, and be available for nurses to make decisions on a strong base of knowledge. Knowledge management has the capacity to have a major impact on the knowledge levels of nurses, with nursing acquiring the capacity to engage in quality improvement cycles based on clean, quality data. This will result in high-level decision making, based on the best available information at the point-of-care, ultimately leading to improved outcomes.

Information technology has the capacity to take nurses into the future as informed, aware knowledge workers ready to meet the challenges. It has the capacity to change nursing as never before, and perhaps the profession will not be recognisable to us in 15 years' time. Whether or not nursing rises to the challenge depends on nursing's and nurses' commitment to the ownership of the process.

REFLECTIVE QUESTIONS

Choose one or more of the following areas of healthcare and then answer the six questions that follow:

- clinical
- management
- research, and/or
- education.

1 What is the problem(s) for which technology might be helpful?
2 Whose problem is it?
3 How will the selected technology help solve the problem?
4 What are the risks/problems associated with the use of this technology?
5 What are the potential clinical/economic benefits?
6 How would you evaluate whether the technology was useful?

RECOMMENDED READINGS

Conrick M 2002 Looking for a needle in a haystack: searching the internet for quality resources. Contemporary Nurse 12(1):49–58

Conrick M, Hovenga E, Cook R, Laracuente T, Morgan T 2004 A framework for nursing informatics in Australia: a strategic paper (commissioned national research report). HISA–NIA, Department of Health and Ageing, Melbourne

Graves J, Corcoran S 1989 The study of nursing informatics. Image: Journal of Nursing Scholarship 21(4):227–231

Marin HF, Carr R 2008 Nursing care systems: enhancing care processes in practice and management. Yearbook of medical informatics, pp 25–8

Walker S, Frean I, Scott P, Conrick M 2003 Classifications and terminologies in residential aged care: an information paper. Department of Health and Ageing, Canberra

RESOURCES

Australian Health Information Council (AHIC) 2007 eHealth future directions briefing paper. AHIC, Canberra

Conrick M 2006 Health informatics: transforming healthcare with technology. Thompson Social Science Press, Melbourne

Health Informatics Society of Australia: www.hisa.org.au/

Nursing Informatics Australia: www.niaonline.org.au/html/about.html

REFERENCES

Armstrong BK, Gillespie JA, Leeder SR, Rubin GL, Russell LM 2007 Challenges in health and healthcare for Australia. Medical Journal of Australia 187(9): 485–489

Australian Council for Safety and Quality in Health Care 2002 Second national report on patient safety: improving medication safety. Third report to the 'Australian health ministers' conference', Canberra

Australian Department of Finance and Administration 2006 ICT investment framework: August 2006. Government Information Management Office, Canberra

Australian Institute of Health and Welfare (AIHW) 2002 Australian hospital statistics 1999–2000. AIHW, Canberra

Australian Institute of Health and Welfare (AIHW) 2004 Knowledgebase redevelopment. AIHW, Canberra

Coats A 2004 Report from the chair. AHIC e-bulletin. Australian Health Information Council, Canberra

Commonwealth of Australia 2003 National electronic decision support taskforce report (final). Department of Health and Ageing, Canberra

Conrick M 2002 Looking for a needle in a haystack: searching the internet for quality resources. Contemporary Nurse 12(1):49–58

Conrick M 2005 The international classification for nursing practice: a tool to support nursing practice? Collegian 12(3):9–13

Conrick M 2006 Health informatics: transforming healthcare with technology. Thompson Social Science Press, Melbourne, pp 5, 296–7

Conrick M, Hovenga E, Cook R, Laracuente T, Morgan T 2004 A framework for nursing informatics in Australia: a strategic paper. HISA–NIA, Department of Health and Ageing, Melbourne

Currell R, Wainwright P, Urquhart C 2002 Nursing record systems: effects on nursing practice and health care outcomes. Cochrane Library Update Software, Oxford

Donaldson P, Conrick M 2004 The effectiveness of using a patient dependency system to develop and audit clinical pathways. HIC2004. HISA, Brisbane

Downer SR, Meara JG, Da Costa AC 2005 Use of SMS text transmission to improve outpatient attendance. Medical Journal of Australia 183(7):366–368

Edirippulige S, Smith AC, Beattie H, Davies E, Wootton R 2007 Pre-registration nurses: an investigation of knowledge, experience and comprehension of e-health. Australian Journal of Advanced Nursing 25(2):78–83

Gahart M, Barsoum G, Dievler A, Saad Khan M, Price R, Sanchez Y, Winslow C 2004 HHS's efforts to promote health information technology and legal barriers to its adoption. Institute of Medicine, Washington DC

Health Informatics Society of Australia 2007 A vision for an Australian healthcare system transformed by health informatics. Health Informatics Society of Australia, Melbourne. Online. Available: www.hisa.org.au/ 7 Aug 2008

Horn S 2001 Quality, clinical practice improvement, and the episode of care. Managed Care Quarterly 9(3):10

Hovenga E, Hindmarsh C 1996a Queensland Health—PAIS validation study report. Queensland Health, Brisbane

Hovenga E, Hindmarsh C 1996b Queensland Health—PAIS validation study: results and issues for nursing cost capture. 'Eighth Casemix conference', Sydney

International Standards Organization (ISO) 1999 ISO 2382–4. Information technology—vocabulary—Part 4: organization of data. ISO, Geneva

Kennedy M 2004 Nursing language: the international classification for nursing practice. Nursing Informatics. HIC2004. HISA, Brisbane

Leonard M, Graham S, Bonocum D 2004 The human factor: the critical importance of effective teamwork and communications in providing safe care. Quality and Safety in Health Care 13(Suppl 1):i85–i90

Lyons A, Richardson S 2003 Clinical decision support in critical care nursing. American Association Critical Care Nurses: Clinical Issues 14(3):295–301

Magrabi F, McDonnell G, Westbrook J, Coiera E 2007 Using an accident model to design safe electronic medication management systems. Medinfo 2007: Proceedings of the 12th world congress on health (medical) informatics; building sustainable health systems, pp 948–52

Meadows G 2002 Nursing informatics: an evolving specialty. Nursing Economist 20(6):300–301

Medic to Medic 2004 Map of medicine. NHS, London

Mercer N 2003 Redevelopment of the AIHW knowledgebase—stage 1. scope and issues paper. AIHW, Canberra

Ong B 2002 Leveraging on information technology to enhance patient care: a doctor's perspective of implementation in a Singapore academic hospital. The Annals Academy of Medicine Singapore 31(6):707–711

Runciman WB, Roughead EE, Semple SJ, Adams RJ 2003 Adverse drug events and medication errors in Australia. International Journal for Quality in Health Care 15:i49–i59

Smith AC 2007 Telemedicine: opportunities and challenges. Expert Review of Medical Devices 4(1):5–7

Smith AC, Scuffham P, Wootton R 2007 The costs and potential savings of a novel telepaediatric service in Queensland. BMC Health Services Research 7:35

Smith AC, Youngberry K, Isles A, McCrossin R, Christie F, Wootton R 2003 The family costs of attending hospital outpatient appointments via videoconference and in person. Journal of Telemedicine and Telecare 9(Suppl. 2):58–61

Staggers N, Thompson C 2002 The evolution of definitions for nursing informatics: a critical analysis and revised definition. Journal of the American Medical Informatics Association May/June 9(3):255–261, 262

Standards Australia 2003 Health concept terminology data base. Draft standard AS5021. Standards Australia, Sydney

Walker S, Frean I, Scott P, Conrick M 2003 Classifications and terminologies in residential aged care: an information paper. Department of Health and Ageing, Canberra

Willis E, Toffoli L, Henderson J, Walter B 2008 Enterprise bargaining: a case study in the de-intensification of nursing work in Australia. Nursing Inquiry 15(2): 148–157

World Health Organization (WHO) 2008 eHealth for health care delivery. Online. Available: www.who.int/eht/eHealthHCD/en/ 24 Oct 2008

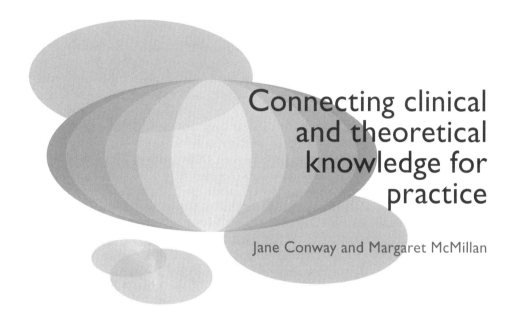

CHAPTER 23

Connecting clinical and theoretical knowledge for practice

Jane Conway and Margaret McMillan

LEARNING OBJECTIVES

Those who have read this chapter should be able to:

- appreciate the interaction between clinical practice and classroom-based learning activities
- identify strategies that maximise learning opportunities in a range of contexts
- explore strategies for acquiring knowledge-ABILITY
- view themselves as autonomous, action-oriented learners
- appreciate the interaction between lifelong learning and professional development, and
- recognise the attributes they possess that will facilitate their practice as graduates.

KEY WORDS

Transition, graduate, accountability, lifelong learning, curriculum, clinical learning, clinical decision making

THE CLINICAL AREA: THE SITE OF NURSING PRACTICE

A confident, competent nursing workforce that has the capacity to provide comprehensive, person-centred care and is part of a cohesive, interprofessional healthcare team is dependent upon the effective transition from being a student to a recent graduate who makes connections between clinical and theoretical knowledge. The curriculum underpinning a nursing program focuses on educating students for clinical practice and uses educational strategies that support the integration of clinical and theoretical knowledge.

Nursing programs globally recognise that the clinical area is an important, if not the most important, area for practice professions such as nursing (Campbell 2003, Lambert & Glacken 2005). Definitions of clinical teaching and learning invariably include some notion that clinical practice is the place where students apply theory in practice, or where contradictions between theory and practice, and nursing and educational values, are highlighted (Campbell 2003). The clinical environment is, in fact, where students begin to develop professional identities as nurses, but it is only the beginning of the pathway to personal confidence and competence. This pathway continues throughout the postgraduate transition year and beyond (Newton & McKenna 2007).

Individuals, employers, supervisors, education bodies and regulatory authorities have a collective responsibility to ensure that the knowledge and skills base from which a nurse operates is not only extensive enough for the roles and functions of a given position, but is also up-to-date, within the law and directed towards client benefit. This provides a series of safeguards, enhances risk management and contributes to quality improvement through promoting application of the principles of ethics, which include doing good, not doing harm, justice and autonomy.

Clinical practice provides the stimulus for students and practitioners alike to use these skills in order to recognise best practice and, if necessary, enhance and modify existing practice. This chapter is designed to encourage students to view clinical and on-campus learning as one entity—a continuum of development and lifelong learning that has the unifying goal of achieving and maintaining competence within the complexities of contemporary practice.

Figure 23.1 depicts the interrelationship between clinical practice knowledge and the theoretical knowledge embedded in nursing-specific frameworks within nursing curricula. This diagram indicates that clinical activity and on-campus learning are interdependent.

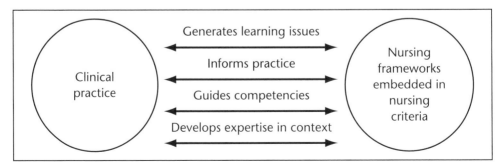

Figure 23.1 The interrelationship between practice and curriculum in nursing programs

The curriculum provides formal structure to a student's learning. However, beyond graduation, nurses are able to create their own curriculum by framing work experiences as learning experiences and drawing upon their abilities as lifelong learners, reflective practitioners and information-literate graduates who appreciate the importance of continuing professional development for fulfilment of the competency standards for nursing practice.

The transition from student to graduate provides an opportunity to launch a career in nursing. This requires the development of the ability to critically examine one's own and others' practice and be accountable for individual action. These abilities are often linked to the idea of being a lifelong learner (Department of Health 2001, National Review of Nursing Education 2002), and are seen as increasingly important to professional nursing practice in the twenty-first century.

The changing nature of health service delivery continues to present challenges to both clinicians and students. In literature related to contemporary health service delivery, it is widely acknowledged that reduced average lengths of stay, an ageing clientele, increased throughput and acuity, developments in healthcare and educational technology, and increasing numbers of learners requiring clinical experience, impact on the clinical learning milieu and the extent to which it consistently fosters the cognitive skills required for professional practice (Jeffries 2008, Lunney 2008, McMillan et al 2004). It is imperative that learners capitalise on events in both clinical and on-campus settings that foster their ability to critically analyse situations, identify underpinning knowledge and ideas, and critically appraise their own professional development. Such critique needs to be managed carefully in order to maintain perspective and avoid overreaction.

Over decades, much has been written about the impact of a purported reality shock that students experience during clinical experience and/or upon entry into the workforce as a graduate. The transition period from graduate to practitioner has been seen as a time during which nurses are socialised into the workplace and its formal and informal rules, protocols, norms and expectations. It has been identified as an exciting, challenging and stressful period (Chang & Hancock 2003). A range of factors contribute to a sense of reality shock, including the need to adjust to the demands of shift work, time pressures associated with assuming a case load, coping with workplace staff shortages, experiencing potential intergenerational differences in work values and ethics, and the need to accept accountability for patient safety and to delegate to and supervise other staff. Etheridge (2007) has reported that new graduates experience a lack of confidence in their interpretation of assessment data and clinical decision making.

The transition from student to graduate has been likened to a grieving response (Halfer & Graf 2006) and is a period whereby the graduate initially focuses (we would say rightly) on themselves and their own development for the first 6 months in the workplace (McKenna & Green 2004). The aspirations of the profession of nursing are for the transition period to be positive and supportive. However, despite these aspirations, new graduates continue to experience fragmentation and frustration as clinical demands conflict with access to support, mentorship and continuing development (Fox et al 2005, Moore 2006).

It is our contention that there is a need to focus on the positive rather than the negative aspects of transition and to acknowledge the extent to which graduates have a repertoire of portable knowledge and skills, which provide a foundation for the development of individual agency as a practitioner. Individual agency is the mechanism that enables knowledge-ABILITY through continuing development of self-insight, a sense of self-efficacy and recognition of the need for self-determination. It is associated with moving beyond the initial and natural sense of alienation experienced in an unfamiliar context to a sense of self-confidence, composure and resilience. Development of self-agency is an iterative rather than lineal process that requires that nurses take responsibility for themselves and their learning. This self-agency requires an ability to create meaning in a given context and to embrace a view of learning as 'volitional, curiosity-based, discovery-driven, and mentor-assisted' (Janik 2005:144) and results in the continuing creation and transformation of perspective, through cognitive and affective engagement in reflective practice (Dirkx 2006).

The capacity to respond appropriately and effectively in nursing practice is dependent upon the extent to which we connect clinical and theoretical knowledge in order to make sense of the situations that students engage with during clinical learning experiences and that graduates encounter during their transition. Such sense making requires what we have termed knowledge-ABILITY. The concept of knowledge-ABILITY requires that learners are able to transfer concepts between the learning cultures typical of on-campus and clinical environments. Without clinical learning experiences which provide the opportunity to integrate classroom theory in 'real-life' practice situations, nursing students may have had little opportunity to develop the lifelong learning skills of critical thinking and reflective practice considered important to professional practice.

In her often cited, seminal work about the development of registered nurses, Benner (1984) has identified that the ability to integrate theory and practice to the point of being able to generalise is essential to development from novice (newly qualified nurse) to more advanced levels of nurse. However, Benner also acknowledges that there are particular challenges in being able to transfer concepts across clinical contexts. Effective clinicians are aware that *context* is the crucial moderator in nursing practice, and have developed mechanisms for managing situations contextually, rather than seeking to manage all situations in the same way.

Such ability to transfer core concepts across situations and modify actions according to context is an indication of 'expert' nursing practice (Benner 1984). Expanding upon this, we believe there is a need for learners to be able to transfer concepts between the learning cultures typical of on-campus and clinical environments. In the remainder of this chapter, we seek to reinforce to readers that throughout their learning as students, they will acquire a set of knowledge and skills in both nursing and learning that are transferable to a range of contexts and which are foundational for professional practice as a nurse.

CONNECTING CLINICAL AND THEORETICAL LEARNING TO BECOME KNOWLEDGE-ABLE

We recognise that, for many student nurses, clinical practice is the goal of nursing education.

Clinical educators, lecturers and clinicians often declare that they have a shared goal of ensuring quality education for nursing students. However, each of these sectors of the nursing community has what, at times, may seem to be very different definitions of nursing and, within that, different expectations of students and graduates. This results in what students may perceive as a lack of alignment between the values of, and experiences in, the education and health service sectors.

While much of this perceived lack of alignment has been attributed to what students and clinicians may hear described as the theory–practice gap (Howatson-Jones 2003), it is our view that nursing education has a single unifying focus—to assist people to be nurses. Being a nurse requires the ability to actively respond with nursing interventions, to think about the clinical judgments made and the consequences of action taken, and to develop a capacity to articulate that thinking to others.

> The principles that underpin learning in the clinical area are used in on-campus learning activities. These are transferable across clinical and theoretical learning contexts.

Contemporary nursing curricula include discipline-specific knowledge, and integration of knowledge from other disciplines to inform the practice of nursing. This differs from previous practices of modifying knowledge from other disciplines to suit nursing situations. Thus, nursing education serves both an epistemological and political purpose, and students should be able to articulate and conceptualise the nature of their discipline and apply their thinking to actual practice.

The overarching structure of all nursing courses is the nursing curriculum, which determines both the outcomes that should be achieved and the processes by which these will be achieved. Nursing education programs include both on-campus and clinical learning experiences, which provide students with opportunities to practise the skills of nursing, to develop and demonstrate their knowledge base about nursing, and to acquire academic skills that support communication of their thinking about nursing. Increasingly, nursing curricula use problem-based teaching strategies to encourage development of the knowledge, skills and behaviours of effective clinicians. This type of learning fosters exploration of 'real-life' situations to enhance critical thinking and clinical decision making (Conway & Little 2003).

Figure 23.2 demonstrates the continual process of conceptualisation and reconceptualisation of nursing, which occurs through situation deconstruction, analysis and reconstruction. These enquiring and processing skills are essential to professional practice and the development of knowledge.

The curriculum should cause students to think about what they do as nurses, why they do what they do, and how they might do it differently. It is these enquiry skills that will cause the student to generate knowledge about nursing. For this reason, it is important that the nursing curriculum raises questions such as: 'What is nursing?' 'What does it mean to nurse?' 'Whom do nurses nurse?' 'Where do nurses nurse?' 'Is nursing the same as caring?' and so on, as well as helping students to learn the task-oriented content of how to nurse.

Conceptualising or thinking about nursing needs to both direct and emerge from practice. It is a process of enquiry in which students work with concepts and form networks of concepts that frame and impact on their practice. It is not our intention to give the impression that qualified nurses should only think about nursing. The goal of

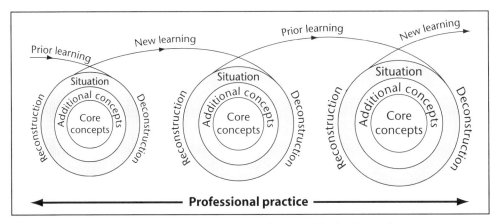

Figure 23.2 Relationship between situation analysis, learning and professional practice

nursing programs is to develop a graduate who can apply concepts to practice, manage complex nursing situations, and accept accountability for practice. Of course, this also demands skills in doing nursing activities.

However, we believe that students should be aware that nursing is about the ability to analyse situations and respond appropriately. How we interpret and analyse situations depends upon how we think about them. As our thinking about nursing develops, the meaning we give to situations changes and learning occurs. We then take this learning with us to the next situation and create new meanings and experiential knowledge.

Experiential knowledge is not merely being exposed to an experience. It is that which emerges when the experience is structured to achieve learning as an outcome of the experience. Therefore, students should use the theoretical base developed from on-campus, university-based activities to frame the clinical experience so that learning, rather than merely experiencing, occurs. Students should ask themselves: 'What is it that I want to achieve from this learning experience and how does this relate to my ability to practise nursing?'

Clinical learning experiences provide nursing students with the opportunity to begin to develop the skills of identifying general principles of practice, transferring these across contexts, and modifying actions based on principles of management. While clinical experience clearly is a powerful motivator for students to learn *how* to nurse, the literature suggests that clinical experiences are an important part of the transfer of learning from the classroom to the practice setting.

How we think about nursing practice shapes *what* we learn from or about practice and how we direct the transition from student to recent graduate and subsequent movement along a career pathway. However, as noted by Heartfield (2006), there are differing representations or constructions of nursing practice dependent on individual, professional, industrial, regulatory and organisational perspectives. Irrespective of perspective and context, 'being a nurse' requires the ability to integrate the knowledge, skills and attitudes of nursing into who we are and how we practise.

Now, more than ever before, contemporary health service delivery demands that nurses demonstrate the full suite of skills representative of the knowledge-ABLE worker. The knowledge-ABLE worker aspires to enhance patient and staff safety, minimise adverse circumstances, promote partnership initiatives, focus on 'fitness-to-function' and acknowledge that health service delivery is dependent upon multiprofessional team effort. Thus, the student nurse as a knowledge-ABLE learner sees connections between clinical and theoretical knowledge of nursing within a broader framework of learning that integrates his or her experience and the outcomes of education for a knowledge-ABLE worker.

Table 23.1 presents the elements of contemporary health service challenges and desired knowledge-ABLE worker responses. The table indicates that although the factors that impact on health service delivery and healthcare work can be viewed in isolation, nurses, as knowledge-ABLE workers, require a multifaceted education to respond meaningfully to the challenges in contemporary health service provision.

Health service challenges	Knowledge-ABLE worker responses
Fragmented patient experience/changing health patterns/chronicity and consumerism	Contributors to systems review
Technology: increased emphasis on clinical and information systems interface	Effective managers of consumer expectations, competing value systems, and tensions in resource allocation
Changing workforce: unaligned skill mix and case mix	Procedurally competent, information fluent personnel
Inappropriate structures and process	Coordinators of throughput and care processes
Changing professional roles and functions	Participants in networked organisation and healthcare teams
Overcoming rigidity in professional frameworks and knowledge bases	Personnel who focus on consumer needs and outcomes, rather than profession-specific outcomes

Table 23.1 Worker responses to a changing health service

HOW TO BEST DEVELOP KNOWLEDGE-ABILITY

Classroom-based learning activity provides us with a relatively safe environment to explore what we know, what we do and who we are as nurses, so that we are more prepared for professional practice situations. Clinical learning activity provides us with the opportunity both to test out what we have learnt in practice and to confront new situations from which we can further our learning. However, we can only learn if we are prepared to do so. It is important that we value learning as much as we value what we have learnt. It is our ability to question ourselves and our practice that enhances our professional development.

In order to learn we need to develop the process skills for lifelong learning (Armstrong et al 2003, Griffitts 2002, Maslin-Prothero & Owen 2001). These process skills are the basis of learning and are transferable across disciplines. In the case of nursing, nursing knowledge provides specific content which, when processed, results in nursing action. That is to say, when we become nurses we have developed general learning skills and we demonstrate our use of these through being able to 'think and act like a nurse'. In order to be lifelong learners in relation to nursing practice, we need to become what has been termed 'reflective practitioners' (Johns 2000). We need to reflect about what we do as nurses, how we respond as nurses and individuals, and what we would do again in a similar situation. We then need to act when a similar situation occurs. The skills of reflective practice unite theoretical and clinical concepts; are both thought-oriented and action-oriented; allow for consideration of the affective aspects of nursing experience, and provide opportunity to explore how the learner as a reflective practitioner felt about the experience. Such an approach is particularly useful in nursing, as it acknowledges human and emotional, as well as intellectual, domains of decision making and encourages self-regulation and autonomy in learning (Morgan et al 2006, Zimmerman 2000).

In Figure 23.3, Gibbs (1988) provides a useful framework for situation analysis that is both thought-oriented and action-oriented, and allows for consideration of the affective aspects of nursing experience and provides opportunity to explore how the learner as a reflective practitioner felt about an experience.

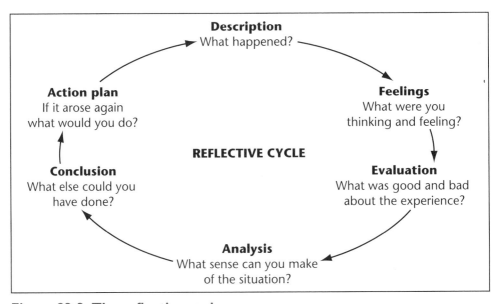

Figure 23.3 The reflective cycle
Source: Gibbs G 1988 Learning by doing: a guide to teaching and learning methods. Further Education Unit, Oxford Polytechnic, Oxford.

Little (1996) has developed a framework of questions that are applicable in both classroom and clinical learning situations that can be used to facilitate reflection. These questions provide a useful guide to developing lifelong learning skills, yet are equally important questions for clinical decision making. The framework recognises that learning is inherently a personal experience and places emphasis on the subjective nature of learning (Griffitts 2002). In order to be accountable for their practice, nurses need to become subjectively engaged in that practice.

Little's approach consists of the sets of questions, related to a range of areas, in the box below.

LITTLE'S (1996) FRAMEWORK OF QUESTIONS

Situation/analysis or decision making
- What information do I have?
- What further information do I need?
- What options/alternatives do I have?
- What should I prioritise?
- What action/s should I take?
- Why?
- Can I justify this action (lawfully, ethically, effectively, theoretically)?

The learning process
- What do I already know?
- How do I know it?
- What do I need to know?
- Where will I find it?
- What resources can I use?
- How will I know I know?
- Why should I learn it?

Perceptions
- What are my feelings?
- What are my beliefs about the situation?
- What are my assumptions?
- How have I derived these beliefs/assumptions?
- How do my feelings/beliefs:
  —affect my interpretation?
  —affect my response?
  —relate to espoused professional values?

Learning processes
- What is the validity of my source?
  —legislation
  —data based on research
  —opinion
  —practice
  —expertise
  —experience

➡

- What is the currency of the knowledge, skills, behaviour?
- What is the support for this view?
  —political/ideological
  —cultural
- What other ideas/concepts/skills does it relate to?
- How does it relate to my view of the world (current understanding)?
- Why do I hold this belief/assumption?
- What are alternative beliefs/assumptions?

The situation revisited
- How does my learning relate to/apply in this situation?
- How does my learning relate to/affect my original ideas?
- What gaps/misconceptions did my learning identify?
- What ideas/skills did my learning confirm?
- What response would I give now in the situation?

Reflection on:

Situation analysis:
- How well did I use the data?
- How well did I define the situation in need of a response?
- How comprehensive were my alternatives?
- How well can I justify my response?

The learning process:
- How valid/relevant were my sources?
- How comprehensive were my sources?
- How effective was my learning?

The group process:
- How well did I contribute?
- What was my role in the group?
- How effective was each member's contribution?
- Did the group remain on task?
- Did the group attend to process (i.e. how people were feeling/responding/behaving)?

This framework of questions is useful because it encourages us to look at situations in context and to focus on learning. It enables us to appreciate that, as learners and professionals who make sound clinical judgments, we are required to interact effectively with others, provide reasoning and support for our actions and decisions, and be aware that we are accountable for our own learning and practice actions.

KNOWLEDGE-ABILITY AS ACTIVE LEARNING

While frameworks for reflection are relevant to a number of practice disciplines, including nursing, there is potential for nurses to utilise the 'learning' components of models such as these selectively and to overlook the critical elements related to action. In responding to the needs of individuals and communities, nursing is both reactive and proactive. As both the guardians of and visionaries for nursing's future, it is important that students be given the opportunity to develop the skills to critically evaluate the nursing practice they observe and to create and consider alternatives to this practice. The imagination of possibilities can only occur when nurses think about nursing. In other words, each of us has a professional responsibility to conceptualise in context. We need to think about what needs to be done for the client and how this impacts on the care situation. There needs to be a relationship established between theory, judgment and action taking.

Ultimately, professional accountability is related to actions, not a capacity to generate ideas. Although theory is important, because it provides a framework for the work nurses do, it is of little consequence unless it results in effective nursing actions. Conversely, practice can become meaningless unless we seek to understand it through conceptualising the practice of nursing. Such integration of theory and practice leads to our moving beyond *becoming* nurses to *being* nurses who integrate our knowing, doing and being to produce what is meaningful, client-focused management of situations. Many educational theorists have highlighted the importance of being reflective practitioners in order to be, both personally and professionally, constantly transformed and emancipated from our previous ways of thinking and acting (Brookfield 1993, Cranton 1994, Friere 1972, Mezirow 1985, Taylor 2008).

Figure 23.4 represents what we perceive to be the relationships between context and lifelong learning processes and curriculum and improved practice. Achieving improved practice requires the process skills of lifelong learning and reflective practice.

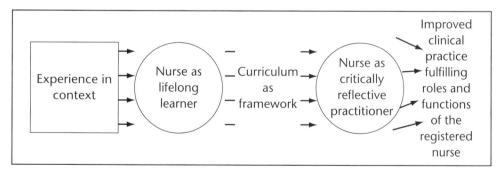

Figure 23.4 An educational equation for improved nursing practice

The knowledge-ABLE nurse develops awareness that the range of factors that impact upon nursing extend beyond the immediate client care situation. Organisational theorists have developed PETS—a schema for examining these political, economic, sociocultural and technological factors. When nurses seek to enhance their knowledge-ABILITY, they should reflect upon the extent to which these factors shape what constitutes nursing service delivery. Figure 23.5 provides an example of the application of PETS to delivery of nursing services.

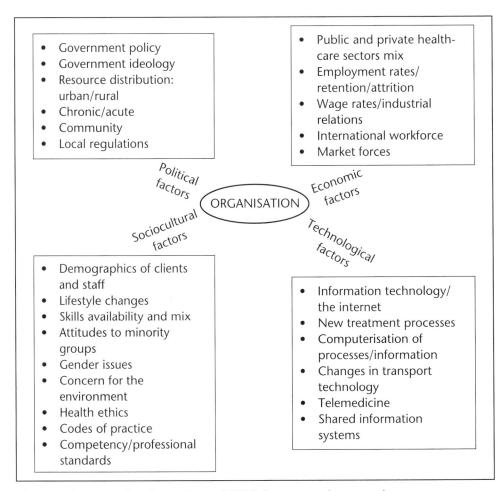

Figure 23.5 Application of the PETS framework to explore professional change in nursing

It has been reported that when nursing students, qualified nurses and their employers are asked to evaluate nursing education, they feel that the time in clinical placements was inadequate and this has led to suggestions that there needs to be an increase in clinical experience as part of undergraduate learning. However, it may well be that an increase in *quality* of the clinical experience is preferable to an increase in *quantity* of clinical placements (Mannix et al 2006). We believe that while clinical educators, lecturers and unit staff share in structuring the clinical experience, students are also accountable for ensuring that they gain a quality clinical experience. This accountability for self-learning links closely with the principles of adult learning and ongoing professional development.

Despite the emphasis on skills such as critical thinking, problem solving and reflective practice in on-campus learning experiences, in clinical settings students are often encouraged to operate routinely and are not challenged to reflect upon their practice in a way that creates intellectual challenge.

We are concerned that the attitude that clinical and classroom learning are separate entities may result in the mistaken perception that there is an insurmountable division between the theoretical and practical aspects of nursing. Students of nursing need to be encouraged to develop skills in reflective practice and situation analysis, not for the purpose of intellectualising or rationalising nursing practice, but for the purpose of identifying and maintaining excellence in clinical practice and meeting the goals of nursing. As a profession, nursing needs to ensure that the culture of healthcare supports and encourages positive, passionate and committed students and graduates who are able to embrace change and shape the profession of nursing for both the current and future contexts in which it will flourish.

Each student has a responsibility to integrate theory and practice experiences. With their colleagues in practice and education, students should seek intellectual challenge. A useful framework for this can be reflective practice models, which facilitate full participation in learning experiences. Underpinning reflective practice is a capacity to intellectualise and appraise one's performance in context.

APPRAISAL AS A STRATEGY FOR KNOWLEDGE-ABILITY

The ability to critically examine our own performance and be accountable for our own actions is essential to professional career development. Transition is often marked by a process of exploration of achievements and aspirations (Flum & Blustein 2000) and requires the ability to conduct a realistic self-appraisal. Appraisal is a process by which people can:

- confirm outcomes of previous experience
- identify areas of strength
- identify areas for development
- remotivate and energise
- help predict and identify personal potential, and
- acknowledge performance against existing standards.

Appraisal is an ongoing process that can be informed by, but is not limited to, the formalised feedback sessions that occur among learners and educators. Appraisal consists of assessing accomplishments and performance to make an informed judgment about strengths and limitations in order to identify areas for improvement. It is a mechanism through which nurses can begin to self-manage their performance development.

Feedback is considered an essential part of the appraisal process. You should seek feedback that is constructive and includes comments about both things you have done well and areas (and suggested strategies) for improvement where necessary. All too often, feedback can be perceived as reactive and punitive, rather than as a vehicle for development through identifying one's own and others' strengths, availing yourself and others of opportunity, and operating within and accepting processes. Appraisal involves both openness and vulnerability. It should be authentic, active, meaningful and constructive for both nurses and those they work with as clients and peers.

GAINING THE MOST FROM EXPERIENCE

In order to optimise learning, it is important that each experience be approached as a way of linking theory and practice, and as an opportunity for further learning and generation of new perspectives. Increasingly, nurses are required to engage in roles beyond that of direct patient caregiver and engage in 'systems level intervention', such as contributor in multidisciplinary teams, researcher and manager, through which they facilitate quality patient care. At the very least, students need to think about how the roles and functions that registered nurses perform have shaped, and been shaped, by the practice situation.

Nursing students should explore roles other than direct caregiver. In most nursing programs the primary emphasis is placed on providing clinical experience in a range of settings (e.g. mental health, acute care and the community). However, it is unclear whether students are encouraged to explore a range of nursing roles and functions while in those settings. In order to prepare for the diversity of practice, students themselves should analyse each situation and try to determine what nursing roles and competencies are applicable. For example, students should ask themselves:

- What is the role of the registered nurse here? Is the registered nurse in this context a 'direct caregiver' or a 'care facilitator'?
- Does the role require skills as a clinician, supervisor, researcher, educator, manager or communicator, or a combination of these?
- If I were to be asked to manage this person's situation, what would I do and why?
- What nursing activities are most important and why?
- What knowledge base is required for sound clinical decision making?
- Where does this knowledge come from?
- How do I know what I know?
- What more could I know?
- How could I find out about this?
- How has my response to this situation been shaped by my beliefs about what practice is?
- What strengths do I have to respond to this situation?
- What are my learning needs in response to this situation?

Asking questions such as these encourages us to explore the diverse roles and functions of nurses and to differentiate between the roles of registered nurses and other levels of nurses.

It also acknowledges that, in order to maintain effectiveness as clinicians, nurses need to learn continually from a range of situations. In order to achieve this, it is essential that someone (including the learner) facilitate their learning towards nursing outcomes. Learners often seek, indeed need, external support, guidance and assessment (Brennan & Hutt 2001, Maslin-Prothero & Owen 2001). Thus, the clinical educator, the university lecturing staff and other personnel can provide feedback and support to students or peers.

Clinical educators and preceptors in practice settings have been reported to fulfil many roles, which seemingly mirror the roles of nurses, including practitioner, administrator, teacher, counsellor, problem solver, manager, assessor, advocate, guide and facilitator (Maslin-Prothero & Owen 2001).

The current trend in education to view educators as 'facilitators', rather than 'givers' of learning, has been well-recognised in nursing education literature. It implies that nurses as educators are increasingly adopting a more student-centred, collaborative model of education. Moreover, the nurse as educator needs to model the way students or peers are expected to approach learning, as well as modelling exemplary nursing practice.

Clinical experiences provide the opportunity for students to observe and participate in nursing practice. Inherent in the notion of effective practice is the ability to make sound clinical judgments based on assessments and reassessments, to collaborate with others, to provide meaningful feedback to colleagues about performances, and to establish and maintain professional relationships. Clinical experiences acclimatise students to the real world of practice and its culture, providing preparation for the reality of practice, which is dynamic and replete with novel situations.

Specifically, we have observed that students and clinicians in the clinical setting are often confused about when students should be observing another's practice and when they should be actively participating in the provision of client care. Understandably, students and clinicians alike want to be opportunistic and seize what they perceive to be limited practice learning opportunities and may, with the very best of intentions, place themselves and the client at risk because they are dealing with situations that are new to them. Our advice would be for the student to always consider the need for optimal client outcomes, to be sure of the core objectives and concepts of the clinical placement, and determine the relationship between these goals and the activity to be performed. If the learning experience is highly desirable, students need to seek advice from the clinical educator about the scope of the student's practice and the need for close supervision.

When students are invited to perform care with which they do not feel comfortable, they might tell the qualified nurse that they are too busy or have other things to do. Sometimes the nurse, who has made an effort to give the student a meaningful learning experience, may interpret this response as disinterest in nursing. In situations such as these, we would suggest that students recognise the nurse's offer as a way to enhance their learning. The student should explain their situation to the senior nurse on duty, confirm that the qualified nurse is ultimately responsible for the client's care, and engage in the activity as far as possible.

THE IMPORTANCE OF OTHER RESOURCES IN LEARNING

We have already made substantial reference to the reciprocity between theoretical and practical frameworks for learning, and identified the importance of focused experiences related to nursing in either classroom or clinical settings.

Classroom learning provides opportunities to explore options and alternatives, to justify thinking and to learn from examples drawn from practice. It also gives students opportunities to develop the scholarly approaches necessary for contemporary nursing practice. An amplified enquiry approach is needed. Skills in clinical judgment are encouraged through the student developing nursing intervention strategies built upon explicit relationships between thought, judgment and action. Knowing about the person for whom students are caring requires a focus on our ability to acquire, recall and process information from a range of sources, including, but not confined to, the immediate care situation.

While this is important learning, in our experience, it is also essential that student nurses are able to access, retrieve and use information from reputable sources, to draw conclusions about implications of ideas for nursing practice, and to communicate these in writing. Increasingly, nursing programs are integrating these skills into the core nursing program and instructing students in information literacy and writing skills (Ku et al 2007). Information literacy and fluency is required in both learning and practice settings.

Additional support in informative literacy and academic writing skills is available to students. Generic assistance to students ranges from short courses to individual consultations to assist in essay writing, including analysing and interpreting questions, planning, structuring and writing essays, referencing and assistance with mathematics for drug calculations. Students also benefit from spending time with the librarian, learning how to use the library effectively, to conduct literature searches, and use databases to access resources (Honey et al 2006, McNeil et al 2003).

While we encourage the use of these support services, we would caution students that they do not provide discipline-specific information. That is to say, staff of these units can assist you in structuring your writing, ensure your grammar and punctuation are correct and inform you about referencing, but they cannot provide the ideas for your work because they do not 'think and act like nurses'. It is important that students seek assistance from lecturing and library staff who are aware of current issues and debates in nursing, to clarify questions and check their understanding of aspects of nursing.

Perhaps the most effective strategy we have seen students use in on-campus learning is the peer learning group, which provides students with a forum for discussion and clarification of their ideas, mutual assistance and support. We would encourage all students to participate in such a learning group. Your nursing department may already provide a web-based support service (such as 'Blackboard' or 'Web CT'), which perhaps you can ask about. This need not necessarily be on campus. The internet has made it possible to access a number of resources, including other students via the worldwide web. Of course, users should be cautious about disclosing personal information and should check the validity of any information obtained via 'the net'.

CONCLUDING THOUGHTS

While there is increasing emphasis on the development of cognitive abilities in nursing, this should not lead to what has been labelled as a dichotomy between clinical skills and theoretical knowledge. Despite claims made by some authors that emphasis on theoretical knowledge in nursing results in a devaluing of clinical skills and, consequently, a devaluation of clinical practice, practical and theoretical nursing knowledge are inevitably and infinitely intertwined. Nursing practice and nursing education have increasingly recognised the need to integrate thinking and doing to create informed action. Discussion of the separation of thinking and doing does little to promote integration of on-campus and clinical learning activity. Students should view their learning to be nurses as occurring in two distinct yet interdependent contexts, the classroom and the clinical setting. Furthermore, they should use their experiences as students to develop foundational knowledge and skills for effective, confident and competent transition to employment.

The past few decades have provided evidence that there is a paradigm shift in education, which now views learning as the construction of meaning in context rather than what to learn and how to do things. Nurse education is about the ability—indeed flexibility—to examine situations, deconstruct them from a number of perspectives, and reconstruct them around core concepts essential to nursing practice. When students engage in reflective practice in a manner that enacts individual agency, they are able to reinforce self-worth, retain confidence and self-esteem, and expand knowledge and skills.

Contemporary nursing practice demands that nurses question and justify decisions in context, and emphasises the ability to think about nursing, as well as the ability to perform nursing actions to best manage nursing situations. The challenge for students is to develop an integrated approach to practice, which values thoughtful, highly skilled and efficient action, and to continue with lifelong learning and professional development—that is, to be knowledge-ABLE rather than simply knowledgable.

REFLECTIVE QUESTIONS

1 How can you become more responsible and accountable for your own learning?

2 How can you plan and evaluate your ongoing professional development?

3 Who can assist you with meeting these needs?

4 What are the strengths you take as a learner and a student of nursing to your future practice?

5 What strategies will you use to develop resilience, confidence and competence as a beginning professional?

RECOMMENDED READINGS

Etheridge S 2007 Learning to think like a nurse: stories from new nurse graduates. Journal of Continuing Education in Nursing 38(1):24–30

Henderson A, Fox R, Armit L 2008 Education in the clinical context: establishing a strategic framework to ensure relevance. Collegian 15(2):63–68

Levett-Jones T, Lathlean J, Maguire J, McMillan M 2007 Belongingness: a critique of the concept and implications for nursing education. Nurse Education Today 27:210–218

Newton J, McKenna L 2007 The transitional journey through the graduate year: a focus group study. International Journal of Nursing Studies 44(7):1231–1237

REFERENCES

Armstrong ML, Johnston BA, Bridges RA, Gessner BA 2003 The impact of graduate education on reading for lifelong learning. Journal of Continuing Education in Nursing 34(1):19–27

Benner P 1984 From novice to expert: excellence and power in clinical nursing practice. Addison Wesley, Menlo Park, California

Brennan AM, Hutt R 2001 The challenges and conflicts of facilitating learning in practice: the experiences of two clinical nurse educators. Nurse Education in Practice 1(4):181–188

Brookfield S 1993 On impostorship, cultural suicide and other dangers: how nurses learn critical thinking. Journal of Continuing Education in Nursing 24(5):197–205

Campbell SL 2003 Cultivating empowerment in nursing today for a strong profession tomorrow. Journal of Nursing Education 42(9):423

Chang E, Hancock K 2003 Role stress and role ambiguity in new nursing graduates in Australia. Nursing and Health Sciences 5:155–163

Conway J, Little P 2003 Adopting PBL as an institutional approach: considerations and challenges. Journal of Excellence in College Teaching 11(2–3):11–26

Cranton P 1994 Understanding and promoting transformative learning: a guide for educators of adults. Jossey-Bass, San Francisco

Department of Health 2001 The NHS plan: a plan for investment, a plan for reform. Department of Health, London

Dirkx JM 2006 Engaging emotions in adult learning: a Jungian perspective on emotion and transformative learning. New Directions for Adult and Continuing Education 109:15–26

Etheridge SA 2007 Learning to think like a nurse: stories from new nurse graduates. Journal of Continuing Education in Nursing 38(1):24–30

Flum H, Blustein DL 2000 Reinvigorating the study of vocational exploration: a framework for research. Journal of Vocational Behavior 56:380–404

Fox R, Henderson A, Malko K 2005 They survive despite the organisational culture not because of it: a longitudinal study of new staff perceptions of what constitutes support during transition to an acute tertiary facility. International Journal of Nursing Practice 11:193–199

Friere P 1972 The pedagogy of oppression. Penguin, Harmondsworth

Gibbs G 1988 Learning by doing: a guide to teaching and learning methods. Further Education Unit. Oxford Polytechnic, Oxford

Griffitts L 2002 Geared to achieve with lifelong learning. Nursing Management 33(11):22–24

Halfer D, Graf E 2006 Graduate nurse perceptions of the work experience. Nursing Economic$ 24(3):150–155

Heartfield M 2006 Specialisation and advanced practice discussion paper. Online. Available: www.nnnet.gov.au/downloads/recsp_paper.pdf

Honey M, North N, Gunn C 2006 Improving library services for graduate nurse students in New Zealand. Health Information and Libraries Journal 23(2):102–109

Howatson-Jones IL 2003 Difficulties in clinical supervision and lifelong learning. Nursing Standard 17(37):37

Janik DS 2005 Unlock the genius within neurobiological trauma, teaching, and transformative learning. Rowman and Littlefield Education, Lanham, Maryland

Jeffries PR 2008 Getting in STEP with simulations: Simulations take educator preparation. Nursing Education Perspectives 29:70–73

Johns C 2000 Becoming a reflective practitioner: a reflective and holistic approach to clinical nursing, practice development and clinical supervision. Blackwell Science, London

Ku Y, Sheu S, Kuo S 2007 Efficacy of integrating information literacy education into a women's health course on information literacy for RN-BSN. Students Journal of Nursing Research 15(1):67–76

Lambert V, Glacken M 2005 Clinical education facilitators: a literature review. Journal of Clinical Nursing 14:664–673

Little P 1996 Questions for learning. Unpublished workshop material. PROBLARC University of Newcastle, Newcastle.

Lunney M 2008 Current knowledge related to intelligence and thinking with implications for the development and use of case studies. International Journal of Nursing Terminologies and Classifications 19(4):158–162

McKenna L, Green C 2004 Experiences and learning during a graduate nurse program: an examination using a focus group approach. Nurse Education in Practice 4(4):258–263

McMillan M, Conway J, FitzGerald M 2004 Issues in workplace, work practice and workforce: the implications for care models and nursing service delivery. Final report of a desktop study commissioned by the Department of Human Services, Melbourne

McNeil BJ, Elfrink VL, Bickford CJ, Pierce ST 2003 Nursing information technology knowledge, skills and preparation of student nurses, nursing faculty and clinicians: a US survey. Journal of Nursing Education 42(8):341

Mannix J, Faga P, Beale B, Jackson D 2006 Towards sustainable models for clinical education in nursing: an on-going conversation. Nurse Education in Practice 6:3–11

Maslin-Prothero S, Owen S 2001 Enhancing your clinical links and credibility: the role of nurse lecturers and teachers in clinical practice. Nurse Education in Practice 1(4):189–195

Mezirow J 1985 A critical theory of self directed learning. New Directions for Continuing Education 25:17–30

Moore C 2006 The transition from student to qualified nurse: a military perspective. British Journal of Nursing 15(10):540–542

Morgan J, Rawlinson M, Weaver M 2006 Facilitating online reflective learning for health and social care professionals. Open Learning 21(2):167–176

National Review of Nursing Education 2002 Our duty of care. Commonwealth of Australia, Canberra

Newton J, McKenna L 2007 The transitional journey through the graduate year: a focus group study. International Journal of Nursing Studies 44(7):1231–1237

Taylor E 2008 Transformative learning theory. New Directions for Adult and Continuing Education 119:5–15

Zimmerman B 2000 Self-regulatory cycles of learning. In: Straka GA (ed.) Conceptions of selfdirected learning, theoretical and conceptual considerations. Waxman, New York, pp 221–34

GLOSSARY

Aboriginal and Torres Strait Islander Health Services; Aboriginal Medical Services: Services that may be established and governed (controlled) by Aboriginal and Torres Strait Islander peoples in their communities or in partnership with Aboriginal and Torres Strait Islander peoples specifically to improve access to health services for Aboriginal and Torres Strait Islanders. They offer diverse services, ranging from general practice and medical services to comprehensive holistic primary healthcare services to meet physical, mental health, social, cultural and environmental health needs.

Acceptability: The test applied to a premise or reason. In order to have a sound argument, a premise must be acceptable to the person evaluating the argument.

Aesthetic: A term defined in the *Australian Concise Oxford Dictionary* (1987) as 'belonging to the appreciation of the beautiful; having such appreciation; in accordance with principles of good taste … philosophy of the beautiful or of art … set of principles of good taste and appreciation of beauty'. An abstract notion used in discussing the artistic aspect of nursing (and its creative expression). In this context, it relates broadly to theoretical and practical aspects of nursing art.

Affective: 'Pertaining to the affections … being affected, mental state, emotions … mental disposition, good will, kindly feeling, love' (*Australian Concise Oxford Dictionary* 1987).

Altruism: 'Regard for others as a principle for action; unselfishness' (*Australian Concise Oxford Dictionary* 1987).

Argument: A conclusion that is supported by a set of reasons intended to provide grounds for the acceptability of the conclusion.

Autonomy: 'Personal freedom; freedom of the will' (*Australian Concise Oxford Dictionary* 1987). Right to self-determination.

Binary: Comprised of two parts. See also dichotomy.

Bioethics: An interdisciplinary field of inquiry characterised by a systematic and critical examination of the moral dimensions of healthcare and other associated fields (e.g. the life sciences) from the standpoint of various ethical perspectives.

Biologism: A particular form of essentialism (see below) in which women's essence is defined in terms of their biological capacities.

Caring: Compassionate or showing concern for others. Can refer to behaviour used by those who belong to a profession such as nursing that involves looking after people's physical, medical and general welfare.

'Close the gap': A campaign to reduce the gap in life expectancy, employment and educational opportunities between Aboriginal and Torres Strait Islander peoples and other Australians.

Community assessment: '[I]ncludes a comprehensive assessment of the determinants of health. Data analysis identifies deviations from expected or acceptable rates of disease, injury, death or disability as well as risk or protective factors' (Stanhope & Lancaster 2008:192).

Conceptual framework: A developing theoretical model that has little empirical support.

Congruency: 'Agreement or consistency' (*Australian Concise Oxford Dictionary* 1987). For example, in examining two or more theoretical views, one may find that there are areas of agreement across the same ground; hence, there is evidence of congruency.

Construct: 'A type of highly abstract and complex concept whose reality base can only be inferred. Constructs are formed from multiple less abstract or more empirical concepts' (Chinn & Jacobs 1983:200).

Critical friend: A trusted colleague who provides feedback on your journal entries.

Critical incident analysis: The use of clinical or personal incidents as a reflective tool.

Critical thinking: The development of a questioning attitude to that which is normally taken for granted.

Cultural competence: 'A set of behaviours, attitudes and policies that come together in a system, agency or among professionals to enable that system, agency or group of professionals to work effectively in cross cultural situations' (National Health and Medical Research Council 2005).

Cultural safety: A philosophy of healthcare specific to working in a cross-cultural situation with Indigenous peoples. It is achieved by personal reflection and understanding of your own culture before you can meaningfully interact with Indigenous people (Ramsden 2002). The Congress of Aboriginal and Torres Strait Islander Nurses (CATSIN) consider cultural safety as essential when providing healthcare to Aboriginal and Torres Strait Islander peoples (Indigenous Nurse Education Working Group 2002).

Deductive reasoning: The process of inferring particulars from general laws or principles.

Dialectic: Defined in the *Australian Concise Oxford Dictionary* (1987) as the 'art of investigating the truth of opinions, testing of truth by discussion [or] logical disputation or criticism dealing with metaphysical contradictions and their solutions; existence or action of opposing forces'.

Dialectical: A process or perspective involving a dialectic. For example, in theory development using a dialectical approach to generation of knowledge, the process could involve debate with presentation of an argument (thesis), which is considered critically and challenged by a counterargument (antithesis), which is considered critically in relation to the thesis and other knowledge, possibly leading to new areas of agreement and understanding (synthesis).

Dichotomy: 'A division (especially sharply defined) into two; result of such division; binary classification', according to the *Australian Concise Oxford Dictionary* (1987). The term can be used to indicate a divide between two theoretical positions, which are polarised or incompatible.

Discourse: An abstract notion used to label a collection of theoretical perspectives within an academic discipline. This may be composed of theses or arguments representing knowledge in the discipline, including areas of agreement and disagreement, fundamental assumptions, values and beliefs, expressed in disciplinary language and symbols. The notion reflects the idea of a conversation using language within these boundaries.

Dissemination: The act of distributing or spreading something, especially information for it to become widespread.

Diversity: A variety of something, such as opinion, colour or style; can refer to ethnic variety, as well as socioeconomic and gender variety, in a group, society or organisation.

Early intervention: Early intervention can mean intervening early through working with parent(s) during pregnancy and infancy or it can mean intervening early during a key transition point or pathway in an individual's life (Edgecombe 2004:143).

Empiricist/logical positivist model: An approach grounded in the belief that the world can be viewed as a machine and that the task of science is to discover the laws by which the machine operated; emphasis on predictability, measurement, and the quantification of observable data.

Epistemology: The theory of knowledge; the origins, nature, methods and limits of human knowledge.

Essentialism: The attribution of a fixed essence to women; that there are given, universal characteristics of women, including biological, psychological and social characteristics, which are not readily amenable to change.

Ethical principalism: The view that moral decisions are best guided by appealing to sound universal moral principles, such as the principles of autonomy, beneficence, nonmaleficence and justice; ethical principalism is one of the most popular approaches used to examine ethical issues in healthcare.

Ethical universalism: The view that there exists one set of universal values/standards that is applicable to all people throughout space and time, regardless of their histories and/or cultural backgrounds (contexts).

Ethics: A branch of philosophic inquiry concerned with understanding and examining the moral life. It seeks rational clarification and justification of basic assumptions and beliefs that people hold about what constitutes right or wrong/ good or bad conduct. Can also be defined as a system of action guiding rules and principles that function by specifying that certain types of conduct are required, prohibited or permitted. The term ethics/ethical may be used interchangeably with the term morality/moral.

Etiquette: A set of behavioural action guides concerned with the maintenance of style and decorum in social settings; often, although mistakenly, confused with ethics/morality.

Evidence: Something that gives a sign or proof of the existence or truth of something, or that helps us to come to a particular conclusion.

Feminisms: The variety of theoretical approaches to the advocacy of equal rights for women, accompanied by a commitment to improve the position of women in society; includes liberal feminism, socialist feminism, radical feminism, postmodern feminism, and so on.

Gender: A social construction that expresses the many areas of social life, as distinguished from biological sex; the socially learned behaviours and expectations that are associated with the two sexes.

Generic: A characteristic that is 'general, not specific or special' (*Australian Concise Oxford Dictionary* 1987).

Grounded theory: A research process designed to lead to generation of theory through study of a particular human situation or context.

Grounds: The degree to which a set of reasons supports a conclusion.

Health policies: 'The strategies and courses of action adopted as being advantageous and expedient to provide within the resources available from a health system that at least maintains, and preferably improves, health' (Hennessy & Spurgeon 2000:6).

Health promotion: 'Health promotion is a broad field of activity ranging from actions that are essentially medically focused and individual (such as individual risk-factor assessment and counselling) to actions aimed at helping people to change their behaviour, and further along to actions that seek to create supportive environments and settings that address a broad range of social and environmental determinants of health' (Marshall 2004:185).

Healthy communities: 'A healthy city [community] is one that is continually creating and improving those physical and social environments and expanding those community resources which enable people to mutually support each other in performing all the functions of life and in developing to their maximum potential' (World Health Organization 1998:13).

Hermeneutics: A process of interpretive analysis, which is concerned with uncovering meaning and a technique for interrogating text. Van Manen states that 'hermeneutics is the theory and practice of interpretation. The word derives from the Greek god Hermes whose task it was to communicate messages from Zeus and other gods to the ordinary mortals' (van Manen 1990:179). Hermeneutics was originally a technique used to interpret religious text, which has made a transition into research activity in the social sciences and humanities. Hermeneutical refers to a process or perspective involving hermeneutics.

Holism: A perspective in which people are seen as made up of biological, psychological, social and spiritual components, which are indivisible.

Hypotheses: Tentative statements of relationships between two or more variables, which have little empirical support. The repeated confirmation of hypotheses changes their status to empirical generalisations (statements with moderate empirical support) and thence to law (statements with overwhelming empirical support).

Iconography: 'Illustration of subject by drawings or figures; book whose essence is pictures; treatise on pictures or statuary; study of portraits esp. of an individual' (*Australian Concise Oxford Dictionary* 1987).

Inductive reasoning: The process of inferring a general law or principle from the observation of particular instances.

Journalling: The technique of recording thoughts and feeling after reflecting on an event.

Magnet hospitals: Hospitals that have certain measurable characteristics, each of which is predicated on recognition of nurses' contribution to patient care and the environment of the healthcare facility. These characteristics include: effective and supportive leadership; nursing staff decision making; commitment to professional clinical nurse qualities; participatory management; autonomy and accountability, and a supportive environment (Buchan 1999).

Managed care: A system that controls the financing and delivery of health services to members who are enrolled in a specific type of healthcare plan.

Masculinist: Pertaining to the masculine; the male gender characteristics derived from social construction and expectation.

Meta: A prefix commonly encountered in theoretical literature. In this context it means 'beyond or higher order' (*Australian Concise Oxford Dictionary* 1987). A meta-paradigm of any discipline is a statement or group of statements identifying the relevant phenomena to the discipline (Fawcett 1984).

Model: A schematic representation of some aspect of reality, which may be empirical or theoretical. Empirical models are replicas of observed realities (e.g. a plastic model of the ear). Theoretical models represent the world in language or mathematical symbols (e.g. nursing's 'grand theories').

Moral/morality: See ethics above.

Moral duty: An act that a person is bound to perform for moral reasons.

Moral obligation: An act that a person is bound to perform for moral reasons; is generally regarded as being weaker than a moral duty and may be overridden by stronger moral duties.

Moral principles: General standards of conduct that make up an ethical system of action guides and which carry particular imperatives (e.g. 'Do no harm').

Moral right: A special interest that a person has and which ought to be protected for moral reasons (e.g. the right to life) (contrast with legal right; e.g. a special interest that a person has and which ought to be protected for legal reasons); moral rights generally entail correlative rights.

Moral rules: Derived from principles and prescribed particular standards of conduct (e.g. 'Always tell the truth'). Rules have less scope than principles; they also do not have the same force and can be overridden by principles.

Naturalism: A form of essentialism in which a fixed nature is assumed for women, not readily amenable to change.

Nursing ethics: The examination of all kinds of ethical and bioethical issues from the perspective of nursing theory and practice which, in turn, rest on the agreed core concepts of nursing: person, culture, care, health, healing, environment and nursing itself.

Occam's Razor: The principle that the simplest explanation is most likely to be the right one.

Paradigm: A paradigm is a term used to describe accepted practices and techniques through which a discipline accumulates and refines its knowledge base.

Patriarchy: The social system in which men dominate, oppress and exploit women, within the spheres of reproduction, sexuality, work, culture and the state.

Phenomenology: Is a philosophy and descriptive research method designed to uncover the essence and meaning of lived experiences—for example, suffering or grieving (Parse 2001). In a phenomenological research study, the focus is on the meaning of the phenomenon under investigation for the research participants who participate in the study.

Philanthropic: 'Loving one's fellow men, benevolent, humane' (*Australian Concise Oxford Dictionary* 1987).

Philosophy (alternative view): 'A way of reflecting not so much on what is true and false but on our relationship to the truth' (Foucault, cited in Lotringer 1989).

Philosophy/philosophic inquiry (conventional view): An argumentative intellectual discipline concerned with the discovery of 'truth' and meaning. Unlike science, which seeks answers to questions that can only be answered by empirical evidence, philosophy seeks answers to questions that cannot be answered by empirical evidence.

Postmodernism: Relates to the critique of modern, capitalist, industrialised society; new political and social strategies, which embrace pluralism and diversity of cultures and values.

Poststructuralism: Refers to a range of theoretical positions in which the mode of knowledge production uses particular theories of language, subjectivity, social processes and institutions to understand existing power relations and to identify areas and strategies for change.

Praxis: Praxis can be seen as the link between reflection and action. Friere (1972) defines praxis as 'reflection and action upon the world in order to transform it' (Cox et al 1991:385).

Premise: A reason offered in support of a conclusion.

Pre-reflection: Preparatory reflection that occurs before the experience.

Preventive ethics: The study and practice of ethics (including ethics education) aimed at preventing (as opposed to remedying) moral problems.

Professional development: Refers to skills and knowledge attained for both personal development and career advancement.

Public health: 'The science and art of promoting health, preventing disease, and prolonging life through the organised efforts of society' (World Health Organization 1998:3).

Qualitative research: Research that focuses on human experiences, including accounts of subjective realities, and conducted in naturalistic settings, involving close, often sustained contact between the researcher and research participants (Denzin & Lincoln 2005, Sarantakos 2005).

Quantitative research: Refers to research that seeks to measure some concept of phenomenon of interest (e.g. blood pressure, pain or student attitudes to learning about research). It is also called positivist, reductionist or empirical. Quantitative research is termed deductive, which means the thinking leads from a known principle to an unknown, and is used to test a particular research hypothesis.

Racism: A 'form of oppression/privilege which exists in a dialectical relationship with antiracism … societal system in which people are divided into races with power unevenly distributed, or produced based on their racial classification' (Paradies 2006:68).

Rationalism: A philosophical position that argues that the only way to truth is through the deliberations of the rational human mind.

Realism: A practical understanding and acceptance of the actual nature of the world, rather than an idealised view of it.

Reductive: From reduction 'in reducing or being reduced; amount by which prices etc are reduced; reduced copy of picture, map etc … to absurdity … so reductive' (*Australian Concise Oxford Dictionary* 1987).

Reflection (also Reflection-on-action): Reflection that occurs after the experience.

Reflective practice: The incorporation of reflection into practice.

Regulatory authorities: Those organisations responsible for the registration of nurses (e.g. the Queensland Nursing Council or the Nurses and Midwives Board of New South Wales).

Relevance: A test applied to a premise or reason. If a premise or reason is relevant, it helps to support the conclusion of the argument.

Self-awareness: A self-conscious state in which attention focuses on oneself, making people more sensitive to their own attitudes and behaviour. Self-awareness theory states that when we focus our attention on ourselves, we evaluate and compare our current behaviour to our internal standards and values. We become self-conscious objective evaluators of ourselves.

Shared governance: A concept based on the principles of partnership, equity, accountability and ownership (Porter-O'Grady 1991). It requires health professionals to be self-directive, effective decision makers, strongly involved in the activities of the organisation at every level of participation, and providing clinical leadership (Porter-O'Grady 1991).

Social capital: 'Social capital represents the degree of social cohesion which exists in communities. It refers to the processes between people which establish networks, norms, and social trust, and facilitate co-ordination and co-operation for mutual benefit' (World Health Organization 1998:19).

Social class: A broad concept encapsulating objective material, position and subjective understandings, and incorporates differing access to power (Walter & Saggers 2007:88).

Social support: 'That assistance available to individuals and groups from within communities which can provide a buffer against adverse life events and living conditions, and can provide a positive resource for enhancing the quality of life' (World Health Organization 1998:20).

Sound: An argument is sound when the premises are acceptable and provide adequate grounds for accepting the conclusion.

Stereotype: A preconceived idea that attributes certain characteristics (in general) to all members of a class or set. The term is often used with a negative connotation when referring to an oversimplified, exaggerated or demeaning assumption that a particular individual possesses the characteristics associated with the class due to his or her membership in it. Stereotypes often form the basis of prejudice and are usually employed to explain real or imaginary differences due to race, gender, religion, disability, sexuality, ethnicity or socioeconomic class, for example.

Theory: A logically consistent set of propositions, which presents a systematic view of some aspect of reality.

Transformative leadership: Leadership provided by a transformational leader who is a catalyst for expanding a holistic perspective, empowering nursing personnel at all levels and maximising use of technology in the movement beyond patient-centred healthcare to patient-directed health outcomes. Such leaders have vision, meet change 'head on', grow from it, and can harness others to support change measures.

Universalism: Refers to the attributions of functions, social categories and activities to which women of all cultures are assigned; asserts what is shared in common by all women.

Validity: An argument is valid when the premises that are offered provide adequate grounds for acceptance of the conclusion.

REFERENCES

Buchan J 1999 Still attractive after all these years? Magnet hospitals in a changing health care environment. Journal of Advanced Nursing 30(1):100–108

Chinn P, Jacobs MK 1983 Theory and nursing: a systematic approach. Mosby, St Louis

Cox H, Hickson P, Taylor B 1991 Exploring reflection: knowing and constructing practice. In: Gray G, Pratt R (eds) Towards a discipline of nursing. Churchill Livingstone, Melbourne, pp 373–89

Denzin NK, Lincoln YS 2005 (eds) Handbook of qualitative research, 3rd edn. Sage, Thousand Oaks, California

Edgecombe G 2004 Child and family nursing and early intervention. Contemporary Nurse 18(1):143–144

Fawcett J 1984 The meta-paradigm of nursing: present status and future refinements. Image: Journal of Nursing Scholarship 16(3):84–86

Friere P 1972 The pedagogy of oppression. Penguin, Harmondsworth

Hennessy D, Spurgeon P 2000 Health policy and nursing. Macmillan Press, London

Indigenous Nurse Education Working Group (INEWG) 2002 Getting 'em 'n' keepin' 'em: report of the Indigenous Nursing Education Working Group to the Commonwealth Department of Health and Ageing Office for Aboriginal and Torres Strait Islander Health, September 2002. INEWG, Canberra

Lotringer S 1989 Foucault live (interviews, 1966–84). Semiotext(e), New York

Marshall B 2004 Health promotion in action: case studies from Australia. In: Keleher H, Murphy B (eds) Understanding health: a determinants approach. Oxford University Press, Melbourne

National Health and Medical Research Council (NHMRC) 2005 Cultural competency in health: a guide for policy, partnership and participation. NHMRC, Canberra

Paradies Y 2006 A systematic review of empirical research on self reported racism. International Journal of Epidemiology 35(4):888–901

Parse RR 2001 Qualitative inquiry: the path of sciencing. Jones & Bartlett, Boston

Porter-O'Grady T 1991 Shared governance for nursing. Association of Operating Room Nurses Journal Feb–Mar, 53(3):691–703

Ramsden I 2002 Cultural safety and nursing education in Aotearoa and Te Waipounamu. Victoria University, Wellington

Sarantakos S 2005 Social research, 3rd edn. Palgrave Macmillan, London

Stanhope M, Lancaster J (eds) 2008 Public health nursing: population-centered health care in the community, 7th edn. Mosby, St Louis

van Manen M 1990 Researching lived experience. State University of New York Press, New York

Walter M, Saggers S 2007 Poverty and social class. In: Carson B, Dunbar T, Chenall R, Baille R (eds) Social determinants of Indigenous health. Allen & Unwin, Sydney

World Health Organization (WHO) 1998 Health promotion glossary. Online. Available: www.wpro.who.int.hpr/docs/glossary.pdf

INDEX